The Impact of Therapy and Pet Animals on Human Stress

The Impact of Therapy and Pet Animals on Human Stress

Edited by

Lori R. Kogan

Colorado State University, USA

CABI

CABI is a trading name of CAB International

CABI
Nosworthy Way
Wallingford
Oxfordshire OX10 8DE
UK

Tel: +44 (0)1491 832111
E-mail: info@cabi.org
Website: www.cabi.org

CABI
200 Portland Street
Boston
MA 02114
USA

Tel: +1 (617)682-9015
E-mail: cabi-nao@cabi.org

A catalogue record for this book is available from the British Library, London, UK.

ISBN-13: 9781800626515 (hardback)
9781800626522 (ePDF)
9781800626539 (ePub)

DOI: 10.1079/9781800626539.0000

Commissioning Editor: Alexandra Lainsbury
Editorial Assistant: Emma McCann
Production Editor: Shankari Wilford

Typeset by Straive, Pondicherry, India

Contents

Original Publication Details

2 The influence of dogs' presence on children's performance on cognitive tests: Implications for clinical practice
Abigail Alfrey

Previously published in Human–Animal Interaction Bulletin 2021
https://doi.org/10.1079/hai.2021.0016

3 Sustained Effects of Animal-Assisted Crisis Response on Stress in School Shooting Survivors
Ariann E. Robino, David M. Feldman, Alyssa N. Stein, Melody A. Schmaltz, Hailey A. Fitzpatrick, Jaime L. Tartar, Frankie Pizzo, Marah Friedman, and Olivia Feldman

Previously published in Human–Animal Interaction Bulletin 2022
https://doi.org/10.1079/hai.2022.0019

4 Psychophysiological effects of human-dog interaction in university students exposed to a stress-induced situation using the Trier Social Stress Test (TSST)
Rafael Martos-Montes, David Ordóñez-Pérez, Jesús Ruiz-Maatallah, and Miriam Martínez-Cobos

Previously published in Human–Animal Interaction Bulletin 2020
https://doi.org/10.1079/hai.2020.0010

5 Effects of Human–Animal Interactions on Affect and Cognition
Elise R. Thayer and Jeffrey R. Stevens

Previously published in Human–Animal Interaction Bulletin 2022
https://doi.org/10.1079/hai.2022.0015

6 Examining the impact of a brief human-canine interaction on stress and attention
Jonathan B. Banks, Caitlin McCoy, and Courtney Trzcinski

Previously published in Human–Animal Interaction Bulletin 2018
https://doi.org/10.1079/hai.2018.0003

7 **Comparing the Effect of Human-Dog Interactions and Progressive Muscle Relaxation on Self-Report and Physiological Measures of Stress**
Nicole L. Beasley, Greg C Elvers, Roger N. Reeb, and Hannah L. Torok

Previously published in Human–Animal Interaction Bulletin 2022
https://doi.org/10.1079/hai.2022.0005

8 **Experimental trial demonstrates effects of animal-assisted stress prevention program on college students' positive and negative emotion**
Patricia Pendry, Alexa M. Carr, Stephanie M. Roeter and Jaymie L. Vandagriff

Previously published in Human–Animal Interaction Bulletin 2019
https://doi.org/10.1079/hai.2018.0004

9 **Effect of Pet Interaction on Stress Reduction and Positive Mood Enhancement among Pet-Owners and Non-Owners**
Aliya Khalid and Saadia Dildar

Previously published in Human–Animal Interaction Bulletin 2019
https://doi.org/10.1079/hai.2019.0005

10 **Oxytocin Responses After Dog and Cat Interactions Depend on Pet Ownership and May Affect Interpersonal Trust**
Benjamin A. Curry, Brianne Donaldson, Moana Vercoe, Matthew Filippo and Paul J. Zak

Previously published in Human–Animal Interaction Bulletin 2015
https://doi.org/10.1079/hai.2015.0008

11 **Effects of Canine-Assisted Intervention on the Mental Health of Higher Education students: a systematic review**
Karen Manville, Mark Coulson, Michele A. Mulqueen, Kirsty Neller, Caroline Searing, Sarah Welland and Gemma Reynolds

Previously published in Human–Animal Interaction Bulletin 2022
https://www.cabidigitallibrary.org/doi/full/10.1079/hai.2022.0012

12 **A mixed-methods examination of an on-campus canine-assisted intervention by gender: Women, men, and gender-diverse individuals' self-reports of stress-reduction and well-being**
John-Tyler Binfet, Freya L.L. Green, Rebecca J.P. Godard, Madisyn M. Szypula, Camille X. Rousseau and Jordy Decker

Previously published in Human–Animal Interactions 2023
https://doi.org/10.1079/hai.2023.0037

13 **Therapy dogs, stress-reduction, and well-being within the detachment: Interviews with law-enforcement personnel**
Freya L. L. Green and John-Tyler Binfet

Previously published in Human–Animal Interaction Bulletin 2021
https://doi.org/10.1079/hai.2021.0018

14 Therapeutic horseback riding as a complementary intervention for military service members with PTSD
Beth A. Lanning, Amelia L. Wilson, Robert Woelk and A. Alexander Beaujean

Previously published in Human–Animal Interaction Bulletin 2018
https://doi.org/10.1079/hai.2018.0013

15 Pets on Campus: Best Friend or Bad Decision?
Lauren Highfill and Miranda Goodman-Wilson

Previously published in Human–Animal Interaction Bulletin 2017
https://doi.org/10.1079/hai.2017.0012

16 The effects of dog-owner relationship on perceived stress and happiness
Mónica Teresa González-Ramírez, René Landero-Hernández and Minerva Vanegas-Farfano

Previously published in Human–Animal Interaction Bulletin 2018
https://doi.org/10.1079/hai.2018.0012

1 Introduction

Lori Kogan
Colorado State University, USA

Mental health is a state of emotional well-being that enables people to cope with the stresses of life, realize their abilities, learn and work well, and contribute to their community. It is an integral component of health that provides the foundation for our abilities to make decisions, build relationships, and shape our world (World Health Organization, 2022). Stress, defined as a state of worry or mental tension caused by a difficult situation, is a natural human response, yet it can negatively impact physical and mental health, and is a major contributor to anxiety and depression (Daviu et al., 2019; Hammen, 2005; Shin & Liberzon, 2010; World Health Organization, 2023).

Stress is central to the human condition. It is a popular topic in the media and there has been an exponential growth in research and public awareness about stress and its effects. Throughout the world, stress is recognized as a leading cause of long-term sickness, accounting for millions of lost working days (World Health Organization, 2022). An annual survey of stress in the USA found that the effects of the COVID-19 pandemic, global conflict, racism and racial injustice, inflation, and climate-related disasters are major stressors for many Americans (American Psychological Association, 2023). A study in the UK found that the rate of self-reported work-related stress, anxiety, or depression has increased over the last several years, with evidence suggesting that this increase is not COVID-19 related. The main causes appear to be workload, lack of managerial support, and role uncertainty (Health and Safety Executive, 2024).

Indeed, stress impacts everyone in all aspects of life. Stress affects health directly through autonomic and neuroendocrine responses, as well as indirectly through changes in health-related behaviors that can contribute to obesity, cardiovascular disease, and cancer risk. Some level of stress, however, is needed to survive; the human body must continually adapt to the changing internal and external environment. At its most basic level, this is known as homeostasis, in which the body regulates its internal physiological states (e.g., body temperature, oxygen supply) to keep it alive. In order to maintain homeostasis, the body releases hormones (e.g., cortisol, adrenaline, and noradrenaline) and switches on the autonomic and central nervous systems to allow the body to adapt and respond to day-to-day activities. The release of these physiological mediators and changes in immune and metabolic parameters (allostasis) are protective and adaptive as long as they switch on and switch off in a balanced way when an environmental challenge or stressor is no longer present (McEwen, 1998). However, when this fails to happen and the physiological response is maintained over time, it can become damaging for health and well-being.

Allostatic load, referenced in several recent HAI studies (e.g., Applebaum et al., 2023a; Wijker et al., 2021), refers to the wear and tear that the body experiences due to repeated and long-term exposure to stress and is characterized by an inefficient switching on and off of stress mediators or the failure of those mediators to respond with an adequate response when needed (e.g., too little or too much cortisol when faced with an acutely stressful encounter) (McEwen, 1998). The long-term impact of excessive stress, or allostatic overload, affects the body at a cardiovascular, metabolic, behavioral, and cellular level (McEwen & Seeman, 1999).

The increasing prevalence of stress-related diseases and disorders, as well as the rising costs for health care to address these issues (deVries & Wilkerson, 2003; Kalia, 2002; Meier et al., 2021), creates the need for affordable and effective treatments to counteract stress. In recent years, research studies have explored different interventions that could positively impact stress levels, including stress management training for adults, children, and college students (Amanvermez et al., 2023; Kraag et al., 2006; Richardson & Rothstein, 2008), social interaction and emotional support (Ditzen et al., 2007; Sparacio et al., 2023), mindfulness programs (Grossman et al., 2004; Querstret et al., 2020), and exposure to nature (Ulrich et al., 1991; Yao et al., 2021).

Animals, as a therapeutic intervention or as pets, have also gained attention as a viable method for reducing stress. Animal-assisted interventions (AAIs) have been defined by the International Association of Human–Animal Interaction Organizations (2018) as recreational, educational, or rehabilitation/therapeutic activities that, due to the presence and mediation of domestic animals, aim to act on pathological situations and on social or educational problems. AAI is a goal-oriented and structured intervention that intentionally includes or incorporates animals in health, education, and human services for the purpose of therapeutic gains in humans (International Association of Human–Animal Interaction Organizations, 2018). AAIs include animal-assisted activity (AAA), animal-assisted therapy (AAT), and animal-assisted education (AAE). AAAs are planned and goal-oriented informal interactions conducted by a human–animal team for motivational, educational, and recreational purposes (Santaniello et al., 2020). AAT is a goal-oriented, planned, and structured therapeutic intervention directed and/or delivered by health, education, or human service professionals, including, for example, psychologists and social workers (International Association of Human–Animal Interaction Organizations, 2018). AAEs are goal-oriented, planned, and structured interventions that act as an educational intervention, directed and/or delivered by educational service professionals (e.g., general or special education teachers), and offered in a group or individual setting (Santaniello et al., 2020).

Numerous studies of human–animal interactions (HAIs) and AAIs have found beneficial effects on adults' and children's health and well-being (Bert et al., 2016; Brelsford et al., 2017; Fine, 2019; Gee et al., 2017; Gee & Mueller, 2019), including a positive effects on stress reduction (Gandenberger et al., 2022; Meints et al., 2022; Rathish et al., 2021). However, other studies have shown mixed evidence or small effects (Kertes et al., 2017; Powell et al., 2020; Schretzmayer et al., 2017). Clearly, more research is needed to understand when, and for whom, HAI and AAI are of benefit in reducing human stress. To this end, this book features a series of studies that explore the impact of AAIs and pets on the stress levels of children and adults.

Many children experience stress and anxiety during cognitive assessments and testing (Roos et al., 2021; Segool et al., 2013). Alfrey's chapter on "The Influence of Dogs' Presence on Children's Performance on Cognitive Tests: Implications for Clinical Practice" offers a review of the literature that explores the effect dogs have on children's performance during cognitive tests. Through the analysis of nine studies, the author suggests that the presence of a dog can reduce children's stress and enhance their cognitive performance. Importantly, none of the assessed studies found the presence of a dog to be detrimental to children's performance. With the caveat that more research is needed, Alfrey surmises that dogs have promising potential in helping to improve the cognitive testing experience for some children by providing a buffer against the test anxiety.

The next chapter explores the effects of AAIs in the form of an animal-assisted crisis response (AACR). "Sustained Effects of Animal-Assisted Crisis Response on Stress in School Shooting Survivors" by Robino et al. analyzes the effect of offering AACR to students following a mass school shooting – a growing social and public health issue (Katsiyannis et al., 2023). AACR involves the use of highly trained and experienced therapy dogs to provide comfort and support to those in need following disasters and crises. AACR teams are trained to respond to both natural disasters (e.g., tornadoes, fires, floods, and earthquakes) and human-made crises (e.g., mass shootings, bombings) (Eaton-Stull, 2020). The increase in natural disasters and school shootings has led to a dramatic increase in requests for AACR interventions (Lackey & Haberstock, 2019). Robino et al.'s chapter details a quantitative study that examines the sustained effects of AACR in a sample of mass shooting survivors. Their results suggest that AACR may be useful in crisis interventions, including a long-lasting positive effect on those who receive this type of intervention.

Several chapters, using a variety of methods, explore the impact of dogs on college students' stress. Martos-Montes et al.'s chapter focuses on a study of the potential benefits of a dog's presence on college students' heart rate, blood pressure, and subjective anxiety levels during a stress-induced task. This task involved giving a short, video-recorded speech after preparing for five minutes. Students were then immediately asked to verbally continue a sequence of numbers by subtracting 13 from the previous total. The experimental group performed these tasks in the presence of a friendly dog and their handler. Martos-Montes et al. found that those exposed to the dog and handler had lower anxiety and heart rate, but not blood pressure, when compared with the experimental group.

The next chapter, "Effects of Human–Animal Interactions on Affect and Cognition" by Thayer and Stevens, explores the impact of dog presence on students' affect and cognitive abilities during cognitive tasks that test long-term memory, attentional control, and working memory. They found that while dog interaction had a positive effect on students' affect (i.e., positive affect, negative affect, anxiety, and stress), it had no effect on executive functioning (i.e., long-term memory, attentional control, or working memory).

Banks et al.'s chapter on "Examining the Impact of a Brief Human–Canine Interaction on Stress and Attention" also explores the effect of a dog's presence during cognitive tasks. In this study, the researchers assessed attention, speed of processing, and mind wandering. They asked students to complete a letter and pattern comparison task, and the Sustained Attention to Response Task (SART). They inserted probes into the SART task to measure the frequency of mind wandering. In addition to measuring attention, speed of processing, and mind wandering, they also assessed perceived stress, anxiety, positive and negative affect, and self-perception of mind wandering. The canine interaction consisted of participants interacting with a dog for ten minutes prior to the testing. Their study found that interacting with a dog during the intervention was related to lower levels of perceived stress and state of anxiety, yet had no effect on sustained attention, mind wandering, or speed of processing.

The next six chapters focus on college students' affect and reported stress levels. The chapter on "Comparing the Effect of Human–Dog Interactions and Progressive Muscle Relaxation on Self-Report and Physiological Measures of Stress" by Beasley et al. compares two interventions – AAI and progressive muscle relaxation – to help reduce students' stress level. During finals week, students were randomly assigned to either 15 minutes with a therapy dog or 15 minutes completing a progressive muscle relaxation task. The researchers measured students' heart rate variability and self-reported stress level before and after the intervention. They found that interacting with the dog helped reduce students' physiological stress as well as subjective stress. In comparison, those in the progressive muscle relaxation group experienced a reduction in subjective stress but no change in heart rate variability.

The chapter "Experimental Trial Demonstrates Effects of Animal-Assisted Stress Prevention Program on College Students' Positive and Negative Emotion" by Pendry et al. also explores the potential benefits of brief (ten minute) animal interaction. The researchers assessed students' self-report of contentment, irritableness, anxiousness, depression, worry, and perceived stress before and after one of three interventions (interaction with dogs and cats from a local humane society, viewing a slide show featuring photos of the same humane society animals, and control/waitlist). They found that interaction with the dogs and/or cats significantly lowered self-reported feelings of anxiety, irritability, and increased contentment, but not moment-to-moment feelings of sadness and depression, when compared with students who watched a silent slide presentation of animal pictures or the control group.

The next chapter in this section investigates the impact of pet ownership among college students who participate in AAI. In this chapter, "Effect of Pet Interaction on Stress Reduction and Positive Mood Enhancement among Pet-Owners and Non-Owners" by Khalid and Dildar, college students' (pet owners (dog or cat) and non-pet owners) stress level and mood were assessed before and after group AAI with either a dog or a cat. They found that while the AAI resulted in stress reduction and positive mood enhancement for both pet-owners and non-owners, pet-owners had greater stress reduction and positive mood enhancement compared with non-pet owners. They also reported no differences between the cat interactions and the dog interactions.

The chapter "Oxytocin Responses After Dog and Cat Interactions Depend on Pet Ownership and May Affect Interpersonal Trust" by Curry et al. explores the physiological effects of HAI and the impact on interpersonal trust. To this end, the researchers tested the effects on college students of interacting with a dog or cat for ten minutes by testing oxytocin (OT), adrenocorticotropic hormone, and cortisol levels before and after animal exposure. After the AAI, participants were asked to make interpersonal monetary decisions to assess trust and trustworthiness toward strangers. The researchers found that OT levels decreased after interactions with both dogs and cats, with a positive correlation between the change in OT after interacting with a dog and lifetime pet exposure. Specifically, they found that participants who had lived with four or more dogs in their lifetimes had a positive increase in OT after interacting with an unknown dog. However, there was a negative correlation between the change in OT after interacting with a cat and cat ownership. They also found that participants who had a reduction in stress hormones after a dog interaction showed increased trust in strangers. They surmised that the human OT response to animals depends on previous pet exposure and that previous pet experience may prime the brain for physiologic attachment, such as an increase in OT, when one interacts with an unknown dog.

The aim of the next chapter in this section was to better understand the impact of canine intervention on the mental health of college students by conducting a systematic review. "Effects of Canine-Assisted Intervention on the Mental Health of Higher Education Students: A Systematic Review" by Manville et al. assesses 33 papers utilizing the Effective Public Health Practice Project Quality Assessment Tool. The authors found that the quality of the studies ranged from weak to moderate. Based on their review, Manville et al. suggest that canine intervention has a positive effect on stress and anxiety levels, as well as social benefits, for college students. The review also notes common limitations of the studies including confounding variables, and a lack of control groups and standardized measures. The authors conclude that canine intervention has an overall positive effect on college students.

In the last chapter in this section, "A Mixed-Methods Examination of an On-Campus Canine-Assisted Intervention by Gender: Women, Men, and Gender-Diverse Individuals' Self-Reports of Stress-Reduction and Well-Being," Binfet et al. explores the impact of participants' gender (i.e., women, men, and gender-diverse) on the effectiveness of AAI. The intervention was a small group setting (three to four participants per dog/handler) and 20 minutes in duration. The men and women could participate in either the group for their gender or the gender-diverse group, and gender-diverse individuals could participate in any of the three groups. The researchers asked participants to complete a survey before and after the intervention that measured well-being (campus connectedness, happiness, positive affect, and optimism) and ill-being (homesickness, loneliness, negative affect, anxiety, and stress). They found that the effect of the intervention did not differ across the gender conditions; all groups demonstrated significantly increased well-being and decreased ill-being after the intervention.

The next two chapters in this book explore the effects of AAI with adult populations, namely law-enforcement personnel and military service members. Law-enforcement jobs involve dangerous and distressing events on a regular basis, leading to an increased risk of mental health problems (Chen & Grupe, 2021; Syed et al., 2020). The chapter on "Therapy Dogs, Stress-Reduction, and Well-Being within the Detachment: Interviews with Law-Enforcement Personnel" by Green and Binfet describes a qualitative study that assessed, through interviews, the impact of canine-assisted intervention in the form of 90-minute weekly visits. The chapter aimed to better understand the perceptions of law-enforcement personnel surrounding workplace stress and the canine-assisted intervention visits. The results of the eight interviews with law-enforcement personnel resulted in four themes: 1) law-enforcement stress and coping mechanisms within the workplace; 2) experiences of the canine-assisted intervention; 3) the role of therapy dogs; and 4) the potential of canine-assisted intervention within law enforcement. Their results suggest that many law-enforcement personnel felt that the canine-assisted intervention was calming and stress relieving, and helped them feel more positive and resilient.

The chapter on "Therapeutic Horseback Riding as a Complementary Intervention for Military Service Members with PTSD" by Lanning et al. explores the potential benefit of an eight-week therapeutic horseback riding program for veterans with combat-related posttraumatic stress disorder (PTSD). PTSD is one of the most frequently diagnosed disorders following trauma exposure for US military personnel (Blais et al., 2021). PTSD affects about 20% of US military veterans and is a major cause of mortality (Haveman-Gould & Newman, 2018). Lanning et al.'s chapter details the impact of an eight-week structured therapeutic riding curriculum that consisted of 90-minute sessions occurring weekly. Most of the participants had completed at least two tours of duty in at least one of the Operations Iraqi Freedom and Enduring Freedom or Operation New Dawn conflicts. The first four weeks of the program included non-riding exercises (e.g., grooming, leading, working with the horse in a round pen, developing a relationship with the horse), and the last four weeks included riding and horsemanship exercises. They found that participants in the therapeutic horseback riding had a clinically meaningful improvement in PTSD symptoms and depression compared with participants in the comparison group (who had treatment as usual), suggesting that therapeutic horseback riding offers an effective therapeutic intervention for military service members.

The next section of the book includes two chapters that explore the potential benefits of pets, one that focuses on college students, and one that assesses pet ownership among adults in the community. While there is no consensus regarding valid and reliable measures of the prevalence of pet ownership (Applebaum et al., 2023b), estimates of the number of US households with pets range from 57% to 67% (American Pet Products Association, 2023; American Veterinary Medical Association, 2017). Pet ownership is at an all-time high in the UK (57%) (Pet Food Manufacturers' Association, 2022), as well as other countries such as New Zealand (64%), Australia (63%), and Germany (47%) (Gates et al., 2019; Mathers et al., 2010; USDA Foreign Agricultural Service, 2022).

Several studies suggest that pet owners feel their pet is a member of the family and report strong attachment (Applebaum et al., 2021; Barker et al., 2020; Bussolari et al., 2021; Kogan et al., 2021b, c). The relationship between an owner and a companion animal often consists of a unique bond, a strong emotional connection that provides security, comfort, and support (Ainsworth, 1989; Meehan et al., 2017). Pets are viewed as family members by most owners (Bowen, 1993; Humane Society of the United States, n.d.; Irvine & Cilia, 2017; Kogan et al., 2022; Laurent-Simpson, 2021; McConnell et al., 2011, 2019; Serpell & Paul, 2011). Numerous studies suggest that pets offer physical and emotional health benefits (Bures, 2021; Carr et al., 2020; Trigg, 2021), including increased well-being (Bao & Schreer, 2016; Brooks et al., 2018; Gee et al., 2021; Hajek & König, 2020; McConnell et al., 2019; McDonald et al., 2021a; Trigg, 2021), and act as a buffer against depression (Cheung & Kam, 2018; Friedmann et al., 2011; Lem et al., 2016; McConnell et al., 2011; Watson & Weinstein, 1993), anxiety (Hussein et al., 2021; Jennings, 1997; Wright et al., 2015), and stressors (Allen et al., 2001; Applebaum et al., 2021; Bussolari et al., 2021; Currin-McCulloch et al., 2021; Friedmann, 2013; Kogan et al., 2021a; McDonald et al., 2021b; Wheeler & Faulkner, 2015; Young et al., 2020).

The first chapter in section 4, "Pets on Campus: Best Friend or Bad Decision?" by Highfill and Goodman-Wilson explores the relationship between pet ownership and psychological benefits among college students. There are a growing number of colleges who have "pet-friendly" housing that allow students to keep dogs and cats in their dorm rooms (Willgohs et al., 2023). This chapter explores the impact of dog or cat ownership by asking college students with or without pets to complete a survey at the beginning and end of the semester assessing depression, perceived stress, and cognitive and somatic anxiety. They found no significant differences between the pet owners and non-pet owners for affective symptomatology and stress. While pet ownership did not lead to any direct difference in depression or anxiety, the authors found that it did serve as a moderator for the relationship between stress and anxiety whereby pet owners with high stress experienced fewer symptoms of somatic anxiety than non-pet owners. They also found that pet owners reported that living with their pet decreased their stress level, they found their pet a source of companionship, and their pet helped them create social connections with peers.

The next chapter exploring pet ownership, “The Effects of Dog–Owner Relationship on Perceived Stress and Happiness” by González-Ramírez et al., studied dog owners in Mexico. The authors asked dog owners to complete an online survey that assessed the dog–owner relationship (Monash Dog Owner Relationship Scale), subjective happiness (Subjective Happiness Scale), perceived stress (Perceived Stress Scale), and negative life events (utilizing one question, “In the last months, have you dealt with a difficult situation that you considered negative or that caused you stress, anxiety, or depression?”). The authors found that the effects of the human–dog relationship on perceived stress differed for men and women, whereby this relationship was significant for women but not for men. They also found that the dog–owner relationship had an effect on perceived stress but not on subjective happiness.

Taken together, these chapters present a broad array of the current research pertaining to the impact of animals on human stress. Through both qualitative and quantitative research that includes dogs, cats, and horses, these studies demonstrate the breadth of research within this important area and offer a solid foundation for the next steps.

References

Ainsworth, M. S. (1989). Attachments beyond infancy. *American Psychologist*, 44(4), 709–716. https://doi.org/10.1037/0003-066X.44.4.709

Allen, K., Shykoff, B. E., & Izzo, J. L. (2001). Pet ownership, but not ace inhibitor therapy, blunts home blood pressure responses to mental stress. *Hypertension (Dallas, Tex.: 1979)*, 38(4), 815–820.

Amanvermez, Y., Rahmadiana, M., Karyotaki, E., de Wit, L., Ebert, D. D., Kessler, R. C., & Cuijpers, P. (2023). Stress management interventions for college students: A systematic review and meta-analysis. *Clinical Psychology: Science and Practice*, 30(4), 423–444. https://doi.org/10.1111/cpsp.12342

American Pet Products Association. (2023). *Pet Industry Data Insights*. https://www.americanpetproducts.org/research-insights/appa-national-pet-owners-survey

American Psychological Association. (2023). *Stress in America 2023: A nation recovering from collective trauma*. https://www.apa.org/news/press/releases/stress/2023/collective-trauma-recovery

American Veterinary Medical Association. (2017). *AVMA Pet Ownership and Demographics Sourcebook*. American Veterinary Medical Association. https://www.avma.org/sites/default/files/resources/AVMA-Pet-Demographics-Executive-Summary.pdf

Applebaum, J. W., Ellison, C., Struckmeyer, L., Zsembik, B. A., & McDonald, S. E. (2021). The impact of pets on everyday Life for older adults during the COVID-19 pandemic. *Frontiers in Public Health*, 9. https://www.frontiersin.org/article/10.3389/fpubh.2021.652610

Applebaum, J. W., McDonald, S. E., & Zsembik, B. A. (2023a). Longitudinal associations between allostatic load, pet ownership, and socioeconomic position among U.S. adults aged 50+. *SSM – Population Health*, 21, 101344. https://doi.org/10.1016/j.ssmph.2023.101344

Applebaum, J. W., Peek, C. W., & Zsembik, B. A. (2023b). Examining U.S. pet ownership using the General Social Survey. *Social Science Journal*, 60(1), 110–119. https://doi.org/10.1080/03623319.2020.1728507

Bao, K. J., & Schreer, G. (2016). Pets and happiness: examining the association between pet ownership and wellbeing. *Anthrozoös*, 29(2), 283–296. https://doi.org/10.1080/08927936.2016.1152721

Barker, S. B., Schubert, C. M., Barker, R. T., Kuo, S. I.-C., Kendler, K. S., & Dick, D. M. (2020). The relationship between pet ownership, social support, and internalizing symptoms in students from the first to fourth year of college. *Applied Developmental Science*, 24(3), 279–293. https://doi.org/10.1080/10888691.2018.1476148

Bert, F., Gualano, M. R., Camussi, E., Pieve, G., Voglino, G., & Siliquini, R. (2016). Animal assisted intervention: A systematic review of benefits and risks. *European Journal of Integrative Medicine*, 8(5), 695–706. https://doi.org/10.1016/j.eujim.2016.05.005

Blais, R. K., Tirone, V., Orlowska, D., Lofgreen, A., Klassen, B., Held, P., Stevens, N., & Zalta, A. K. (2021). Self-reported PTSD symptoms and social support in U.S. military service members and veterans: A meta-analysis. *European Journal of Psychotraumatology*, 12(1), 1851078. https://doi.org/10.1080/20008198.2020.1851078

Bowen, M. (1993). *Family Therapy in Clinical Practice*. Jason Aronson.

Brelsford, V. L., Meints, K., Gee, N. R., & Pfeffer, K. (2017). Animal-assisted interventions in the classroom – A systematic REVIEW. *International Journal of Environmental Research and Public Health*, 14(7), Article 7. https://doi.org/10.3390/ijerph14070669

Brooks, H. L., Rushton, K., Lovell, K., Bee, P., Walker, L., Grant, L., & Rogers, A. (2018). The power of support from companion animals for people living with mental health problems: A systematic review and narrative synthesis of the evidence. *BMC Psychiatry*, 18(1), 31. https://doi.org/10.1186/s12888-018-1613-2

Bures, R. M. (2021). Integrating pets into the family life cycle. In R. M. Bures & N. R. Gee (Eds.), *Well-Being Over the Life Course: Incorporating Human–Animal Interaction* (pp. 11–23). Springer International Publishing. https://doi.org/10.1007/978-3-030-64085-9_2

Bussolari, C., Currin-McCulloch, J., Packman, W., Kogan, L., & Erdman, P. (2021). "I couldn't have asked for a better quarantine partner!": Experiences with companion dogs during Covid-19. *Animals*, 11(2), Article 2. https://doi.org/10.3390/ani11020330

Carr, D. C., Taylor, M. G., Gee, N. R., & Sachs-Ericsson, N. (2020). Psychological health benefits of companion animals following a social loss. *The Gerontologist*, 60(3), 428–438. https://doi.org/10.1093/geront/gnz109

Chen, S., & Grupe, D. W. (2021). Trait mindfulness moderates the association between stressor exposure and perceived stress in law enforcement officers. *Mindfulness*, 12(9), 2325–2338. https://doi.org/10.1007/s12671-021-01707-4

Cheung, C., & Kam, P. K. (2018). Conditions for pets to prevent depression in older adults. *Aging & Mental Health*, 22(12), 1627–1633. https://doi.org/10.1080/13607863.2017.1385723

Currin-McCulloch, J., Bussolari, C., Packman, W., Kogan, L. R., & Erdman, P. (2021). Grounded by purrs and petting: Experiences with companion cats during COVID-19. *Human Animal Interaction Bulletin*, 11(2), 1–15.

Daviu, N., Bruchas, M. R., Moghaddam, B., Sandi, C., & Beyeler, A. (2019). Neurobiological links between stress and anxiety. *Neurobiology of Stress*, 11, 100191. https://doi.org/10.1016/j.ynstr.2019.100191

deVries, M. W., & Wilkerson, B. (2003). Stress, work and mental health: A global perspective. *Acta Neuropsychiatrica*, 15(1), 44–53. https://doi.org/10.1034/j.1601-5215.2003.00017.x

Ditzen, B., Neumann, I. D., Bodenmann, G., von Dawans, B., Turner, R. A., Ehlert, U., & Heinrichs, M. (2007). Effects of different kinds of couple interaction on cortisol and heart rate responses to stress in women. *Psychoneuroendocrinology*, 32(5), 565–574. https://doi.org/10.1016/j.psyneuen.2007.03.011

Eaton-Stull, Y. M. (2020). *Animal-Assisted Crisis Response*. Oxford University Press. https://naswpress.org/shopping_product_detail.asp?pid=53648

Fine, A. H. (2019). *Handbook on Animal-Assisted Therapy: Foundations and Guidelines for Animal-Assisted Interventions*. Academic Press.

Friedmann, E. (2013). The role of pets in enhancing human well-being: Physiological effects. In *The Waltham Book of Human-Animal Interaction: Benefits and Responsibilities of Pet Ownership*. Elsevier.

Friedmann, E., Thomas, S. A., & Son, H. (2011). Pets, depression and long-term survival in community living patients following myocardial infarction. *Anthrozoös*, 24(3), 273–285. https://doi.org/10.2752/175303711X13045914865268

Gandenberger, J., Flynn, E., Moratto, E., Wendt, A., & Morris, K. N. (2022). Molecular biomarkers of adult human and dog stress during canine-assisted interventions: A systematic scoping review. *Animals*, 12(5), Article 5. https://doi.org/10.3390/ani12050651

Gates, M., Walker, J., Zito, S., & Dale, A. (2019). Cross-sectional survey of pet ownership, veterinary service utilisation, and pet-related expenditures in New Zealand. *New Zealand Veterinary Journal*, 67(6), 306–314. https://doi.org/10.1080/00480169.2019.1645626

Gee, N. R., Fine, A. H., & McCardle, P. (2017). *How Animals Help Students Learn: Research and Practice for Educators and Mental-Health Professionals*. Taylor & Francis.

Gee, N. R., & Mueller, M. K. (2019). A systematic review of research on pet ownership and animal interactions among older adults. *Anthrozoös*, 32(2), 183–207. https://doi.org/10.1080/08927936.2019.1569903

Gee, N. R., Rodriguez, K. E., Fine, A. H., & Trammell, J. P. (2021). Dogs supporting human health and well-being: a biopsychosocial approach. *Frontiers in Veterinary Science*, 8. https://doi.org/10.3389/fvets.2021.630465

Grossman, P., Niemann, L., Schmidt, S., & Walach, H. (2004). Mindfulness-based stress reduction and health benefits: A meta-analysis. *Journal of Psychosomatic Research*, 57(1), 35–43. https://doi.org/10.1016/S0022-3999(03)00573-7

Hajek, A., & König, H.-H. (2020). How do cat owners, dog owners and individuals without pets differ in terms of psychosocial outcomes among individuals in old age without a partner? *Aging & Mental Health*, 24(10), 1613–1619. https://doi.org/10.1080/13607863.2019.1647137

Hammen, C. (2005). Stress and depression. *Annual Review of Clinical Psychology*, 1(1), 293–319. https://doi.org/10.1146/annurev.clinpsy.1.102803.143938

Haveman-Gould, B., & Newman, C. (2018). Post-traumatic stress disorder in veterans: Treatments and risk factors for nonadherence. *Journal of the American Academy of Physician Assistants*, 31(11), 21. https://doi.org/10.1097/01.JAA.0000546474.26324.05

Health and Safety Executive. (2024). *Work-related Stress, Anxiety or Depression Statistics in Great Britain, 2019*. https://humanfactors101.files.wordpress.com/2021/01/work-related-stress-anxiety-or-depression-humanfactors101.com_.pdf

Humane Society of the United States (n.d.). *Pets by the numbers*. HumanePro. https://humanepro.org/page/pets-by-the-numbers

Hussein, S., Soliman, W., & Khalifa, A. (2021). Benefits of pet's ownership, a review based on health perspectives. *Journal of Internal Medicine and Emergency Research*, 2(1), 1–9.

International Association of Human–Animal Interaction Organizations. (2018). *White Paper on Animal-assisted Interventions*. International Association of Human–Animal Interaction Organizations. https://iahaio.org/best-practice/white-paper-on-animal-assisted-interventions/

Irvine, L., & Cilia, L. (2017). More-than-human families: Pets, people, and practices in multispecies households. *Sociology Compass*, 11(2), e12455. https://doi.org/10.1111/soc4.12455

Jennings, L. B. (1997). Potential benefits of pet ownership in health promotion. *Journal of Holistic Nursing*, 15(4), 358–372. https://doi.org/10.1177/089801019701500404

Kalia, M. (2002). Assessing the economic impact of stress – The modern day hidden epidemic. *Metabolism: Clinical and Experimental*, 51(6 Suppl. 1), 49–53. https://doi.org/10.1053/meta.2002.33193

Katsiyannis, A., Rapa, L. J., Whitford, D. K., & Scott, S. N. (2023). An examination of US school mass shootings, 2017–2022: findings and implications. *Advances in Neurodevelopmental Disorders*, 7(1), 66–76. https://doi.org/10.1007/s41252-022-00277-3

Kertes, D. A., Liu, J., Hall, N. J., Hadad, N. A., Wynne, C. D. L., & Bhatt, S. S. (2017). Effect of pet dogs on children's perceived stress and cortisol stress response. *Social Development*, 26(2), 382–401. https://doi.org/10.1111/sode.12203

Kogan, L. R., Currin-McCulloch, J., Bussolari, C., Packman, W., & Erdman, P. (2021a). The psychosocial influence of companion animals on positive and negative affect during the COVID-19 Pandemic. *Animals*, 11(7), Article 7. https://doi.org/10.3390/ani11072084

Kogan, L. R., Erdman, P., Bussolari, C., Currin-McCulloch, J., & Packman, W. (2021b). The initial months of COVID-19: Dog owners' veterinary-related concerns. *Frontiers in Veterinary Science*, 8. https://doi.org/10.3389/fvets.2021.629121

Kogan, L.R., Erdman, P., Currin-McCulloch, J., Bussolari, C., & Packman, W. (2021c). The impact of COVID on cat guardians: Veterinary issues. *Animals*, 11(3), Article 3. https://doi.org/10.3390/ani11030603

Kogan, L. R., Wallace, J. E., Hellyer, P. W., & Carr, E. C. J. (2022). Canine caregivers: Paradoxical challenges and rewards. *Animals*, 12(9), Article 9. https://doi.org/10.3390/ani12091074

Kraag, G., Zeegers, M. P., Kok, G., Hosman, C., & Abu-Saad, H. H. (2006). School programs targeting stress management in children and adolescents: A meta-analysis. *Journal of School Psychology*, 44(6), 449–472. https://doi.org/10.1016/j.jsp.2006.07.001

Lackey, R., & Haberstock, G. (2019). Animal-assisted crisis response: Offering opportunity for human resiliency during and after traumatic incidents. In P. Tedeschi & M. A. Jenkins (Eds.), *Transforming Trauma: Resilience and Healing Through Our Connections With Animals*. Purdue University Press. https://doi.org/10.2307/j.ctv2x00vgg

Laurent-Simpson, A. (2021). *Just Like Family: How Companion Animals Joined the Household*. NYU Press.

Lem, M., Coe, J. B., Haley, D. B., Stone, E., & O'Grady, W. (2016). The protective association between pet ownership and depression among street-involved youth: A cross-sectional study. *Anthrozoös*, 29(1), 123–136. https://doi.org/10.1080/08927936.2015.1082772

Mathers, M., Canterford, L., Olds, T., Waters, E., & Wake, M. (2010). Pet ownership and adolescent health: Cross-sectional population study. *Journal of Paediatrics and Child Health*, 46(12), 729–735. https://doi.org/10.1111/j.1440-1754.2010.01830.x

McConnell, A. R., Brown, C. M., Shoda, T. M., Stayton, L. E., & Martin, C. E. (2011). Friends with benefits: On the positive consequences of pet ownership. *Journal of Personality and Social Psychology*, 101(6), 1239–1252. https://doi.org/10.1037/a0024506

McConnell, A. R., Lloyd, E. P., & Humphrey, B. T. (2019). We are family: Viewing pets as family members improves wellbeing. *Anthrozoös*, 32(4), 459–470. https://doi.org/10.1080/08927936.2019.1621516

McDonald, S. E., Matijczak, A., Nicotera, N., Applebaum, J.W., Kremer, L., Natoli, G., O'Ryan, R., Booth, L.J., Murphy, J.L., Tomlinson, C.A., & Kattari, S.K. (2021a). "He was like, my ride or die": Sexual and gender minority emerging adults' perspectives on living with pets during the transition to adulthood. *Emerging Adulthood,* 10, 1008–1025. https://doi.org/doi:10.1177/21676968211025340

McDonald, S. E., O'Connor, K. E., Matijczak, A., Tomlinson, C. A., Applebaum, J. W., Murphy, J. L., & Zsembik, B. A. (2021b). Attachment to pets moderates transitions in latent patterns of mental health following the onset of the COVID-19 pandemic: Results of a survey of U.S. adults. *Animals*, 11(3), Article 3. https://doi.org/10.3390/ani11030895

McEwen, B. S. (1998). Stress, adaptation, and disease: Allostasis and allostatic load. *Annals of the New York Academy of Sciences*, 840(1), 33–44. https://doi.org/10.1111/j.1749-6632.1998.tb09546.x

McEwen, B. S., & Seeman, T. (1999). Protective and damaging effects of mediators of stress. Elaborating and testing the concepts of allostasis and allostatic load. *Annals of the New York Academy of Sciences*, 896, 30–47. https://doi.org/10.1111/j.1749-6632.1999.tb08103.x

Meehan, M., Massavelli, B., & Pachana, N. (2017). Using attachment theory and social support theory to examine and measure pets as sources of social support and attachment figures. *Anthrozoös*, 30(2), 273–289. https://doi.org/10.1080/08927936.2017.1311050

Meier, M., Wirz, L., Dickinson, P., & Pruessner, J. C. (2021). Laughter yoga reduces the cortisol response to acute stress in healthy individuals. *Stress*, 24(1), 44–52. https://doi.org/10.1080/10253890.2020.1766018

Meints, K., Brelsford, V. L., Dimolareva, M., Maréchal, L., Pennington, K., Rowan, E., & Gee, N. R. (2022). Can dogs reduce stress levels in school children? Effects of dog-assisted interventions on salivary cortisol in children with and without special educational needs using randomized controlled trials. *PLOS ONE*, 17(6), e0269333. https://doi.org/10.1371/journal.pone.0269333

Pet Food Manufacturers' Association. (2022, April). *NEW Pet Population Data Highlights Pet Peak But The Number Of Owners Giving Up Their Pet Is Huge Concern.* Pet Food Manufacturers' Association. https://www.ukpetfood.org/resource/new-pfma-pet-population-data-highlights-pet-peak-but-the-number-of-owners-giving-up-their-pet-is-huge-concern.html

Powell, L., Edwards, K. M., Michael, S., McGreevy, P., Bauman, A., Guastella, A. J., Drayton, B., & Stamatakis, E. (2020). Effects of human–dog interactions on salivary oxytocin concentrations and heart rate variability: A four-condition cross-over trial. *Anthrozoös*, 33(1), 37–52. https://doi.org/10.1080/08927936.2020.1694310

Querstret, D., Morison, L., Dickinson, S., Cropley, M., & John, M. (2020). Mindfulness-based stress reduction and mindfulness-based cognitive therapy for psychological health and well-being in nonclinical samples: A systematic review and meta-analysis. *International Journal of Stress Management*, 27(4), 394–411. https://doi.org/10.1037/str0000165

Rathish, D., Rajapakse, R. P. V. J., & Weerakoon, K. G. A. D. (2021). The role of cortisol in the association of canine-companionship with blood pressure, glucose, and lipids: A systematic review. *High Blood Pressure & Cardiovascular Prevention*, 28(5), 447–455. https://doi.org/10.1007/s40292-021-00469-3

Richardson, K. M., & Rothstein, H. R. (2008). Effects of occupational stress management intervention programs: A meta-analysis. *Journal of Occupational Health Psychology*, 13(1), 69–93. https://doi.org/10.1037/1076-8998.13.1.69

Roos, A.-L., Goetz, T., Voracek, M., Krannich, M., Bieg, M., Jarrell, A., & Pekrun, R. (2021). Test anxiety and physiological arousal: A systematic review and meta-analysis. *Educational Psychology Review*, 33(2), 579–618. https://doi.org/10.1007/s10648-020-09543-z

Santaniello, A., Dicé, F., Claudia Carratú, R., Amato, A., Fioretti, A., & Menna, L. F. (2020). Methodological and terminological issues in animal-assisted interventions: An umbrella review of systematic reviews. *Animals*, 10(5), Article 5. https://doi.org/10.3390/ani10050759

Schretzmayer, L., Kotrschal, K., & Beetz, A. (2017). Minor immediate effects of a dog on children's reading performance and physiology. *Frontiers in Veterinary Science*, 4. https://www.frontiersin.org/articles/10.3389/fvets.2017.00090

Segool, N. K., Carlson, J. S., Goforth, A. N., von der Embse, N., & Barterian, J. A. (2013). Heightened test anxiety among young children: Elementary school students' anxious responses to high-stakes testing. *Psychology in the Schools*, 50(5), 489–499. https://doi.org/10.1002/pits.21689

Serpell, J. A., & Paul, E. S. (2011). Pets in the family: An evolutionary perspective. In T. K. Shackelford & C. Salmon (Eds.), *The Oxford Handbook of Evolutionary Family Psychology* (pp. 298–310). https://doi.org/10.1093/oxfordhb/9780195396690.013.0017

Shin, L. M., & Liberzon, I. (2010). The neurocircuitry of fear, stress, and anxiety disorders. *Neuropsychopharmacology*, 35(1), Article 1. https://doi.org/10.1038/npp.2009.83

Sparacio, A., Ropovik, I., Jiga-Boy, G., Cem Lağap, A., & IJzerman, H. (2023). Stress regulation via being in nature and social support in adults, a meta-analysis. *Collabra: Psychology*, 9(1), 77343. https://doi.org/10.1525/collabra.77343

Syed, S., Ashwick, R., Schlosser, M., Jones, R., Rowe, S., & Billings, J. (2020). Global prevalence and risk factors for mental health problems in police personnel: A systematic review and meta-analysis. *Occupational and Environmental Medicine*, 77(11), 737–747. https://doi.org/10.1136/oemed-2020-106498

Trigg, J. (2021). Examining the role of pets in cancer survivors' physical and mental wellbeing. *Journal of Psychosocial Oncology*, 40(6), 834–853. https://doi.org/10.1080/07347332.2021.1936337

Ulrich, R. S., Simons, R. F., Losito, B. D., Fiorito, E., Miles, M. A., & Zelson, M. (1991). Stress recovery during exposure to natural and urban environments. *Journal of Environmental Psychology*, 11(3), 201–230. https://doi.org/10.1016/S0272-4944(05)80184-7

USDA Foreign Agricultural Service. (2022). *Germany: Increased Pet Ownership in Germany due to COVID-19 Lockdowns*. USDA Foreign Agricultural Service. https://fas.usda.gov/data/germany-increased-pet-ownership-germany-due-covid-19-lockdowns

Watson, N. L., & Weinstein, M. L. (1993). Pet ownership in relation to depression, anxiety, and anger in working women. *Anthrozoös*, 6(2), 135–138. https://doi.org/10.2752/089279393787002295

Wheeler, E. A., & Faulkner, M. E. (2015). The "pet effect": Physiological calming in the presence of canines. *Society & Animals*, 23(5), 425–438. https://doi.org/10.1163/15685306-12341374

Wijker, C., Kupper, N., Leontjevas, R., Spek, A., & Enders-Slegers, M.-J. (2021). The effects of Animal Assisted Therapy on autonomic and endocrine activity in adults with autism spectrum disorder: A randomized controlled trial. *General Hospital Psychiatry*, 72, 36–44. https://doi.org/10.1016/j.genhosppsych.2021.05.003

Willgohs, K., Williams, J., Crisostomo, I., Keck, K., Young-Erdos, C., & Highfill, L. (2023). College canines: Investigating the behavioral and physiological impacts of various college-housing environments on companion dogs. *American Journal of Undergraduate Research*, 20(2), 87–95. https://doi.org/10.33697/ajur.2023.090

World Health Organization. (2022, June). *Mental health*. World Health Organization. https://www.who.int/news-room/fact-sheets/detail/mental-health-strengthening-our-response

World Health Organization. (2023, February). *Stress*. World Health Organization. https://www.who.int/news-room/questions-and-answers/item/stress

Wright, H., Hall, S., Hames, A., Hardiman, J., Mills, R., PAWS Project Team, & Mills, D. (2015). Pet dogs improve family functioning and reduce anxiety in children with autism spectrum disorder. *Anthrozoös*, 28(4), 611–624. https://doi.org/10.1080/08927936.2015.1070003

Yao, W., Zhang, X., & Gong, Q. (2021). The effect of exposure to the natural environment on stress reduction: A meta-analysis. *Urban Forestry & Urban Greening*, 57, 126932. https://doi.org/10.1016/j.ufug.2020.126932

Young, J., Pritchard, R., Nottle, C., & Banwell, H. (2020). Pets, touch, and COVID-19: Health benefits from non-human touch through times of stress. *Journal of Behavioral Economics for Policy*, 4(2), 25–33.

2 The Influence of Dogs' Presence on Children's Performance on Cognitive Tests: Implications for Clinical Practice

Abigail Alfrey
Salomons Institute for Applied Psychology, Canterbury Christ Church University

Abstract

Evidence suggests that cognitive assessments can evoke feelings of stress for some children, potentially inhibiting cognitive performance and undermining the validity of results. Dogs have been found to be an unobtrusive form of social support for children in other settings, potentially offering a solution to this problem. The aim of this paper was to critically review the literature to explore what effect, if any, dogs may have on children's performance on cognitive tests, and consider implications for clinical practice. To do so, five databases were systematically searched and returns were screened for eligibility. Studies were collectively described and then appraised using a common appraisal framework. Nine studies exploring the relationship between dogs and cognitive functioning in children (≤18 years) were identified in the literature search. All used an experimental methodology and were of good to fair quality. Together, results indicated that the presence of a dog could reduce stress and enhance cognitive performance across various domains, lending experimental evidence to support the idea that dogs may support children undergoing cognitive assessments. Further trials are now required to explore the generalizability of these associations to clinical settings and implications for test validity. Further implications for policy and practice are discussed.

Keywords: Dogs, children, cognitive assessment, cognitive performance, clinical psychology

Funding

This research did not receive any specific grant from funding agencies in the public, commercial, or not-for-profit sectors.

Cognitive Assessments in Children's Mental Health Services

In the UK, clinical psychologists working in child and adolescent mental health services (CAMHS) sometimes conduct cognitive assessments. These are used to profile examinees' strengths and weaknesses to provide tailored support specific to their needs (Lezak et al., 2012). For instance, results can inform Education, Health and Care Plans[1] (EHCPs), reasonable adjustments in education (see Equality and Human Rights Commission, 2015), and gatekeeping into specialist services.

Despite this rationale, for some children (defined here as people below 18 years of age), testing can be experienced as a stressful process. Testing commonly requires examinees to perform challenging tasks for a sustained period of time,

Corresponding author email: Abigail.alfrey1@nhs.net

often with an unfamiliar adult in an unfamiliar environment, which some children can find difficult - particularly those with pre-existing psychological difficulties and/or insecure attachment styles (Diamond, 2015), a group over-represented in clinical populations (Palitsky et al., 2013). Bayrak et al. (2018) found that insecurely attached individuals have reduced access to adaptive coping strategies when faced with a stressful situation, and thus greater vulnerability to stress. Children's awareness of the contingencies resting upon their performance could further influence feelings of stress (Howard, 2020).

An increase in stress levels has potential ramifications upon the validity of the assessment results. Cognitive assessments can only be helpful insofar as they provide an accurate representation of the examinee's abilities, yet substantial evidence relates test anxiety to reduced test performance for children (see von der Embse et al., 2018 for review). This may be related to the finding that anxiety impedes the functioning of the prefrontal cortex (Park & Moghaddam, 2017). Given the prefrontal cortex's role in "the maintenance of attention, the monitoring of information in working memory, and the coordination of goal-directed behaviors" (Teffer & Semendeferi, 2012, p. 192), few cognitive tests could be seen to evade this inhibitory effect. This casts question over the usefulness of test results when examinees experience test anxiety.

The finding that test anxiety can have an inhibitory effect on cognitive performance presents a dilemma for clinicians and service providers, because the standardised delivery format of the tests (see Lezak et al., 2012) means that emotional support is generally unavailable. For instance, clinicians are advised against permitting a parent or carer into the testing room with the child in case they were to be distracting or provide assistance. Likewise, most test protocols follow a scripted format that does not allow much feedback from the examiner that could put the examinee at ease (e.g. Wechsler & Kaplan, 2015).

It follows, therefore, that services might be improved by considering ways in which the testing *environment* could be altered to reduce stress or anxiety for children that experience testing in this way. Such improvements could improve the quality of care given to examinees, by increasing confidence in the validity of their assessment results, whilst also demonstrating the services' person-centred and compassionate values (National Health Service [NHS], 2018).

Dogs

In 2007, Deborah Wells summarised the multifarious ways in which dogs can positively influence humans' physical and mental health. More recent research supports and extends her claims: for instance, the finding that human-canine touch mutually increases oxytocin and dopamine, and decreases cortisol and blood pressure (Handlin et al., 2012; Pop et al., 2014).

Numerous papers have explored how dogs can improve children's experiences of the criminal justice system (e.g. Sandoval, 2010; Spruin et al., 2019); dentistry (e.g. Vincent et al., 2019); and physical health settings (e.g. Lindström Nilsson et al., 2019); as well as school reading performance (Hall et al., 2016). Similarly, Jones et al.'s (2019) review found that dogs positively impacted both engagement and outcomes in psychological therapy, supporting earlier claims that dogs can support children who find it difficult to engage in therapy (Levinson, 1962) or act out aggressive impulses (Eggiman, 2006). Further, several studies suggest that dogs improve the acceptability of psychological interventions (Jones et al., 2019), and service users rate and respond to therapists more positively in the presence of a dog (Isenstein, 2018; Schneider & Harley, 2006). Should this effect generalise to cognitive testing, this may serve to enhance engagement with the assessment process, the assessing psychologist, and the service alike.

Despite this proliferation of research, to date, it appears that little research been conducted looking at the impact of dogs on children's test anxiety and its predicted impact on test performance – although Crossman et al. (2020) did find that interacting with a dog reduced anxiety among children more generally. In contrast, studies among adult populations suggest that dogs can reduce university students' biological stress markers prior to examination (McDonald et al., 2017), as well as self-reported wellbeing around the time of exams (Ward-Griffin et al., 2018). This may go some way to explain the finding that interacting with dogs prior to testing can positively influence outcomes for nursing students (e.g. Young, 2012): If dogs can indeed reduce test anxiety and/or stress (at least for some people), and anxiety impedes cognitive performance, it follows that some examinee's cognitive performance, and their experience thereof, could be enhanced by the presence of a dog - a naïve model through which the impact of dogs on children's test anxiety might be understood.

Terminology. As the field of animal-assisted interventions has developed, so too has the language used to describe the different ways in which dogs have been introduced to support humans, and Assistance Dogs International (2019) provide a helpful glossary of these key terms, which includes the following:

> Therapy dog: a pet dog that is trained to provide affection, comfort, and love to those it interacts with in many different settings. Therapy dog owners may [...] visit with their animals to facilities in which the team is welcomed or may be practitioners who utilize the dog in a professional setting.
> Facility dog: a specially trained dog that is working with a volunteer or professional who is trained by a program. The work of a facility dog can include visitations or professional therapy in one or more locations.

As both therapy and facility dogs might be relevant to supporting children undergoing cognitive assessments, the broader term of "dogs" or "canines" is used in this work.

This review: overview and objectives

There is evidence to suggest that the presence of a dog may positively affect the experience of cognitive testing for some children, potentially optimising validity whilst providing compassionate, effective care in line with NHS values. However, it seems equally possible that the converse could be true: dogs may prove distracting to examinees and/or examiners, and thus undermine the validity of the tests; and could likewise raise anxiety or distress in the case of examinees with fears or allergies relating to dogs (Terras, 2006). It is also possible that dogs' presence could benefit performance to a degree that lends advantage, compromising the established validity and reliability of tests, which are currently normed without dogs (Institute of Medicine, 2015). As such, the purpose of this review was to critically summarise the literature so as to explore the questions "what influence might a dogs' presence have on children's performance on cognitive tests" and "what implications might this have for clinical practice in the CAMHS context?".

Method

Literature Search

Five databases were searched (ASSIA, CINAHL, OpenDissertations, PsychINFO, and Web of Science) to capture psychological, medical, and social/community based literature, as well as unpublished dissertations. Searches were limited to "title only" to capture the most relevant literature. Due to the exploratory nature of this research all articles published before 24th May 2020 were searched, limited to English language papers.

The database search query used was: TI = ((child* OR adolescen* OR teenage* OR "young person" OR "young people" OR student* OR pupil* OR pe?diatric*) AND ("cognitive function*" OR "cognitive test*" OR "cognitive assessment*" OR "psychometric test*" OR "psychometric assessment*" OR "neuropsychometric test*" OR neuropsychometry OR "neuropsychometric assessment*" OR "intelligence test*" OR "intelligence assessment" OR memor* OR "cognitive neuropsycholog*" OR "executive function*" OR "processing speed" OR "verbal fluency" OR perform* OR concentrat*) AND (dog OR canine OR "canine-assisted" OR "dog-assisted" OR "therapy dog" OR "assistance dog" OR "facility dog" OR "human-animal interaction" OR "animal-assisted")).

To capture any missed literature, the reference lists of relevant articles were manually searched and ResearchGate was used to identify missed work by key authors. Linkedin was used to request the full-text of a paper unavailable online, but unfortunately, no response was received. Three British university digital research archives (Canterbury Christ Church University, King's College London and the University of Edinburgh), a specialist human-animal research repository ("HABRI"), and Google were also searched using combinations of the above terms to capture any other missed or "grey" literature.

Selection and review process

Database searching retrieved 50 articles, and manual searching contributed a further 12. Duplicates were removed before articles were screened for eligibility. For inclusion, articles had to be text-based and investigate dogs, children (≤18 years) and cognitive performance; all other articles were excluded. Fig. 2.1 summarises this process and outlines the number of papers identified at each stage of the search.

Findings

Approach

In total, nine studies were reviewed, all of which used quantitative methodologies. Due to the heterogeneity of the populations, experimental aims, and designs employed, meta-analysis was not possible. Studies were appraised for quality individually using the Specialist Unit for Review Evidence's (SURE, 2018) assessment framework for experimental studies to inform the degree of confidence attributable to the findings. Then, to provide a summary view of the literature, studies were collectively described and appraised. Study identifiers, key extracted data, and quality summaries are presented in Table 2.1.

Study description

Studies Identified. The nine studies were conducted in three laboratories: Two that sampled across both Austria and Germany, six in the USA, and one in Switzerland. All were published between 2007-2014 in three journals (Anthrozoös, Frontiers in Psychology, and the Human–Animal Interaction Bulletin).

Aims. All of the studies sought to assess the impact of a real dog on some aspect of children's cognitive functioning as compared to one or more control groups. Studies covered all six of the cognitive domains specified in DSM-5's taxonomy (Sachdev et al., 2014; see Table 2.1), including attention (Studies 5, 8 & 9), executive functioning (Study 4), language (Studies 6 & 8), memory (Study 3, 4, 6, 7, 8, & 9), motor-perceptual skills (Study 7), and the HPA axis (stress-response pathway; Studies 1 & 2).

Participants. Participants' ages ranged from 3-14 years. Seven studies (Studies 3-9) included male and female participants, whereas two studies recruited only males (Studies 1 and 2). Children's cognitive ability varied across studies: Studies 1 and 2 recruited children who attended mainstream and special educational establishments with insecure-avoidant or disorganised attachment styles, Studies 3-8 recruited a mixture of developmentally delayed and typically developing preschool children from integrated classrooms (where developmentally delayed and typically developing children are educated in the same programme), and Study 9 only recruited typically developing children attending a mainstream school.

Design and Setting. All studies used an experimental design. Studies 1 and 2 used independent measures; Studies 3-8 used repeated measures; and Study 9 used a randomised controlled crossover design. Studies 1 and 2 used an unfamiliar classroom, Studies 3-8 used a laboratory setting near to the participants' school; and Study 9 did not report the setting. Room set-up was well described across studies.

Intervention and Procedure. Studies 1 and 2 allocated participants randomly to one of three experimental conditions: a real dog, a friendly human, or a toy dog. Participants were assessed using the Trier Social Stress Test for Children (TSST-C) and were free to interact with their allocated "social supporter" throughout the task. Salivary cortisol and self-reported mood was measured at five time points: before the test, after a period of time with the children's "social supporter", after the test, after debrief, and after a period of relaxation.

In Studies 3-8, children were randomised to different starting conditions, usually consisting of a real dog, a toy dog, and a human confederate. Children were assigned a task and asked to perform it in each condition in a randomised order, thus acting as their own controls. Studies 3-6 included picture sorting, matching, or recall. Studies 7 and 8 involved an obstacle course, in which the participant copied, mirrored or raced their "co-performer" (dog, toy or confederate).

In Study 9, participants were randomly allocated to either a real dog or robot dog condition. Participants interacted with their "dog" for

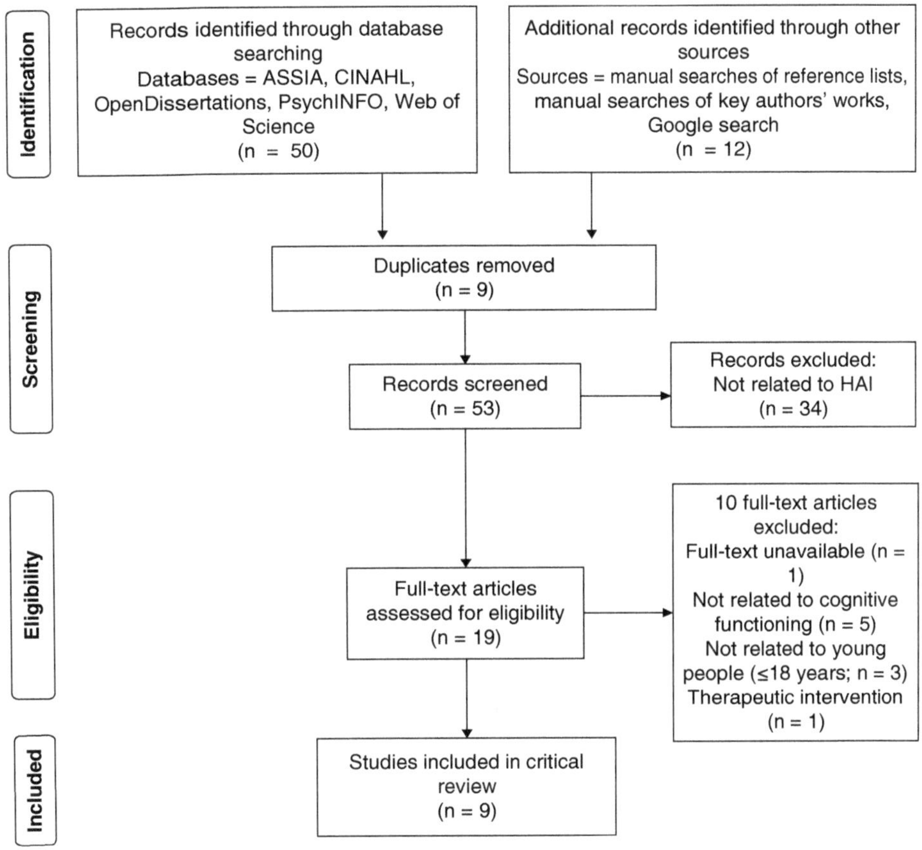

Fig. 2.1. PRISMA flow diagram (Moher, Liberati, Tetzlaff, & Altman, 2009)

15 minutes prior to performing a series of cognitive tasks including a digit span task, a cancellation screen, a continuous performance test and a divided attention test. The "dog" lay by their feet during testing. Each participant completed the tasks in both conditions, acting as their own control. Passive infrared hemoencephalography (PIR HEG) was used as a biological correlate of attention during these tests.

Outcomes and Authors' Conclusions. In Studies 1 and 2 it was reported that participants in the real dog condition spent significantly more time interacting with their "social supporter" prior to the test, and significantly less time interacting during the test, than those allocated to the toy dog condition. Only participants in the real dog condition had significantly lower salivary cortisol levels after the test. Time spent stroking the real dog, but not the toy dog, before the test was positively associated with drop in cortisol level. Changes in self-reported mood were not significant. The authors concluded that physical contact with a dog was the most effective form of social support for participants, and that it did not distract children during testing.

Studies 3-8 found a main effect for participants in the dog condition for all tasks. For matching and sorting tasks (Studies 3-6), children in the dog condition were significantly faster and more accurate. An anecdotal finding was that "the children didn't have to like [...] the dog to benefit from his presence" (Gee et al., 2012a, p. 299). For the motor tasks (Studies 7 & 8), it was found that participants' adherence to instructions for modelled tasks was significantly better in the dog condition, but no significant

Table 2.1. Study Characteristics and Subjective Quality Assessment

No	Authors (Date), Country/Countries	Experimental design	Domain(s)*/ neurocognitive pathway assessed	Sample (Gender, age range)	Key Findings Related to Presence of Dog During Testing	Quality**
1	Beetz, Julius, Turner & Kotrschal (2012), Germany & Austria	Independent measures	HPA axis	M=47, 7–11yrs	Significantly associated with reduced cortisol levels	Good
2	Beetz, Kotrschal, Turner, Hediger, Uvnas-Mober & Julius (2011), Germany & Austria	Independent measures	HPA axis	M=31, 7–12yrs	Significantly associated with reduced cortisol levels	Good
3	Gee, Belcher, Grabski, DeJesus & Riley (2012), USA	Repeated measures	Memory	M=11, F=9, 3–5yrs	Significantly associated with increased speed and accuracy	Good
4	Gee, Church & Altobelli (2010), USA	Repeated measures	Executive function & memory	M=7, F=5, 3–5yrs	Significantly associated with improved task performance	Fair
5	Gee, Crist & Carr (2010), USA	Repeated measures	Attention	M=6, F=6, 3–5yrs	Significantly associated with improved task performance	Good
6	Gee, Gould, Johnson & Wagner (2012), USA	Repeated measures	Memory & language	F=10, M=7, 3–5yrs	Significantly associated with improved task performance	Good
7	Gee, Harris & Johnson (2007), USA	Repeated measures	Memory & perceptual-motor function	F=4, M=10, 4–6yrs	Significantly associated with improved task performance	Fair
8	Gee, Sherlock, Bennett & Harris (2009), USA	Repeated measures	Memory, attention & language	F=3, M=8, 3–5yrs	Significantly associated with increased speed	Fair
9	Hediger & Turner (2014), Switzerland	Randomised controlled crossover trial	Memory & attention	M=13, F=11, 10–14yrs	Non-significant improvement on some tasks; significant learning effect on some tasks	Good

* Follows the six-domain taxonomy specified in DSM-5 (Sachdev et al., 2014)

** Study quality was appraised using the SURE (2018) framework; full notation available by request differences were found in the mirroring or race conditions. Tasks were completed more quickly in the dog condition, without compromising accuracy. The authors conclude that the dog aided cognitive performance and was not a distraction.

The authors of Study 9 reported a non-significant trend towards improvement in the real dog condition on the digit span and cancellation screen tests, but no clear difference in the continuous performance or divided attention tests. In the digit span and divided attention tests the presence of the dog was associated with significantly improved test scores in the second test condition. The authors suggest that the presence of the dog improved the participants' ability to learn how to perform these tests, perhaps via increased attention and/or concentration. PIR HEG data indicated that attention was reduced in the robot dog, but not the real dog, conditions, and concluded that real dogs are not a distraction but robotic dogs can be.

Study Appraisal

Study Focus. All of the studies addressed a clearly focused hypothesis exploring the impact of the presence of a real dog on a specified aspect of children's cognitive performance as compared to one or more control groups. They all used a clearly defined population, and all but Study 1 reported the setting and room set-up, contributing to good replicability. However, only Study 9 reported a clear exclusion criterion.

Design. All studies were small-scale exploratory experiments. Most were well controlled, accounting for potential sources of bias and confounding variables – such as room temperature where the PIR HEG was used (Study 9). However, no studies separated proximity to the dog from interaction with it and in Study 5 the dog's role varied among tasks. As such, providers seeking to integrate dogs into assessments may be unclear as to how to effectively achieve this aim.

All but Study 7 used a human confederate as a control group; six also used a toy dog condition (2, 3, 4, 5, & 8) and Study 9 used a robot dog. In most studies (3, 4, 5, 6, 7, 8 & 9) participants acted as their own controls. Studies 1 and 2 randomly allocated children to different groups, though the process of randomisation was not described. Indeed, only Studies 3 and 6 described the process of randomization, which appropriately used a random number generator, lending confidence to these findings.

Studies 1-6 and 8-9 used active control groups, and only Study 7 used an inactive control. Active control groups are encouraged when testing a novel intervention against an established intervention (see Karlsson & Bergmark, 2015), but toys, robots and human social supporters do not have a well-established effect in the cognitive testing literature. As such, this omission means that it is not possible to see whether examinees could also derive significant benefit from these alternative, and perhaps more pragmatic, interventions.

Intervention. In general, interventions and comparisons were well described and appropriate to the study aims. Aside from the intervention, groups were treated equally. Study procedures and protocols were standardised in all studies. Studies were generally very well described and therefore highly replicable. Sufficient effort was made to avoid order effects where a within-subjects design was used. The demographics of dog(s) handlers and/or human confederates (where used) was often inadequately attended to, however. Some studies did report age range (Studies 1, 2, 4, & 5), gender (Studies 1-6), familiarity with the participants (Studies 3, 4, 5, 6, & 8), demeanour (Studies 1 & 2), and/or responsibility for safety (Study 9). Five studies also provided information about the experimenter, generally limited to gender (Studies 1, 2, 3, 5 & 6). As experimenter demographics have been linked to findings in studies of children's cognitive performance, differences could affect both outcomes and replicability (e.g. Chapman et al., 2018).

In contrast, good consideration was given to dog characteristics. All but Study 2 reported the number of dogs that participated in the study, their breed(s), and their certification status. Study 2 reported only certification status. Evidence suggests that dog breed explains some of the variability in human-canine bonding and communication (Konno et al., 2016) and is thus an important control variable.

Ethics. Just five studies (1, 2, 3, 6, & 9) reported that they received formal ethical approval from a committee. This is concerning, particularly given the vulnerability of the participants, the task demands, and the inherent risks of human–animal interaction. SPSS Statistics (version 23.0) was used to analyse these figures, revealing that year of publication and reporting of ethics was positively correlated ($rs = 0.885$, $p = 0.002$), indicating increased rigour in contemporary publishing standards.

Likewise, only Study 9, the most recent of the studies, received ethical approval from an animal ethics committee. Of the remaining studies, five described how ethical concerns were managed (Studies 3, 5, 6, 7, & 8), three of which in detail sufficient to satisfy the guidelines specified in the International Association of Human–Animal Interaction Organizations' (IAHAIO's) Prague Declaration (1998; Studies 3, 6 & 8). Glenk (2017) reviewed the impact of canine-assisted interventions on dog welfare and found that dogs frequently experience stress in work of this kind. For these reasons, the lack of consideration of animal ethics is also concerning.

Sample. Studies 1-8 recruited children of mixed neurocognitive status, with some participants being developmentally delayed, and others typically developing. Children with special educational needs are more likely to experience difficulties when performing cognitive tasks, and evidence suggests that they are also more likely to experience mental health difficulties (Rose et al., 2009), which could be reflected by higher sensitivity to stress. Studies were adequately powered to run main comparisons but had insufficient power to detect within group differences such as developmental status. A larger sample size was needed to know what impact this had, particularly as anecdotal evidence from studies supported the idea that developmentally delayed children derived more benefit from the dogs than the typically developing children did – a notion supported by the weaker associations found in Study 9, which used a mainstream school sample.

Aside from this, participants appeared to be similar at baseline with regards to key characteristics, such as age and attitudes towards dogs. However, only Studies 4 and 7 reported demographic data such as cultural heritage, which could, plausibly, influence attitudes to dogs (Turner, 2010). Indeed, the authors of Study 3 state that some participants responded differently to the dog than others, yet as heritage and faith background were not reported it is not possible to know whether these variables could account for this. Greater focus on participant demographics could have been informative and, with larger samples, may have enabled meaningful comparisons.

In short, the heterogeneity of participant characteristics can be considered a limitation given the small sample size of these studies. Lack of statistical power precluded between-group comparisons, making the detection of demographic effects difficult. Where this was attempted (Study 6) results were not significant. Presenting results case-by-case, rather than averaging across heterogeneous populations, may have cast light upon differences attributable to uncontrolled variables such as such as attitudes towards dogs or cognitive ability. Nonetheless, the large effect sizes found in several studies, despite this small sample size, indicates compelling evidence for a meaningful real-world effect (Cohen, 1988).

Measures. All studies used psychometric or behavioural outputs. Study 9 used four well-validated measures from established assessment batteries, including subtests from the Wechsler Intelligence Scale for Children (WISC; Wechsler & Kaplan, 2015) and the Candit (2001) battery. Five studies used bespoke rating scales (Studies 1, 2, 5, 8, & 9). Measures were well described in the text, but only two reported inter-rater reliability (Studies 5 & 8) and only Study 2 offered internal consistency scores for psychometric measures, without which it is difficult to discern whether the phenomenon under study was reliably captured. In Studies 1 and 2, self-report tools comprised the Self-Assessment Manikin (SAM; Bradley & Lang, 1994) and Visual Analogue Scales (VAS; Bond & Lader, 1974), both of which have a precedent in the child literature. However, as the authors acknowledged, the SAM uses a single item to assess each mood state and may lack sensitivity, perhaps explaining the null results.

Two studies also used physiological measures: salivary cortisol and PIR HEG. Salivary cortisol has long been used in research exploring stress responses and the methodology is documented to be valid and reliable (Kirschbaum & Hellhammer, 1994). The process by which cortisol samples were obtained, stored, and analysed was reported in sufficient depth. In contrast, PIR HEG is an emergent technology. It does have a clinical precedent which has further developed since the reviewed study was published (e.g. Serra-Sala et al., 2016), and its mechanism of action is described by Shoshev (2017). However, few randomised controlled trials have been published and thus it requires further validation, thus results should be interpreted cautiously.

Data Analysis. For all studies, the experimental designs used precluded the use of participant and investigator blinding, making data blinding important. However, no studies reported that this took place, potentially introducing bias into the analysis, such as expectancy effects. Similarly, no studies reported a pre-specified statistical analysis plan, which may also have introduced bias into the analysis, potentially leading to multiple *post-hoc* comparisons that could jeopardise statistical validity.

Nonetheless, in general, studies were well analysed and results were clearly reported. Statistical methods used were adequately described and appropriate; with all studies reporting effect sizes, although no studies reported confidence intervals. Primary outcomes were clear in all studies and it appeared that all of the important outcomes were assessed; sources of bias were well accounted for and author conclusions were adequately supported by the data.

Critical synthesis

By synthesising the findings from the reviewed studies it becomes possible to understand not only *if* dogs influence cognitive functioning in children, but also *how*. This information, when integrated into the naïve model, whereby interacting with a dog reduces stress, thereby improving cognitive performance, provides a model with far greater explanatory power (Fig. 2.2). This model can be tested and refined in future research to further understand the factors influencing the relationship between dogs and children's cognitive functioning.

Consistent with predictions from the naïve model, Gee and colleagues' series of studies (3-8) indicate that when a dog is available during a demanding task, cognitive performance is enhanced across domains. These findings held when clinical assessment tools were used in Hediger and Turner's (2014) study of memory and attention. Taken together, these studies indicate that dogs improve examinees' ability to attend to the task at hand, which subsequently improves cognitive performance.

Initially this finding might be perplexing: given the high salience of a dog's presence one might predict that children would be more interested in the dog than the task at hand. However,

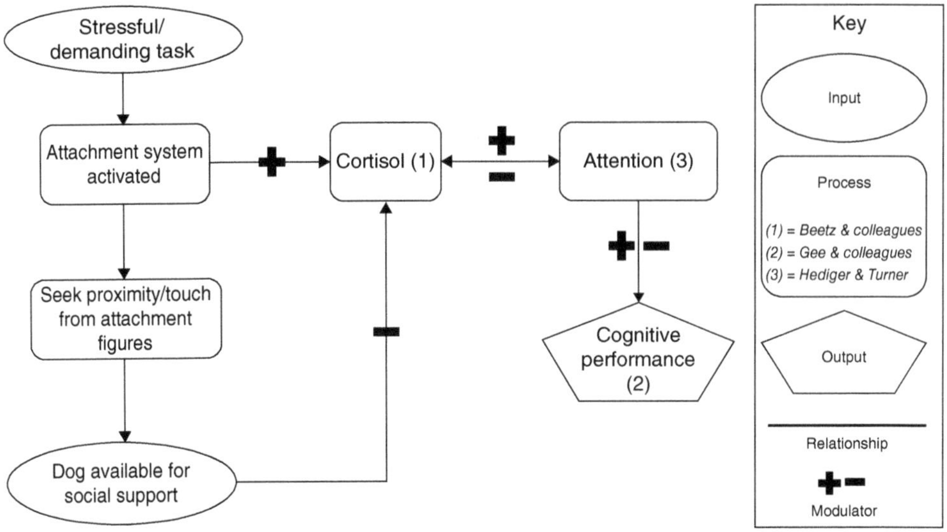

Fig. 2.2. Emergent model from critical synthesis detailing possible impact of dog on cognitive assessment

attachment theory, as explored in Beetz and colleagues' (2011, 2012) studies, offers an explanation. This theory predicts that in stressful situations children seek comfort from a social supporter (Bowlby, 1982). Beetz and colleagues (2011, 2012) found that salivary cortisol was inversely related to the time participants spent physically interacting with dogs, and thus argue that dogs provide a form of social support.

Thought to be the "fight-or-flight" hormone, cortisol is commonly believed to prime mammals to attend to threat and to seek safety (Montoya et al., 2015). Attention towards higher-order cognitive tasks that do not serve this purpose, as are typically measured by cognitive assessments, would therefore be limited. This is consistent with findings that "[e]ven quite mild acute uncontrollable stress can cause a rapid and dramatic loss of prefrontal cognitive abilities" (Arnsten, 2009, p. 410). As such, it appears that physical interaction with dogs modulates children's cortisol response to stressful situations, and in so doing, modulates cognitive performance.

Discussion

Findings

Nine experimental studies were reviewed, providing tentative evidence that dogs can improve children's performance across a range of cognitive domains, including attention, executive functioning, memory, language, and perceptual-motor function, as well as influencing the stress-response pathway. None of the studies found the presence of a dog to be detrimental to children's performance, and several reported that the dog's presence was acceptable to the children. Taken together, this supports the notion that, for some, dogs could offer an effective means by which to improve the cognitive testing experience.

Some confidence can be placed in these results as all studies were of good to fair quality, and methodologically weaker studies yielded findings consistent with the stronger studies. Consistency in findings despite the diversity of interventions, measures and methods of analysis used adds further confidence to these conclusions (Patton, 1999). Systemic bias cannot be discounted, given the small pool of laboratories and journals; however, the findings are also concordant with the adult literature. For instance, in one study, Trammel (2017) found that interacting with a therapy dog prior to sitting an examination significantly reduced university students' self-reported stress levels and significantly improved their exam performance.

Critiquing the model

The emergent model (Fig. 2.2) uses attachment theory and findings from experimental psychology that high levels of cortisol impede cognitive functioning to explain the amalgamated findings of the studies. Compellingly, the model accords with broader literature that support the idea that dogs can be attachment figures for humans (Kurdek, 2008); that stress activates attachment-seeking behaviour, and attachment figures reduce stress via proximity and pleasant touch (Bowlby, 1982); and that pleasant touch releases mood-boosting hormones such as oxytocin (Morrison, 2016). Beetz and colleagues' findings that only the real dog condition (compared with the toy dog and unfamiliar human conditions) significantly influenced cortisol levels supports the primacy of attachment in this process beyond pleasant touch alone (Beetz et al., 2011, 2012).

Amalgamating the results in this way may be an incomplete explanation of the way in which dogs influence cognitive performance, however. For instance, whereas touch is indicated as a means to activate the attachment system under an attachment-based model, evidence from the broader human–animal interaction literature base indicates that proximity may suffice. This finding has real-world implications for the clinical setting. Emergent evidence suggests that dogs' and humans' heart-rate variability synchronises over short distances (Horton, 2016), an effect well-documented in the equine-assisted therapy literature (e.g. Lanata et al., 2016). Evolutionary anthropologists argue that humans and dogs have hunted together for many thousands of years (Schleidt & Shalter, 2003), and intuitively the mutual detection of stress signals would augment this process. However, Grossberg et al. (1988) found no effect of proximity to a dog on heart rate or blood pressure during a stressful arithmetic task, and Beetz et al. (2011, 2012) found positive associations between time spent touching the dog and salivary cortisol levels, casting doubt upon this theory. Nevertheless, as none of the nine studies formally separated touch from proximity this hypothesis cannot be discounted.

Another explanation meriting further consideration is that interacting with a dog improves mood, which improves performance via a positive feedback loop, based upon the theory of self-fulfilling prophecy (Merton, 1948), wherein mood enhances self-belief, and self-belief modulates performance. This helps to explain Hediger and Turner's (2014) finding that the robot dog also somewhat improved cognitive performance, and is supported by evidence from Odendaal and Meintjes (2003) that interacting with a dog was associated with increased dopamine. However, six of the reviewed studies used toy dogs as controls with very limited effects on task performance, and one study recruiting very young children reported that the toy dog appeared distracting to participants, casting doubt upon the theory of self-fulfilling prophecy as the primary effector of change.

Relevance to a clinical context

The reviewed papers provide some preliminary but encouraging evidence to support the use of dogs to help anxious children while taking cognitive assessments. However, as none of the studies were conducted in true-to-life clinical settings, with common cognitive tests used with a clinical population, generalizability to the CAMHS environment can only be cautiously inferred. Nonetheless, several features of the studies can be seen to strengthen the likelihood of their generalizability.

Firstly, although none of the studies included clinical populations, Studies 1 and 2 explicitly recruited participants with insecure attachment styles, which may plausibly represent a proportion of CAMHS service users. The majority of the studies also included language or developmentally delayed children (Studies 1-8), who are more likely to be cognitively assessed in CAMHS than neurotypical children. Study 9 used typically developing school children without identified distress or behavioural difficulties, therefore Hediger and Turner's (2014) findings are the least generalizable to the CAMHS setting in this regard – though, noticeably, this study also found the least compelling evidence for the benefit of a dog.

Secondly, although only Study 9 included formal cognitive assessment tasks used in CAMHS, some generalizability can be inferred from the remaining studies by considering overlaps between the task demands in each setting. For instance, Studies 1 and 2 used mathematical tasks that could be seen as invoking similar demands as the arithmetic sub-test on the WISC. Similarly, the motor skills recruited in Studies 4 and 5 would, arguably, be essential for tasks such as the Block Design component of the WISC, sorting tests (e.g. the Tower of Toronto, the Peg Moving Task), and many processing speed tests (e.g. Trail Making, Cancellation, or Symbol Search). Likewise, the object and picture recognition tasks used in Study 5 bear close resemblance to several standardised memory tests such as the Facial Recognition Test (see Lezak et al., 2012, for test details).

More generally, one could argue that the tasks of attending to, retaining, and acting upon spoken instructions, as assessed by Studies 3, 5 and 8, are a fundamental part of most, if not all, cognitive testing experiences. In studies assessing adherence to task instructions, the fewest prompts were necessary for children in the dog condition, and most for children in the human confederate condition. This has practical importance for the CAMHS testing environment in which an examiner would usually give children verbal instructions. A "no intervention" control group would have been a useful addition to Studies 1-6, 8 and 9, allowing more direct comparison with standard practice in the CAMHS setting.

Implications for future research

These results provide impetus for further research, particularly to assess how applicable the findings may be to the CAMHS cognitive testing environment. Future studies could aim to replicate the reviewed studies with larger samples, clinical populations, a broader age range, and standardised assessment batteries. The use of a "treatment as usual" condition alongside active control groups would make a helpful comparator given that this is an emergent evidence base. If stress-reducing effects can also be found from toys or robots these may offer more pragmatic solutions for services (see O'Cathain et al., 2015), though as some studies noted these to be distracting to children this would require further exploration.

Importantly, experience-close, qualitative accounts would help to understand the perceived impact of dogs on testing from service-users' perspectives. Likewise, it could be important to exploring the potentially competing needs of the children accessing the CAMHS environment, some of whom may find comfort in dogs, and others of whom may find them off-putting, potentially discouraging attendance. Other matters, such as allergies and the dog's welfare, may also need to be explored (Hodgson et al., 2015).

These results also have ramifications for test validity. If dogs can improve cognitive performance, this could, potentially, move the overall distribution of scores and invalidate established norms. Re-validating tests to accommodate dogs (or other interventions) for some children but not others could be a lengthy and complicated process, deserving focused attention should this area develop further. Mediation analyses (Baron & Kenny, 1986) may help establish to what extent improvement in the presence of a dog is a function of anxiety, indicating which children might benefit from a dog, and lending a possible starting point for this enterprise.

Implications for policy and practice

Although further research is merited, these results provide preliminary support for the idea that dogs could help to improve the cognitive testing experience for some children, potentially providing a buffer against the test anxiety that cognitive assessments can sometimes induce, which may, in turn, influence the validity of examinees' results. This holds important implications for clinical practice and policy development; wherein there is an ethical mandate to provide safe, effective, good quality care that *at the very least* does no harm (NHS, 2018). Service providers might, therefore, begin preliminary explorations as to how these ideas can be applied in clinical settings. For instance, small-scale service development projects could be designed to survey attitudes and preferences among service users and professionals. Service providers could consider piloting dog-assisted cognitive assessments in low-stakes situations to explore the clinical impact of the initiative, and to explore the feasibility of the intervention from an organisational perspective. Such studies might also illuminate pragmatic challenges to the implementation of these interventions in the NHS system that would require thought before larger-scale projects and policy changes can be instigated. It is of note that contemporary child-centred justice approaches lend a precedent to this work (see e.g. Spruin et al., 2020) and may offer a helpful starting point for mental health and allied services' development.

Limitations of this review

This main limitation of this review is the small number of studies that met the inclusion criteria, which were conducted in just three laboratories and have heterogeneous samples. Caution should therefore be applied when interpreting the results and applying these to clinical settings. Broadening the search to include papers written in languages other than English might retrieve a greater number of studies eligible for inclusion in future reviews. In addition, whilst taking a critical stance, this review did not include two researchers to appraise the studies, which may have biased the balance given to the results (see May et al., 2016). Additionally, due to time limits, it was not possible to contact authors working in the field directly to retrieve unpublished work, thus the positive findings reported here may represent the "file drawer" effect, wherein null results go unpublished. Nonetheless, the abstract of one unpublished Doctoral dissertation (Becker, 2014) likewise found positive effects of dogs on children's cognitive performance. These limitations notwithstanding, as the first study of its kind, this review may serve to propel further research from which stronger conclusions may be drawn.

Conclusion

Nine studies were critically reviewed. Studies were heterogeneous in design, but consistent in their results and of good to fair quality, offering limited but meaningful evidence to support the use of dogs in cognitive assessments. An attachment-based model was developed to explain these findings, and future research is required to test and refine this model. Such research would benefit from larger samples derived from clinical populations and using standardised cognitive tests to show how these results generalise to the clinical setting. Ambitious and progressive services could consider piloting the inclusion of dogs in assessments to meet the ethical mandate for compassionate care whilst furthering the empirical cause.

Note

[1] See https://www.gov.uk/children-with-special-educational-needs/extra-SEN-help for further information

References

Assistance Dogs International (2019). Glossary. https://assistancedogsinternational.org/resources/adi-terms-definitions/

Arnsten, A. F. T. (2009). Stress signalling pathways that impair prefrontal cortex structure and function. *Nature Reviews Neuroscience*, 10, 410–422. https://doi.org/10.1038/nrn2648.Stress

Baron, R. M., & Kenny, D. A. (1986). The moderator–mediator variable distinction in social psychological research: Conceptual, strategic, and statistical considerations. *Journal of Personality and Social Psychology*, 51(6), 1173–1182. https://doi.org/10.1037//0022-3514.51.6.1173

Bayrak, R., Güler, M., & Şahin, N. H. (2018). The mediating role of self-concept and coping strategies on the relationship between attachment styles and perceived stress. *Europe's Journal of Psychology*, 14(4), 897–913. https://doi.org/10.5964/ejop.v14i4.1508

Becker, J. L. (2014). *Presence of a dog on executive functioning and stress in children with emotional disorders* [unpublished Doctoral dissertation]. Fordham University.

Beetz, A., Kotrschal, K., Turner, D. C., Hediger, K., Uvnäs-Moberg, K., & Julius, H. (2011). The effect of a real dog, toy dog and friendly person on insecurely attached children during a stressful task: An exploratory study. *Anthrozoös*, 24(4), 349–368. https://doi.org/10.2752/175303711X13159027359746

Beetz, A., Julius, H., Turner, D., & Kotrschal, K. (2012). Effects of social support by a dog on stress modulation in male children with insecure attachment. *Frontiers in Psychology*, 3, Article 352. https://doi.org/10.3389/fpsyg.2012.00352

Bond, A., & Lader, M. (1974). The use of analogue scales in rating subjective feelings. *British Journal of Medical Psychology*, 47, 211–218. https://doi.org/10.1111/j.2044-8341.1974.tb02285.x

Bowlby, J. (1982). *Attachment and loss: Vol. 1. Attachment* (2nd ed.). Basic Books.

Bradley, M., & Lang, P. J. (1994). Measuring emotion: The Self-Assessment Manikin and the semantic differential. *Journal of Behavior Therapy and Experimental Psychiatry*, 25(1), 49–59. https://doi.org/10.1016/0005-7916(94)90063-9

Candit. (2001). Computergestützte diagnostik [user manual]. www.candit.com

Chapman, C. D., Benedict, C., & Schiöth, H. B. (2018). Experimenter gender and replicability in science. *Science Advances*, 4(1), 1–7. https://doi.org/10.1016/j.biopsych.2018.02.715

Cohen, J. (1988). *Statistical Power Analysis for the Behavioral Sciences* (2nd ed.). Routledge.

Crossman, M. K., Kazdin, A. E., Matijczak, A., Kitt, E. R., & Santos, L. R. (2020). The influence of interactions with dogs on affect, anxiety, and arousal in children. *Journal of Clinical Child & Adolescent Psychology*, 49(4), 535–548. https://doi.org/10.1080/15374416.2018.1520119

Diamond, L. M. (2015). Stress and attachment. In J. A. Simpson & W. S. Rholes (Eds.) *Attachment theory and research: New directions and emerging themes.* (pp. 97–123). New York, NY: Guilford Press.

Eggiman, J. (2006). Cognitive-Behavioral Therapy: A case report - Animal-Assisted Therapy. *Topics in Advanced Practice Nursing*, 6(3), 1–7. https://www.janeeggiman.com

Equality and Human Rights Commission (2015). *Reasonable adjustments for disabled pupils: Guidance for schools in England.* www.equalityhumanrights.com

Gee, N. R., Belcher, J. M., Grabski, J. L., DeJesus, M., & Riley, W. (2012a). The presence of a therapy dog results in improved object recognition performance in preschool children. *Anthrozoös*, 25(3), 289–300. https://doi.org/10.2752/175303712X13403555186172

Gee, N. R., Church, M. T., & Altobelli, C. L. (2010). Preschoolers make fewer errors on an object categorization task in the presence of a dog. *Anthrozoös*, 23(3), 223–230. https://doi.org/10.2752/175303710X12750451258896

Gee, N. R., Crist, E. N., & Carr, D. N. (2010). Preschool children require fewer instructional prompts to perform a memory task in the presence of a dog. *Anthrozoös*, 23(2), 173–184. https://doi.org/10.2752/175303710X12682332910051

Gee, N. R., Gould, J. K., Swanson, C. C., & Wagner, A. K. (2012b). Preschoolers categorize animate objects better in the presence of a dog. *Anthrozoös*, 25(2), 187–198. https://doi.org/10.2752/175303712X13316289505387

Gee, N. R., Harris, S. L., & Johnson, K. L. (2007). The role of therapy dogs in speed and accuracy to complete motor skills tasks for preschool children. *Anthrozoös*, 20(4), 375–386. https://doi.org/10.2752/089279307X245509

Gee, N. R., Sherlock, T. R., Bennett, E. A., & Harris, S. L. (2009). Preschoolers' adherence to instructions as a function of presence of a dog and motor skills task. *Anthrozoös*, 22(3), 267–276. https://doi.org/10.2752/175303709X457603

Glenk, L. M. (2017). Current perspectives on therapy dog welfare in animal-assisted interventions. *Animals*, 7(7), 1–17. https://doi.org/10.3390/ani7020007

Grossberg, J. M., Alf, E. F., & Vormbrock, J. K. (1988). Does pet dog presence reduce human cardiovascular responses to stress? *Anthrozoös*, 2, 38–44. https://doi.org/10.2752/089279389787058253

Hall, S. S., Gee, N. R., & Mills, D. S. (2016). Children reading to dogs: A systematic review of the literature. *PLoS ONE*, 11(2), 1–22. https://doi.org/10.1371/journal.pone.0149759

Handlin, L., Nilsson, A., Ejdebäck, M., Hydbring-Sandberg, E., & Uvnäs-Moberg, K. (2012). Psychological characteristics of the human–dog relationship and oxytocin and cortisol levels. *Anthrozoös*, 25(2), 215–228. https://doi.org/10.2752/175303712X13316289505468

Hediger, K., & Turner, D. C. (2014). Can dogs increase children's attention and concentration performance? A randomised controlled trial. *Human Animal Interaction Bulletin*, 2(2), 21–39. https://www.researchgate.net/profile/Karin_Hediger/publication/286190655_Can_Dogs_increase_children's_attention_and_concentration_performance_A_randomised_controlled_trial/links/5666b69108ae418a786f510f.pdf

Hodgson, K., Barton, L., Darling, M., Antao, V., Kim, F. A., & Monavvari, A. (2015). Pets' impact on your patients' health: leveraging benefits and mitigating risk. *The Journal of the American Board of Family Medicine*, 28(4), 526–534. https://doi.org/10.3122/jabfm.2015.04.140254

Horton, H. (2016, May 4). A dog's heart beats in sync with its owner's, says new study. *The Telegraph*. https://www.thetelegraph.co.uk

Howard, E. (2020). A review of the literature concerning anxiety for educational assessments. Ofqual. https://assets.publishing.service.gov.uk/government/uploads/system/uploads/attachment_data/file/865832/A_review_of_the_literature_concerning_anxiety_for_educational_assessment.pdf

International Association of Human-Animal Interaction Organisations (IAHAIO; 1998). Prague Declaration. https://iahaio.org/prague-declaration/

Institute of Medicine (2015). *Psychological Testing in the Service of Disability Determination.* The National Academies Press. https://doi.org/10.17226/21704

Isenstein, S. (2018). *Man's best friend is a therapist's best friend: How the presence of a dog influences therapists and others' perceptions of them* [Unpublished Master's dissertation]. University of Toronto.

Jones, M. G., Rice, S. M., & Cotton, S. M. (2019). Incorporating animal-assisted therapy in mental health treatments for adolescents : A systematic review of canine assisted psychotherapy, *PLoS ONE, 14(1),* 1–27. https://doi.org/10.1371/ journal.pone.0210761

Karlsson, P., & Bergmark, A. (2015). Compared with what? An analysis of control-group types in Cochrane and Campbell reviews of psychosocial treatment efficacy with substance use disorders. *Addiction*, 110(3), 420–428. https://doi.org/10.1111/add.12799

Kirschbaum, C., & Hellhammer, D. H. (1994). Salivary cortisol in psychoneuroendocrine research: Recent developments and applications. *Psychoneuroendocrinology*, 19(4), 313–333. https://doi.org/10.1016/0306-4530(94)90013-2

Konno, A., Romero, T., Inoue-Murayama, M., Saito, A., & Hasegawa, T. (2016). Dog breed differences in visual communication with humans. *PLoS ONE*, 11(10), 1–14. https://doi.org/10.1371/journal.pone.0164760

Kurdek, L. A. (2008). Pet dogs as attachment figures. *Journal of Social and Personal Relationships*, 25, 247–266. https://doi.org/10.1177/0265407507087958

Lanata, A., Guidi, A., Valenza, G., Baragli, P., & Scilingo, E. P. (2016). "Quantitative heartbeat coupling measures in human-horse interaction". Proceedings from EMBS's 38th Annual International Conference of the IEEE Engineering in Medicine and Biology Society. Florida. https://doi.org/10.1109/EMBC.2016.7591286

Levinson, B. M. (1962). The dog as a "co-therapist." *Mental Hygiene*, 179, 46–59.

Lezak, M. D., Howieson, D. B., Bigler, E. D., & Tranel, D. (2012). *Neuropsychological assessment* (5th ed.). Oxford University Press.

Lindström Nilsson, M., Funkquist, E. L., Edner, A., & Engvall, G. (2020). Children report positive experiences of animal-assisted therapy in paediatric hospital care. *Acta Paediatrica*, 109(5), 1049–1056. https://doi.org/10.1111/apa.15047

May, D. K., Seivert, N. P., Cano, A., Casey, R. J., & Johnson, A. (2016). Animal-assisted therapy for youth: A systematic methodological critique. *Applied Developmental Science*, 22, 139–153. https://doi.org/10.1080/10888691.2016.1234935

McDonald, S., McDonald, E., & Roberts, A. (2017). Effects of novel dog exposure on college students' stress prior to examination. *North American Journal of Psychology*, 19(2), 477–484.

Merton, R. K. (1948). The Self-Fulfilling Prophecy. *The Antioch Review*, 8, 193–210. https://doi.org/10.2307/4609267

Moher, D., Liberati, A., Tetzlaff, J., & Altman, D. G. (2009). Preferred reporting items for systematic reviews and meta-analyses: The PRISMA statement. *PLoS Medicine*, 6(7), 1–6. https://doi.org/10.1371/journal.pmed.1000097

Montoya, E. R., van Honk, J., Bos, P. A., & Terburg, D. (2015). Dissociated neural effects of cortisol depending on threat escapability. *Human Brain Mapping*, 36(11), 4304–4316. https://doi.org/10.1002/hbm.22918

Morrison, I. (2016). Keep calm and cuddle on: Social touch as a stress buffer. *Adaptive Human Behavior and Physiology*, 2, 344–362. https://doi.org/10.1007/s40750-016-0052-x

National Health Service (NHS; 2018). Principles and values that guide the NHS. https://www.nhs.uk/using-the-nhs/about-the-nhs/principles-and-values/

O'Cathain, A., Hoddinott, P., Lewin, S., Thomas, K. J., Young, B., Adamson, J., ... Donovan, J. L. (2015). Maximising the impact of qualitative research in feasibility studies for randomised controlled trials: Guidance for researchers. *Pilot and Feasibility Studies*, 1(32), 1–13. https://doi.org/10.1186/s40814-015-0026-y

Odendaal, J. S. J., & Meintjes, R. A. (2003). Neurophysiological correlates of affiliative behaviour between humans and dogs. *Veterinary Journal*, 165, 296–301. https://doi.org/10.1016/S1090-0233(02)00237-X

Palitsky, D., Mota, N., Afifi, T. O., Downs, A. C., & Sareen, J. (2013). The association between adult attachment style, mental disorders, and suicidality: findings from a population-based study. *The Journal of Nervous and Mental Disease*, 201(7), 579–586. https://doi.org/10.1097/NMD.0b013e31829829ab

Park, J., & Moghaddam, B. (2017). Impact of anxiety on prefrontal cortex encoding of cognitive flexibility. *Neuroscience*, 345, 193–202. https://doi.org/10.1016/j.neuroscience.2016.06.013

Patton, M. Q. (1999). Enhancing the quality and credibility of qualitative analysis. *Health Services Research*, 34(5 Pt 2), 1189–1208. http://www.ncbi.nlm.nih.gov/pubmed/10591279%0Ahttp://www.pubmedcentral.nih.gov/articlerender.fcgi?artid=PMC1089059

Pop, D., Rusu, A. S., & Constantinescu, R. (2014). Physiological effects of human-animal positive interaction in dogs: Review of the literature. *Bulletin University of Agricultural Sciences and Veterinary Medicine*, 71(2), 102–110. https://doi.org/10.15835/buasvmcn-asb:1039

Rose, R., Howley, M., Fergusson, A., & Jament, J. (2009). Mental health and special educational needs: Exploring a complex relationship. *British Journal of Special Education*, 36(1), 3–8. https://doi.org/10.1111/j.1467-8578.2008.00409.x

Sachdev, P. S., Blacker, D., Blazer, D. G., Ganguli, M., Jeste, D. V., Paulsen, J. S., & Petersen, R. C. (2014). Classifying neurocognitive disorders: The DSM-5 approach. *Nature Reviews Neurology*, 10(11), 634–642. https://doi.org/10.1038/nrneurol.2014.181

Sandoval, G. N. (2010). Court facility dogs — Easing the apprehensive witness. *The Colorado Lawyer*, 39(4), 17–23. https://www.childrenslawoffice.com

Schleidt, W. M., & Shalter, M. D. (2003). Co-evolution of humans and canids: An alternative view of dog domestication: Homo Homini Lupus? *Evolution and Cognition*, 9, 57–72. https://www.nldogs.com

Schneider, M. S., & Harley, L. P. (2006). How dogs influence the evaluation of psychotherapists. *Anthrozoös*, 19(2), 128–143. http://dx.doi.org/10.2752/089279306785593784

Serra-Sala, M., Timoneda-Gallart, C., & Perez-Alvarez, F. (2016). Clinical usefulness of hemoencephalography beyond the neurofeedback. *Neuropsychiatric Disease and Treatment*, 12, 1173–1180. https://doi.org/10.2147/NDT.S105476

Shoshev, M. (2017). Hemoencephalography neurofeedback – Mechanism of action. *Trakia Journal of Sciences*, 15(4), 354–358. https://doi.org/10.15547/tjs.2017.04.016

Specialist Unit for Review Evidence (SURE). (2018). *Questions to assist with the critical appraisal of randomised controlled trials and other experimental studies*. http://www.cardiff.ac.uk/specialist-unit-for-review-evidence/resources/critical-appraisal-checklists

Spruin, E., Mozova, K., Dempster, T., & Freeman, R. (2020). The use of facility dogs to bridge the justice gap for survivors of sexual offending. *Social Sciences*, 9(6), 96. https://doi.org/10.3390/socsci9060096

Spruin, E., Mozova, K., Franz, A., Mitchell, S., Fernandez, A., Dempster, T., & Holt, N. (2019). The use of therapy dogs to support court users in the waiting room. *International Criminal Justice Review*, 29, 1–20. https://doi.org/10.1177/1057567719827063

Teffer, K., & Semendeferi, K. (2012). Human prefrontal cortex: Evolution, development, and pathology. *Progress in Brain Research*, 195, 191–218. https://doi.org/10.1016/B978-0-444-53860-4.00009-X

Terras, K. (2006). The value of a dog in a classroom of children with severe emotional disorders. *Anthrozoös*, 19(1), 35–49. https://doi.org/10.2752/089279306785593919

Trammell, J. P. (2017). The effect of therapy dogs on exam stress and memory. *Anthrozoös*, 30(4), 607–621. https://doi.org/10.1080/08927936.2017.1370244

Turner, D. C. (2010, July). "Attitudes toward animals: A cross-cultural, international comparison". Proceedings from IAHAIO's 12th International Conference on Human-Animal Interactions. Stockholm.

Vincent, A., Sterman, J., & Bussert, K. (2019). Paws for smiles at the dentist: Exploring the biological impact of human-animal interaction. Proceedings from IAHAIO's *15th Triennial Conference*. Brewster, NY.

von der Embse, N., Jester, D., Roy, D., & Post, J. (2018). Test anxiety effects, predictors, and correlates: A 30-year meta-analytic review. *Journal of Affective Disorders*, 227, 483–493. https://doi.org/10.1016/j.jad.2017.11.048

Ward-Griffin, E., Klaiber, P., Collins, H. K., Owens, R. L., Coren, S., & Chen, F. S. (2018). Petting away pre-exam stress: The effect of therapy dog sessions on student well-being. *Stress and Health*, 34(3), 468–473. https://doi.org/10.1002/smi.2804

Wechsler, D., & Kaplan, E. (2015). *WISC-V Integrated Technical and Interpretive Manual.* Pearson.

Wells, D. L. (2007). Domestic dogs and human health: An overview. *British Journal of Health Psychology*, 12(Pt. 1), 145–156. https://doi.org/10.1348/135910706X103284

Young, J. S. (2012). Pet therapy: Dogs de-stress students. *Journal of Christian Nursing*, 29(4), 217–221. https://doi.org/10.1097/CNJ.0b013e31826701a7

3 Sustained Effects of Animal-Assisted Crisis Response on Stress in School Shooting Survivors

Ariann E. Robino[1]*, David M. Feldman[2], Alyssa N. Stein[2], Melody A. Schmaltz[2], Hailey A. Fitzpatrick[2], Jaime L. Tartar[2], Frankie Pizzo[2], Marah Friedman[2] and Olivia Feldman[3]

[1]*Deloitte Consulting;* [2]*College of Psychology, Nova Southeastern University;* [3]*Unaffiliated*

Abstract

Animal-assisted crisis response (AACR) is an intervention that harnesses the human-animal bond for therapeutic benefit through specially trained animal-handler teams deployed to provide comfort following a mass traumatic event. During the months and years following the shooting at Marjory Stoneman Douglas High School on February 14, 2018, therapy animals joined the campus community to promote healing and stress reduction. The purpose of this quantitative study was to examine the sustained effects on bonding and stress in a sample of survivors of the tragedy who participated in animal-assisted crisis response. Data was collected through a quasi-experimental study of three intervention groups (i.e., discussion of AACR, viewing photos related to AACR, and engaging with therapy animals). Cortisol analysis indicated a reduction in stress post-intervention across groups with the largest difference in the therapy animal interaction group. Implications for AACR and addressing the psychological effects of mass traumas are provided.

Keywords: animal-assisted crisis response, animal-assisted intervention, human-animal bond, therapy animals

In the wake of a crisis, there are several possible psychological and physiological reactions that an individual may experience, including changes in sleep patterns, body aches, isolation (Substance Abuse and Mental Health Services Administration, 2021). Traditionally, affected individuals are encouraged to speak with crisis hotlines that are staffed with mental health professionals who are equipped with crisis-specific training (e.g., suicide prevention) (Greenstein, 2017). According to the National Alliance on Mental Illness (n. d.), in addition to this form of support, trauma-informed and recovery-focused crisis stabilization programs, such as Psychological First Aid (PFA; Brymer et al., 2006), are effective in providing care to the impacted individuals. Built upon the concept of human resilience, PFA is an evidence-informed approach that aims to reduce acute stress symptoms and facilitate recovery following exposure to a traumatic event such as a natural disaster, public health emergency, or personal crisis (Brymer et al.,

---

Corresponding author: arobino@deloitte.com
The authors would like to thank the City of Parkland and Mayor Rich Walker, Canine-Assisted Therapy Inc., and Judy Beldon-Feldman.

2006). Specifically, PFA utilizes five elements of psychological response to inform and guide helpers to connect, stabilize, educate, and assist survivors of disaster and crisis. This is achieved through providing safety, emotional support, information, and access to social support systems (Brymer et al., 2006).

In recent years, a complementary modality known as *animal-assisted crisis response* (AACR) has been added to the list of resources available to those who have survived a traumatic event. AACR is defined as a form of animal-assisted activities that provides comfort to those who have been affected by natural, human-caused, or technological disasters (Pet Partners, 2021). It is important to note that AACR is not a form of professional mental health treatment; rather, it is used to complement traditional methods of crisis intervention (Bua, 2013; Robinson, 2004). This method of crisis response aims to provide individuals a safe environment and time with a trained and registered therapy animal. Handlers of the therapy animals are required to undergo training, evaluation, and continuing education practices to ensure they can adequately respond in emotionally charged environments (Lackey & Haberstock, 2019). Although there is minimal research on the effects of AACR, available studies indicate a reduction in psychological and physiological symptoms as measured from before and after an interaction with a therapy animal (Eaton-Stull & Flynn, 2015; Eaton-Stull & Sewall, 2019). To date, AACR has been incorporated to facilitate healing for individuals who have experienced a crisis such as grief, suicide, a mass shooting, or natural disaster (Eaton-Stull & Flynn, 2020). During the months and years following the shooting at Marjory Stoneman Douglas High School on February 14, 2018, therapy animals joined the campus community to promote healing and stress reduction. Their unique bond with these therapy animals provides an opportunity to understand more strongly the relationships and impacts of AACR.

Human-animal bond

AACR is focused on providing support and comfort for survivors of crisis events by leveraging the human-animal bond (Gordon, 2013). The American Veterinary Medical Association (2021) defines the human-animal bond as "a mutually beneficial and dynamic relationship between people and animals that is influenced by behaviors essential to the health and wellbeing of both" (para 1). Research has demonstrated the positive effects the human-animal bond can have on humans' physiological responses to stress (Handlin et al., 2019; Human-Animal Bond Research Institute, 2020; Levin et al., 2013), and these findings may be consistent with stress induced following crisis events. One neurobiological pathway that is likely involved in this process is the hypothalamic-pituitary-adrenal (HPA) axis, which regulates the body's stress response (Kirschbaum & Hellhammer, 1989). To measure activation of the HPA axis, researchers often take salivary cortisol samples as salivary cortisol is considered a reliable measure of physiological stress in human and non-human animals (Balters et al., 2020). At the time of an aversive event, stress produces a variety of behavioral and physiological responses to enable individuals to protect themselves by adapting to the situation. Immediately following the aversive event, the HPA axis is activated, which causes an increase in corticosteroids. Severe stress, such as during and in the aftermath of a crisis event, can cause the HPA axis to become dysregulated, which can lead to an excessive release of corticosteroids. Due to the ongoing development of children and adolescents' brains, this population is particularly vulnerable to the effects of hormone overproduction and dysregulation of the HPA axis (Suzuki et al., 2014).

Childhood trauma is associated with long-standing effects on cortisol responses to stress in adulthood (Suzuki et al., 2014). While childhood trauma can have a significant impact on regulation of cortisol and the HPA-axis, research has demonstrated that human-canine interaction can positively influence HPA-axis and cortisol activity (Rodriguez et al., 2018). Adults have been shown to secrete less cortisol when interacting with dogs, suggesting that dogs have a calming effect on humans through this bonding experience (Odendaal & Meintjes, 2003). Furthermore, the simple presence of dogs may have a stronger effect than interactions with other humans during or after aversive events. Beetz et al. (2011) found that children interacting with a real dog exhibited lower salivary cortisol levels during stressful situations than children that interacted with a friendly human or a toy dog. Moreover, these researchers found that increased interaction with the dog through petting/stroking resulted in less pronounced stress responses; which suggests that the stress-reducing effect of the dog depended on the child's engagement with the dog through sensory contact (Beetz et al., 2011). These findings are supported by prior research that found animate touch, specifically via petting both hard-shelled animals (e.g., turtles) and soft animals (e.g., rabbits) as opposed to petting a toy turtle and rabbit, can result in reduced levels of state-anxiety, a type of anxiety experienced in response to a situation perceived to be threatening or dangerous (Shiloh et al., 2003; VandenBos, 2007). Additionally, Polheber and Matchock (2014) found that college students who spent time with a therapy trained dog before engaging in a stressful task had lower levels of cortisol after and a lower heart rate during the stressful event compared to participants that were accompanied by a human friend. In this body of literature, the human-animal bond component to human-animal interactions appears to significantly improve one's physiological response to stress after experiencing a stressful or traumatic event as measured by salivary cortisol samples.

In addition, humans can experience positive physiological benefits from interacting with dogs as the interaction initiates the release of oxytocin, a hormone associated with the feeling of comfort and well-being (O'Haire et al., 2019). Oxytocin can facilitate positive effects of social interaction (i.e., increased trust) and inhibit stress-related activity (i.e., posttraumatic stress symptoms including hyperarousal, anxiety, and interpersonal difficulties) (MacDonald & MacDonald, 2010). It has been found in previous research that children who were accompanied by a dog to a doctor's visit experienced less behavioral distress, lower systolic blood pressure, lower heart rate, and reduced cortisol than children who were not accompanied by a dog (Nagengast et al., 1997; Vincent, 2019). Altogether, the current research suggests that children and adolescents can experience beneficial effects through human-animal interactions following exposure to a stressful event.

Animals and adolescents

Owning a pet during adolescence can not only provide a sense of comfort, but it has been found that attachment to these pets foster a deeper sense of trust in the adolescent (Piper & Uttley, 2019). This can assist in relationship building and the ability to socialize for the individual as they move into adulthood. The human-animal bond can also positively impact adolescents' development. For example, pet ownership during adolescence has been associated with higher levels of self-esteem, autonomy, and self-concept (Purewal et al., 2017). Caring for a pet during adolescence can also be seen as a buffer against feelings of loneliness, which can further moderate suicidal ideation and behavior (Black, 2009). As emotional support is a significant factor in how effectively an adolescent can manage a challenging situation and its aftermath (Cassels et al., 2017; Piper, 2014), the possibility of animals providing a level of support cannot go unrecognized. Adolescents may experience concern regarding stigma associated with mental health, and this may negatively impact their professional help-seeking behaviors (Lawrence et al., 2015). Therefore, inclusion of animals in the aftermath of a crisis event for adolescents may significantly increase engagement in a therapeutic process. For example, animal-assisted therapy has been found to produce significantly higher retention and attendance rates for adolescents than standard psychological treatments (Jones et al., 2019). Considering trauma-focused mental health treatment is often associated with high rates of drop-out (Berke et al., 2019), animal-assisted interventions, such as animal-assisted crisis response, may considerably help individuals in the aftermath of a traumatic event.

This idea can be applied to an even more specific population: adolescents who have experienced a traumatic event. Following the event, there may be many overwhelming emotions that surface for the adolescent. These emotions can be challenging to talk about in traditional settings, especially for a child or teenager. In effort to provide a safe place where adolescents can talk about their experiences, animal-assisted interventions may be incorporated to decrease an individual's level of physiological stress. For example, researchers found that children who had an animal present during a forensic interview regarding child sexual abuse had lower levels of stress (e.g., lower heart rate) during the interview (Krause-Parello et al., 2018). This is an important finding as it demonstrates that the presence of an animal in the interview room facilitated the reduction in the child's physiological stress response, which in turn increased the child's level of comfort, permitting them to communicate more openly about their traumatic experiences. Moreover, incorporating animal-assisted interventions with trauma survivors can elicit improvements that are natural to the human-animal bond.

Animal-assisted crisis response

Survivors of trauma and crisis events frequently report experiencing a heightened state of alertness, difficulty relaxing, social isolation, a lack of safety and security, numbness, intrusive thoughts, and flashbacks. In addition, individuals who have experienced these responses to trauma often feel ostracized, stigmatized, and alone (O'Haire et al., 2019). In the immediate aftermath of a crisis, the incorporation of animals into crisis response can help facilitate recovery in several ways, including a more rapid development of rapport by creating a bridge between the survivor and helper, providing a safe and calming presence, reducing the need for verbal communication, encouraging physical movement, and facilitating present minded thinking by providing a reality-oriented focus for survivors (Greenbaum, 2006). Research has found that interacting with an animal can reduce and mitigate the physiological stress response (Beetz et al., 2012), restore a sense of calmness and security (Taylor et al., 2013; Yount et al., 2012), reduce self-reported fear and anxiety (Barker et al., 2003, 2015; Lass-Hennemann et al., 2014), and thus modulate overall arousal in individuals exposed to trauma.

As mentioned previously, individuals exposed to a traumatic event often experience an array of reactions that are both psychological and physiological. Further complicating a survivor's experience, research has found that repeated exposure to trauma can have a significant and cumulative impact on an individual's mental health and increase their risk for PTSD, suicide, and substance abuse (Glenn, 2017). A study that examined the effects of cumulative traumatic stress on emergency personnel involved in responding to the 9/11 terrorist attack in New York City produced findings that have implications for the field of AACR (Alvarez & Hunt, 2005). Due to the nature of their job, first responders are a unique population who are chronically exposed to both direct and vicarious trauma. Among the emergency personnel participants was a group of canine search-and-rescue (SAR) teams who had never assisted in a man-made disaster of this caliber, with so few survivors, and with such a large death toll (Alvarez & Hunt, 2005). Interestingly, results from this study indicated that, although deployed SAR handlers endorsed elevated rates of psychological distress and symptoms of PTSD, the levels of PTSD symptom severity, as endorsed on self-report measures, were lower than the rates reported in previous studies of non-canine handler first responders (Alvarez & Hunt, 2005). Researchers have speculated that search-and-rescue animal handlers might be more resilient than other first responders due to the protective effect animals can have on moderating traumatic stress, the development of PTSD, and depression (Allen et al., 2002; Arambasic et al., 2000).

Purpose of the study

Given the increasing popularity of animal-assisted interventions overall (Fine et al., 2019) and AACR specifically (Lackey & Haberstock, 2019), this study was conducted to examine how the bonds that develop through AACR sustain over time. We also wanted to explore the context in which these bonds influence stress response in survivors of a traumatic event who directly engaged in AACR. This interest resulted in two research questions and hypotheses:

1. What is the effect of therapy animals on bonding and stress in survivors of the shooting at Marjory Stoneman Douglas High?

Hypothesis: Survivors of the shooting at Marjory Stoneman Douglas High will experience high levels of self-reported bonding and decreased levels of stress after interaction with therapy animals.

2. What are the differences in bonding and stress levels in survivors of the shooting at Marjory Stoneman Douglas High based on type of therapy animal exposure?

Hypothesis: Survivors of the shooting at Marjory Stoneman Douglas High will experience similar levels of bonding and stress reduction regardless of type of therapy animal exposure with greater bonding and reduced stress upon direct therapy animal interaction compared to only discussion and/or visual stimuli.

Methods

Participants

Eleven survivors of the shooting at Marjory Stoneman Douglas High (MSDH) participated in the quasi-experimental study. All participants were above the age of 18 ($M = 18.73$). Six participants identified as female and four identified as male. Participants were in varying grade levels with 27.3% ($n = 3$) reporting as seniors in high school, 45% ($n = 5$) reporting as freshmen in college, and 27.3% ($n = 3$) reporting as sophomores in college. Most participants identified as White/Caucasian (45.5%; $n = 5$) with the remaining identifying as Hispanic/Latino (18.2%; $n = 2$), Black/African-American (9.1%; $n = 1$), Asian (9.1%; $n = 1$), and bi-racial (18.2%; $n = 2$). Most participants lived with a dog (72.7%; $n = 8$), and over half had interacted with a therapy dog in the past year (54.6%; $n = 6$).

Measures

Perceived stress scale

The Perceived Stress Scale (PSS; Cohen et al., 1983) is a 10-item Likert scale measure used to assess an individual's perception of their baseline stress levels. Participants indicate how often they have felt or thought a certain way over the past month on a scale of 0–4 (0 = *Never* to 4 = *Very Often*). Four items on the scale require reverse-scoring. Higher scores on the PSS indicate higher levels of perceived stress. The PSS has been used often in both research and clinical settings (Answer et al., 2020; Chew et al., 2020; Crutcher et al., 2018). In addition, the PSS has also been used to assess changes in young adults' perceived stress levels upon exposure to a therapy animal (Fiocco & Hunse, 2017). It was found to have acceptable reliability in the current study ($\alpha = 0.77$).

Impact of events scale-revised

Prior to completing the Impact of Events Scale-Revised (IES-R; Weiss & Marmar, 1997), participants were asked to reflect upon the tragedy at their high school when answering the items to assess for immediate symptoms of trauma. The IES-R is a 22-item Likert scale instrument (1 = *Not at all* to 5 = *Extremely*) that assess participants' subjective trauma response (i.e., intrusion, avoidance, hyperarousal) to the event. It has been found to appropriately differentiate between traumatized and non-traumatized populations (McCabe, 2019). The IES-R demonstrated appropriate internal consistency in other studies (Craparo et al., 2013; Norhayati & Aniza, 2014; Uver, 2020). It was also highly reliable in this study ($\alpha = 0.95$).

Center for the study of animal wellness pet bonding

The Center for the Study of Animal Wellness Pet Bonding Scale (CSAWPBS; Johnson & Meadows, 2003) was used to assess for participants' perceptions of their bond with the therapy animal following the exposure. It is a 28-item instrument that measures participants' attachment to the animal and their feelings of reciprocal acceptance. Items are answered using a 5-point Likert scale (*1* = *more often true* to *5* = *more often false*). One item must be reverse scored. Lower scores indicate greater degree of bonding as perceived by the human participant. During scale development, the CSAWPBS was found to be internally consistent ($\alpha = 0.89$); the present study found identical reliability ($\alpha = 0.89$).

Demographics form

Participants also completed a demographics form. Demographics collected included age, gender identity, grade in school, race/ethnicity, religious affiliation, approximate date of last encounter with a therapy animal, and dog guardianship status.

Physiological stress measures

To monitor for changes in physiological responses to stress, participants' saliva, heart rate, and blood pressure were obtained. All three measures are commonly used biological indicators of stress (Iqbal et al., 2021; Morris et al., 2016) as well as in human-animal interaction research (Beetz et al., 2012; Ng et al., 2014; Pendry & Vandagriff, 2019). Blood pressure and heart rate were obtained through a wrist monitor. Individual tubes were used to collect saliva at separate time points. Saliva was collected from each participant by unstimulated passive drool for salivary cortisol analysis (participants drooled directly into a 1.5 mL microcentrifuge tube through a small sterile cylinder). Samples were stored in a freezer following participant testing at −20°C. Cortisol was quantified through the use of a commercially available human enzyme immunoassay (EIA) kit (Salimetrics LLC, USA) which has a 0.91correlation with serum and a sensitivity < 0.007 μg/dL. Interpolated concentrations are in μg/dL. The samples were read on a BioTek ELx800 plate reader (BioTek Instruments, Inc. Winooski, VT).

Procedure

IRB approval was obtained from the authors' institution prior to participant recruitment by word-of-mouth and through key informants within the Parkland/MSDHS community. To ensure ethical safeguards, all participants were over the age of 18 and provided an information sheet to distribute to their parents describing the context of the study with referrals for mental health resources. In addition, two mental health professions and five mental health masters and doctoral-level trainees were on-site of the study all times. The study was developed in consultation with mental health professionals, a neuroscientist, a survivor of the shooting, parents of students who experienced the event, and Parkland/MSDHS community members. At the time of the study, three years had passed since the event to remove recency of the experience. As a condition of the IRB approval, permission to conduct the study on-location was obtained from Parkland City Hall; due to COVID-19 restrictions and to maintain fidelity to the interventions, the study was conducted outdoors with staggered start times for each participant group. Figures 3.1, 3.2, and 3.3 provide graphics of how the study was conducted within these limitations. All groups completed data collection at pre and post points with interventions based on their randomly assigned group. The first group (Discussion Group; Fig. 3.1) participated in a guided discussion on their experiences with the therapy animals after the shooting at their school. The second group (Photo Group; Fig. 3.2) reviewed photos of the therapy animals from their school. The third group (Therapy Animal Group; Fig. 3.3) participated in a direct interaction with therapy animals that had visited their school. Participants of the first two groups were provided a time that they could return to the site of the study to engage with therapy animals, if interested.

Participants were reminded at multiple points during data collection that they could withdraw at any time as a component of ongoing informed consent. Participants completed a consent form, a demographics form, the Perceived Stress Scale to evaluate baseline stress level, and the Impact of Events-Scale to evaluate the presence of trauma symptoms. Participants then provided measurements of their blood pressure, heart rate, and cortisol through saliva. Saliva samples were wiped with a paper towel to avoid contamination and were immediately placed in a bag of ice to preserve the sample. After this, participants participated in one of the previously described therapy animal-related interventions for approximately 20 minutes. After the intervention, participants completed the Center for the Study of Animal Wellness Pet Bonding Scale. The study concluded with another collection of blood pressure, heart rate, and cortisol through saliva. Again, saliva samples were wiped with a paper towel to avoid contamination and were immediately placed in a bag of ice to preserve the sample. This study took approximately 1 hour per participant group. Licensed mental health practitioners trained in crisis intervention were in attendance in the event participants needed de-escalation. Participants were provided with a Project Information Sheet for Parents that encouraged them to monitor their child following their participation in this study and alert the researchers to any concerns. Contact information was provided in the event parents needed any mental health referrals or had any questions.

For the Therapy Animal Group, the handler of the dog was responsible for monitoring the dog's fatigue, stress levels, and overall ability to participate. The three dog-handler teams were volunteers recruited from Canine-Assisted Therapy (CAT), a local therapy animal organization from which multiple therapy animal teams were dispatched in response to the need at MSDHS. To register as a therapy dog team with CAT, the organization requires that the dog is at least one year old, under the guardianship of the handler for at least six months, has passed the American Kennel Club Canine Good Citizen Test within the past two years, in good health and current on

Group 1 (Discussion Group)

1) Group 1 participants arrived on site at 9:00 AM.
2) Upon arrival, participants were paired with a research assistant who guided the participant to one of the three data collection sites arranged around the building.
3) Each participant completed pre-intervention self-report measures and data was collected (blood pressure, heart rate, and cortisol via saliva sample) to establish participant baseline.
4) After the intervention, participants completed post-intervention self-report measures and data was collected a second time (blood pressure, heart rate, and cortisol via saliva sample).
5) Once data collection was complete, each participant was directed to the exit which was intentionally located away from the entrance to maintain fidelity to the intervention and compliance with COVID-19 social distancing guidelines. All group 1 participants were cleared from the site by 9:45 AM.

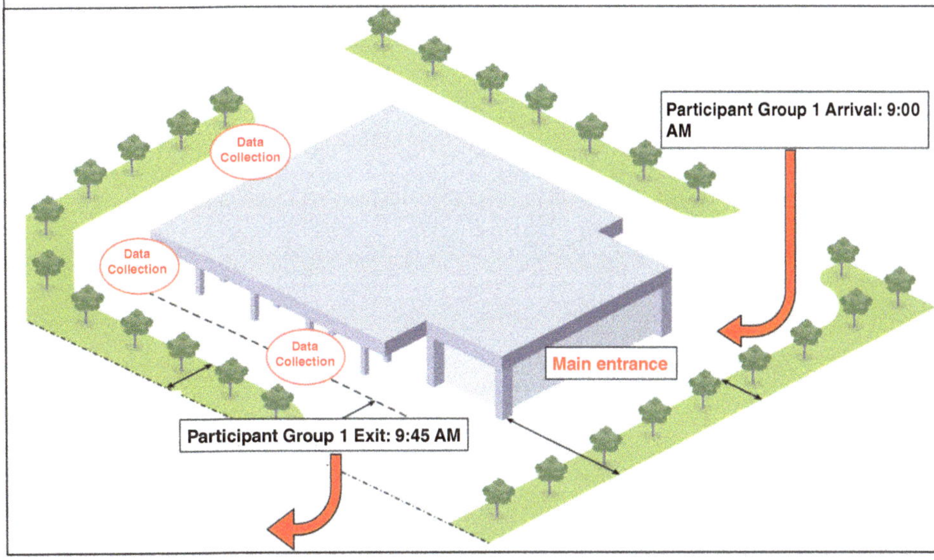

Fig. 3.1. Discussion Group Protocol.

vaccinations, and non-reactive to strangers and other dogs while enjoying the work. CAT handler dog teams undergo an evaluation and certification process (Canine-Assisted Therapy, 2022) once the pre-requisite qualifications are met. Handlers also receive background screening and a series of mentoring sessions prior to independent volunteering. The first team consisted of a handler with an active therapy dog registration with CAT and a female Italian Greyhound/ Golden Retriever mixed breed who worked as a therapy dog for approximately four years. The second team consisted of a handler with an active therapy dog registration with CAT and a female Golden Retriever who worked as a therapy dog for approximately six years. The third team consisted of a handler with an active therapy dog registration with CAT and a Shih Tzu/Yorkie mixed breed who worked as a therapy dog for approximately five years.

Analysis

Data was analyzed using SPSS. Descriptive statistics were obtained for the PSS, IES-R, and CSWAPB. For cortisol analyses, all samples were run in duplicate, and the average values were analyzed. A paired samples t-test was conducted to examine overall cortisol differences pre and post animal

Group 2 (Photo Group)

1) Group 2 participants arrived on site at 10:00 AM.
2) Upon arrival, participants were paired with a research assistant who guided the participant to one of the three data collection sites arranged around the building.
3) Each participant completed pre-intervention self-report measures and data was collected (blood pressure, heart rate, and cortisol via saliva sample) to establish participant baseline.
4) After the intervention, participants completed post-intervention self-report measures and data was collected a second time (blood pressure, heart rate, and cortisol via saliva sample).
5) Once data located was complete, each participant was directed to the exit which was intentionally located away from the sites entrance to maintain fidelity to the intervention and compliance with COVID-19 social distancing guidlines. All group 2 participants were cleared from the site by 10:45 AM.

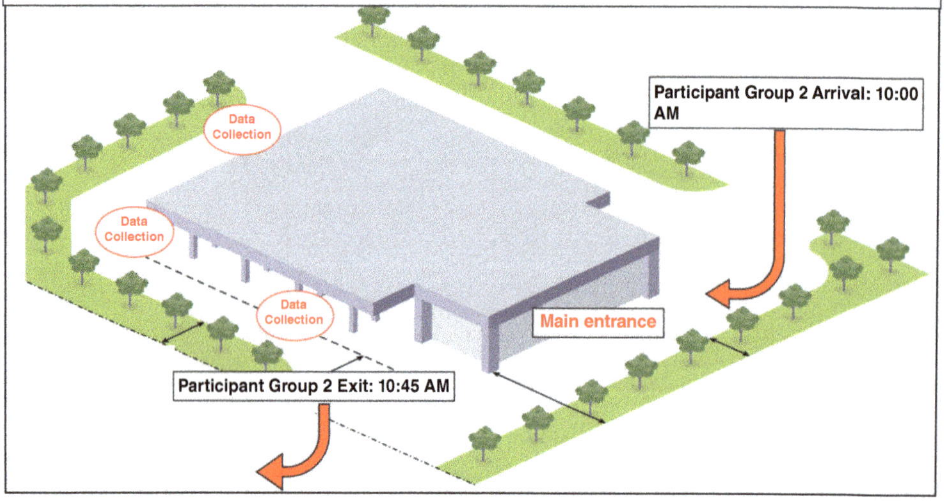

Fig. 3.2. Photo Group Protocol.

intervention. Correlations were run to establish the strength of the relationship between the pre and post-test. Differences between blood pressure and heart rate levels were also examined through t-test. A regression was conducted to determine if bonding was a predictor of change in stress levels. An ANOVA was conducted to explore the differences between the groups of intervention conditions.

Results

To assess the presence of stress and trauma symptoms, descriptive analyses were obtained using the PSS and IES-R. The average PSS score (M = 21.22; SD = 2.41) indicated moderate levels of stress at the time of data collection. The average IES-R score (M = 26.17; SD = 17.35) indicated the presence of some PTSD symptoms in response to the shooting at their high school, although not at levels probable for a diagnosis of PTSD (Weiss & Marmar, 1997).

Research question 1

To answer the first research question, the paired samples t-test revealed a statistically significant difference in cortisol levels between collection prior to the intervention and after the intervention, $t(10) = 2.72$, $p < 0.05$. Fig. 3.4 provides a visual representation of each participants' cortisol levels pre and post therapy animal intervention;

Group 3 (Therapy Animal Group)

1) Group 3 participants arrived on site at 11:00 AM.
2) Upon arrival, participants were paired with a research assistant who guided the participant to one of the three data collection sites arranged around the building.
3) Each participant completed pre-intervention self-report measures and data was collected (blood pressure, heart rate, and cortisol via saliva sample) to establish participant baseline.
4) Therapy animal teams arrived on site at 11:15 AM after pre-intervention data was complete.
5) After the intervention, participants completed post-intervention self-report measures and data was collected a second time (blood pressure, heart rate, and cortisol via saliva sample).
6) Once data collection was complete, each participant was directed to the exit which was intentionally located away from the site entrance to maintain fidelity to the intervention and compliance with COVID-19 social distancing guidelines.

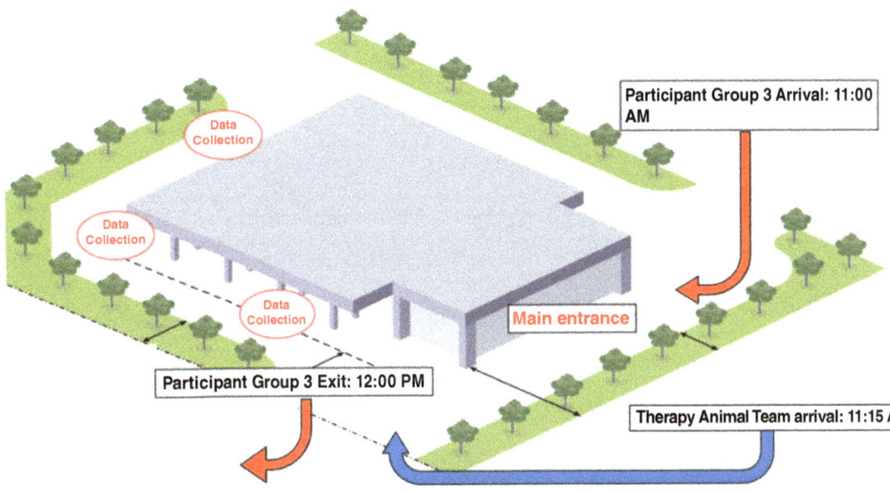

Fig. 3.3. Therapy Animal Group Protocol.

Fig. 3.5 provides a visual representation of the overall change in cortisol levels pre and post therapy animal intervention. To examine further the strength of the relationship between the pre and post results, a Pearson Product correlation was run; all paired samples of systolic blood pressure, diastolic blood pressure, heart rate, and cortisol were strongly correlated ($r = 0.67$, $r = 0.72$, $r = 0.85$, $r = 0.92$, respectively). An additional correlation was conducted to examine the type of relationship and post-cortisol level. Results revealed a strong negative relationship between the type of intervention and cortisol levels after intervention ($r = -0.70$). Due to how the interventions were coded in the data set, this indicated that, the greater degree of exposure to a therapy animal (i.e., discussion, photos, interaction), the stronger relationship to decreased cortisol level. There was no statistically significant difference between blood pressure and heart rate pre and post intervention. The average bonding score was $M = 58.6$, $SD = 13.6$. When used as a predictor in the regression analysis, there was no predictive relationship between the bonding score and cortisol levels.

Research question 2

To answer the second research question, an ANOVA was conducted to examine the differences between groups. There was a statistically significant difference in post-intervention cortisol levels between

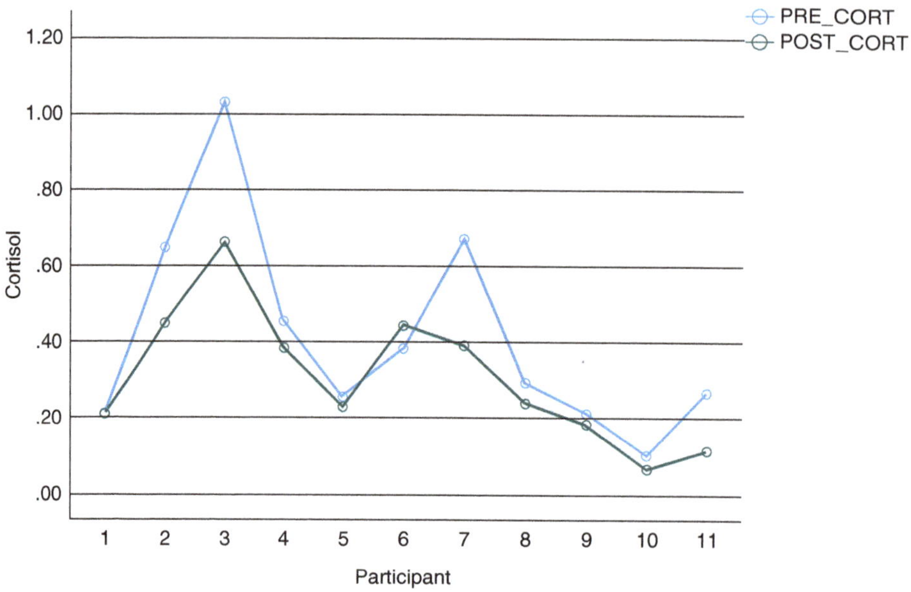

Fig. 3.4. Pre/Post Cortisol By Participant During Therapy Animal Intervention.

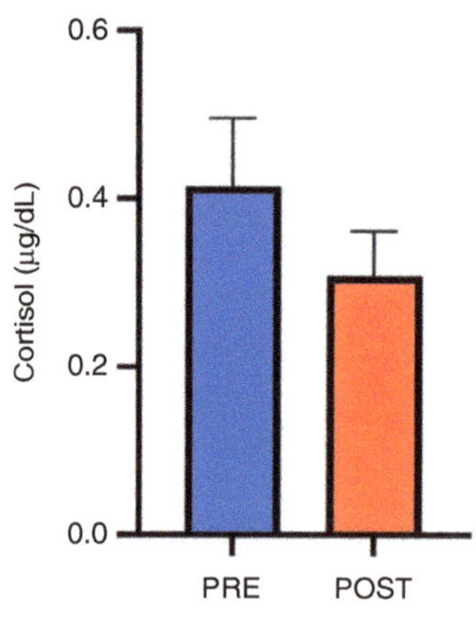

Fig. 3.5. Pre/Post Cortisol Overall During Therapy Animal Intervention.

groups ($F(2, 8) = 4.45$, $p < 0.05$). A Bonferroni post-hoc test revealed differences in post-intervention cortisol levels between the Discussion Group and Therapy Animal Group ($p < 0.10$). No other differences between groups were uncovered, including between the Photo Group and other intervention groups. There was also no statistically significant difference in the bond across interventions.

Discussion

The results of this study suggest that the utilization of AACR may be incorporated as a beneficial option in crisis intervention and have long lasting effects on individuals who have experienced this type of intervention. Previous research has shown the positive effects of AACR for both mental and physiological health, specifically in students in the same age group as the participants (Barker et al., 2016; Binfet & Passmore, 2016; Robino et al., 2021). As was expected, those students that had direct interactions with the therapy dogs did experience lower levels of stress as indicated by cortisol levels and a high degree of bonding as measured by the CSAWPBS, and increased levels of bonding as was indicated by cortisol levels.

The cortisol levels at baseline were relatively high at 0.42 μg/dL. This is consistent with previous work showing that cortisol is chronically elevated following a traumatic experience

(Bremner, 2006). For comparison, an acute psychological stress results in average cortisol levels that are 0.32 μg/dL in a group of young adults (average age = 22). Following the therapeutic intervention, the average cortisol levels dropped to 0.31 μg/dL. This is also consistent with previous studies which showed that therapeutic intervention following traumatic experiences can significantly reduce cortisol levels in adolescents. For example, therapeutic intervention has been shown to reduce cortisol levels in war-affected adolescents (Dajani et al., 2018) and adolescent refugees with PTSD (Budde et al., 2018).

Most importantly, significant differences were observed between type of exposure and cortisol level. Specifically, those that were exposed to physical interactions with the therapy dogs showed greater reduction in cortisol than did those who were only exposed to photos or discussion of the therapy dogs. As these were students who had previously been exposed to therapy dogs in the aftermath of a traumatic event it suggests that 1) the therapy dogs had an impact on stress and stress management, and 2) the effects were long-lasting. Although there was not a significant reduction in heart rate or blood pressure, it is possible that the conditions of the study (i.e., outdoors in a public space and fast-paced environment) and the low sample size might have contributed to this finding.

This study indicates that the effects of animal-assisted crisis intervention are both long-term and evidenced by both physical and self-reported measures. These bonds appeared most significant when the students were interacting with the therapy dogs, but were also evident when talking about, or looking at their photos. It is important to note that these student survivors were interacting, talking about, or looking at photos of several of the actual dogs that had been present for crisis response in the days, weeks, and months following the mass shooting at MSD.

When the small sample size is considered, it is even more interesting how profound the differences in the interactions were and what they implicate for the inclusion of animal- assisted crisis intervention and animal-assisted therapy in other situations, venues, and with other populations. Certainly, such inclusion as a means of stress reduction during difficult therapeutic interventions or victim/witness testimony in court is implied, as well as in post-crisis situations such as natural or man-made disasters, sexual assault, or other traumatic events.

Also important to note is that moderate stress levels are to be expected when working with young adults, specifically in the context which prompts them to recall a traumatic time in their life. Research has demonstrated that recollecting and discussing traumatic memories can cause an individual to feel anxious and fearful for the impact of traumatic stress often generates physiological responses of which individuals cannot control, causing the body to flood with stress hormones such as cortisol (Joëls & Barum, 2009). This study promotes the possibility that human-animal interactions might be a useful buffer to stress for young adults. Overall, young adults experience general stress outside of recalling traumatic events due to the nature of this developmental stage (Matud et al., 2020); therefore, this creates therapeutic implications for working with this population even beyond those who have experienced a crisis.

Limitations

This study was challenged by several limitations. First, the sample size was low due to the nature of the population which consisted of students over 18 who had attended Marjory Stoneman Douglas High School at the time of the 2018 mass shooting. The COVID-19 pandemic also proved to be a challenge as the study required face-to-face contact with the therapy animals and their handlers, the collection of saliva, and physical contact with the participants for blood pressure data. Also affected were such logistical concerns such as availability of space, masking, social distancing, and the timeframe of the study.

Future research

There are several areas where future studies could provide additional information on this subject. As this was a small sample size it would be important to investigate if the same results would be found with a larger and more diverse populations. All of the subjects in this study were survivors of the same tragic event (a mass shooting while in high school) and it would be valuable to see if similar results would be found with other types of tragic or traumatic events. The participants were, on average, 18 years old and majority female. Future studies with a more diverse subject pool would provide broader applicability as to how individuals respond to human-animal interactions in the wake of a traumatic event. In addition, given the findings in cortisol observed here, future work should also consider examining changes in negative feedback regulation of the HPA axis and possible heightened physiological stress responses in adolescents who experience traumatic events.

Conclusion

The purpose of this study was to evaluate stress effects and bonding that develop and are sustained through AACR. Previous studies have shown beneficial and long-lasting effects on individuals of a variety of age groups who experienced this type of intervention. Current findings appear to support these data and suggest that AACR is an effective way to aid students dealing with school-related crisis and trauma. Not only does AACR provide support for these students immediately following these types of events, but then it could provide stress reduction years later. This also supports the idea of human–animal bonding as indicated by cortisol levels measured during direct interactions with the therapy dogs. Despite the small sample size, significant effects on cortisol levels were noted between the different levels of human interactions with the therapy dogs. Consequently, the further and continued incorporation of AACR is indicated and should be further studied related to immediate, short-term, and long-term effects for those dealing with crisis and trauma.

References

Allen, K., Blascovich, J., & Mendes, W. B. (2002). Cardiovascular reactivity in the presence of pets, friends, and spouses: The truth about cats and dogs. *Psychosomatic Medicine,* 64, 727–739.

Alvarez, J., & Hunt, M. (2005). Risk and resilience in canine search and rescue handlers after 9/11. *Journal of Traumatic Stress,* 18(5), 497-505. https://doi.org/10.1002/jts.20058

American Veterinary Medical Association. (2021). *Human-animal bond.* https://www.avma.org/one-health/human-animal-bond

Answer, S., Manzar, M. D., Alghadir, A. H., Salahuddin, M., Abdul Hameed, U. (2020). Psychometric analysis of the Perceived Stress Scale among healthy university students. *Neuropsychiatric Disease and Treatment,* 16, 2389-2396. https://doi.org/10.2147/NDT.S268582

Arambasic, L., Kerestes, G., Kuterovac-Jagodic, G., & Vizek-Vidovic, V. (2000). The role of pet ownership as a possible buffer variable in traumatic experiences. *Studia Psychologica,* 42, 135–146.

Balters, S., Geeseman, J. W., Tveten, A.K., Hildre, H. P., Ju, W., & Steinert, M. (2020). Mayday, mayday, mayday: Using salivary cortisol to detect crisis (and eustress!) in critical incident training. *International Journal of Industrial Ergonomics,* 78, 102975. https://doi.org/10.1016/j.ergon.2020.102975

Barker, S. B., Barker, R. T., McCain, N. L., & Schubert, C. M. (2016). A randomized cross-over exploratory study of the effect of visiting therapy dogs on college student stress before final exams. *Anthrozoos*, 29(1), 35–46. https://doi.org/10.1080/08927936.2015.1069988

Barker, S. B., Knisely, J. S., Schubert, C. M., Green, J. D., & Ameringer, S. (2015). The effect of an animal-assisted intervention on anxiety and pain in hospitalized children. *Anthrozoös*, 28(1), 101–112.

Barker, S. B., Pandurangi, A. K., & Best, A. M. (2003). Effects of animal-assisted therapy on patients' anxiety, fear, and depression before ECT. *The Journal of ECT*, 19(1), 38–44.

Beetz, A., Kotrschal, K., Hediger, K., Turner, D., Uvnäs-Moberg, K., & Julius, H. (2011). The effect of a real dog, toy dog and friendly person on insecurely attached children during a stressful task: An exploratory study. *Anthrozoös*, 24(4), 349–368.

Beetz, A., Uvnäs-Moberg, K., Julius, H., & Kotrschal, K. (2012). Psychosocial and psychophysiological effects of human-animal interactions: the possible role of oxytocin. *Frontiers in Psychology*, 3, 234. https://doi.org/10.3389/fpsyg.2012.00234

Berke, D. S., Kline, N. K., Wachen, J. S., McLean, C. P., Yarvis, J. S., Mintz, J., ... & STRONG STAR Consortium. (2019). Predictors of attendance and dropout in three randomized controlled trials of PTSD treatment for active duty service members. *Behaviour Research and Therapy*, 118, 7-17.

Binfet, J. T., & Passmore, H. A. (2016). Hounds and homesickness: The effects of an animal-assisted therapeutic intervention for first-year university students. *Anthrozoös*, 29(3), 441–454. https://doi.org/10.1080/08927936.2016.1181364

Black, K. (2009). *Exploring adolescent loneliness and companion animal attachment* (Unpublished doctoral dissertation). https://digitalrepository.unm.edu/cgi/viewcontent.cgi?article=1029&context=nurs_etds

Bremner, J. D. (2006). Traumatic stress: Effects on the brain. *Dialogues in Clinical Neuroscience*, 8(4). https://doi.org/10.31887/DCNS.2006.8.4/jbremner

Brymer, M., Jacobs, A., Layne, C., Pynoos, R., Ruzek, J., Steinberg, A., Vern-berg, E., & Watson, P. (2006). *Psychological first aid: Field operations guide* (2nd ed.). National Child Traumatic Stress Network & National Center for PTSD. https://www.nctsn.org/sites/default/files/resources/pfa_field_operations_guide.pdf

Bua, F. (2013). *A qualitative investigation into dogs serving on animal assisted crisis response (AACR) teams: Advances in crisis counseling* (Unpublished doctoral dissertation). http://arrow.latrobe.edu.au:8080/vital/access/manager/Repository/latrobe:35600

Budde, H., Akko, D. P., Ainamani, H. E., Murillo-Rodríguez, E., & Weierstall, R. (2018). The impact of an exercise training intervention on cortisol levels and post-traumatic stress disorder in juveniles from an Ugandan refugee settlement: Study protocol for a randomized control trial. *Trials*, 19(1), 1-11.

Canine-Assisted Therapy. (2022). *Become a pet therapy team.* https://catdogs.org/become- a-pet-therapy-team/

Cassels, M. T., White, N., Gee, N., & Hughes, C. (2017). One of the family? Measuring young adolescents' relationships with pets and siblings. *Journal of Applied Developmental Psychology*, 49, 12-20.

Chew, Q. H., Chia, F. L., Ng, W. K., Lee, W., Tan, P., Wong, C. S., Puah, S. H., Shelat, V. G., Seah, E. D., Huey, C., Phua, E. J., & Sim, K. (2020). Perceived stress, stigma, traumatic stress levels and coping responses amongst residents in training across multiple specialties during COVID-19 pandemic: A longitudinal study. *International Journal of Environmental Research and Public Health*, 17(18), 6572. https://doi.org/10.3390/ijerph17186572

Cohen, S., Kamarck, T., & Mermelstein, R. (1983). A global measure of perceived stress. *Journal of Health and Social Behavior,* 24(4), 385–396. https://doi.org/10.2307/2136404

Craparo, G., Faraci, P., Rotondo, G., & Gori, A. (2013). The Impact of Event Scale – Revised: psychometric properties of the Italian version in a sample of flood victims. *Neuropsychiatric disease and treatment*, 9, 1427–1432. https://doi.org/10.2147/NDT.S51793

Crutcher, B., Moran, R. N., & Covassin, T. (2018). Examining the relationship between social support satisfaction and perceived stress and depression in athletic training students. *Athletic Training Education Journal*, 13(2), 168-174. https://doi.org/10.4085/1302168

Dajani, R., Hadfield, K., van Uum, S., Greff, M., & Panter-Brick, C. (2018). Hair cortisol concentrations in war-affected adolescents: A prospective intervention trial. *Psychoneuroendocrinology*, 89, 138-146.

Eaton-Stull, Y. M., & Flynn, B. (2020). Introduction to animal-assisted crisis response. In Y. M. Eaton-Stull (Eds), *Animal-assisted crisis response: Specialized crisis intervention for individuals affected by disasters and crises* (pp. 3-13). NASW Press.

Eaton-Stull, Y., & Flynn, B. (2015). Animal-assisted crisis response. In K.R. Yeager & A.R. Roberts (Eds), *Crisis Intervention Handbook: Assessment, Treatment & Research, 4th edition* (pp. 599-606). Oxford University Press.

Eaton-Stull, Y., & Sewall, C. (2019). Canine complements to Psychological First Aid. *Human Animal Interaction Bulletin, 7(2).*

Fiocco, A. J., & Hunse, A. M. (2017). The buffer effect of therapy dog exposure on stress reactivity in undergraduate students. *International Journal of Environmental Research and Public Health*, 14(7), 707. https://doi.org/10.3390/ijerph14070707

Fine, A. H., Beck, A. M., & Ng, Z. (2019). The state of animal-assisted interventions: Addressing the contemporary issues that will shape the future. *International Journal of Environmental Research and Public Health*, 16(20), 3997. https://doi.org/10.3390/ijerph16203997ff

Glenn, T. (2017). *First responder resilience: Caring for public servants*. Rising Phoenix Press, LLC.

Gordon, J. (2013, January 4). Hope AACR pets bring smiles to victims of Hurricane Sandy. *Karen Pryor Clicker Training.* https://www.clickertraining.com/node/3904

Greenbaum S. D. (2006). Introduction to working with animal assisted crisis response animal handler teams. *International Journal of Emergency Mental Health*, 8(1), 49–63.

Greenstein, L. (2017, September 20). How to help someone in crisis. *National Alliance on Mental Illness.* https://www.nami.org/Blogs/NAMI-Blog/September-2017/How-to-Help-Someone-in-Crisis.

Handlin, L., Nilsson, A., Lidfors, L., Petersson, M., & Uvnas-Moberg, K. (2018). The effects of a therapy dog on the blood pressure and heart rate of older residents in a nursing home. *Anthrozoos,* 31(5), 567-576. https://doi.org/10.1080/08927936.2018.1505268

Human-Animal Bond Research Institute. (2020, March 31). *Top 5 benefits of the human-animal bond.* https://habri.org/blog/top-5-benefits-of-the-human-animal-bond/

Iqbal, T., Elahi, A., Redon, P., Vazquez, P., Wijns, W., & Shahzad, A. (2021) A review of biophysiological and biochemical indicators of stress for connected and preventive healthcare. *Diagnostics,* 11, 556. https://doi.org/10.3390/ diagnostics11030556

Joëls, M., & Baram, T. Z. (2009). The neuro-symphony of stress. *Nature reviews. Neuroscience*, 10(6), 459–466. https://doi.org/10.1038/nrn2632

Johnson, R. A., & Meadows, R. L. (2003). Center for the Study of Animal Wellness (CSAW) Pet Bonding Scale. In D. C. Anderson (Ed.), *Assessing the human-animal bond: A compendium of actual measures* (pp. 7-9). Purdue University Press.

Jones, M. G., Rice, S. M., & Cotton, S. M. (2019). Incorporating animal-assisted therapy in mental health treatments for adolescents: A systematic review of canine assisted psychotherapy. *PloS One,* 14(1), e0210761

Kirschbaum, C., & Hellhammer, D. H. (1989). Salivary cortisol in psychobiological research: An overview. *Neuropsychobiology,* 22(3), 150–169. https://doi.org/10.1159/000118611

Krause-Parello, C. A., Thames, M., Ray, C. M., & Kolassa, J. (2018). Examining the effects of a service-trained facility dog in stress in children undergoing forensic interview for allegations of child sexual abuse. *Journal of Child Sex Abuse,* 3, 305.

Lackey, R. & Haberstock, G. (2019). Animal-assisted crisis response: Offering opportunity for human resiliency during and after traumatic incidents. In P. Tedeschi (Ed.), *Transforming trauma: Resilience and healing through our connections with animals* (pp. 373-394). Purdue University Press.

Lass-Hennemann, J., Peyk, P., Streb, M., Holz, E., & Michael, T. (2014). Presence of a dog reduces subjective but not physiological stress responses to an analog trauma. *Frontiers in Psychology*, 5, 1010.

Lawrence, D., Johnson, S., Hafekost, J., Boterhoven de Haan, K., Sawyer, M., Ainley, J., & Zubrick, S. R. (2015). *The mental health of children and adolescents: Report on the second Australian child and adolescent survey of mental health and wellbeing.* Department of Health, Canberra.

Levin, G. N., Allen, K., Braun, L. T., Christian, H. E., Friedmann, E., Taubert, K. A., Thomas, S. A., Wells, D. L., & Lange, R. A. (2013). Pet ownership and cardiovascular risk: A scientific statement from the American Heart Association. *Circulation,* 127(23), 2353-2363. https://doi.org/10.1161/CIR.0b013e31829201e1

MacDonald, K., & MacDonald, T. M. (2010). The peptide that binds: A systematic review of oxytocin and its prosocial effects in humans. *Harvard Review of Psychiatry*, 18(1), 1–21.

Matud, M. P., Díaz, A., Bethencourt, J. M., & Ibáñez, I. (2020). Stress and psychological distress in emerging adulthood: A gender analysis. *Journal of Clinical Medicine*, 9(9), 2859. https://doi.org/10.3390/jcm9092859

McCabe, D. (2019). The Impact of Event Scale-Revised (IES-R). *Best Practices in Nursing Care to Older Adults,* 19. https://hign.org/sites/default/files/2020-06/Try_This_General_Assessment_19.pdf

Morris, M. C., Hellman, N., Abelson, J. L., & Rao, U. (2016). Cortisol, heart rate, and blood pressure as early markers of PTSD risk: A systematic review and meta- analysis. *Clinical psychology review*, 49, 79–91. https://doi.org/10.1016/j.cpr.2016.09.001

Nagengast, S. L., Baun, M. M., Megel, M., & Leibowitz, J. M. (1997). The effects of the presence of a companion animal on physiological arousal and behavioral distress in children during a physical examination. *Journal of Pediatric Nursing*, 12(6), 323–330.

National Alliance on Mental Illness. (n.d.). *Crisis response.* https://www.nami.org/Advocacy/Policy-Priorities/Responding-to-Crises/Crisis- Response.

Ng, Z. Y., Pierce, B. J., Otto, C. M., Buechner-Maxwell, V. A., Siracusa, C., & Werre, S.R. (2014). The effect of dog–human interaction on cortisol and behavior in registered animal-assisted activity dogs. *Applied Animal Behaviour Science*, 159, 69-81. https://doi.org/10.1016/j.applanim.2014.07.009

Norhayati, M. N., & Aniza, A. A. (2014). Psychometric properties of the Malay version of Impact of Event Scale - Revised (IES-R). *International Journal of Collaborative Research on Internal Medicine and Public Health,* 6(2), 39-51.

O'Haire, M. E., Philip Tedeschi, M. S. S. W., Jenkins, M. A., Braden, S. R., & Rodriguez, K. E. (2019). The impact of human-animal interaction in trauma recovery. *New Direct Human Animal Bond*, 15, 15-53.

Odendaal, J., & Meintjes, R. (2003). Neurophysiological correlates of affiliative behaviour between humans and dogs. *The Veterinary Journal*, 165(3), 296–301.

Pendry, P., & Vandagriff, J. L. (2019). Animal visitation program (AVP) reduces cortisol levels of university students: A randomized controlled trial. *AERA* Open. https://doi.org/10.1177/2332858419852592

Pet Partners. (2021). *Animal-assisted crisis response*. https://petpartners.org/act/aacr/

Piper, L. J. (2014). *The Practice of Animal-Assisted Psychotherapy: An Innovative Model for Facilitating Mental Wellness*. BookBaby.

Piper, L. J., & Uttley, C. M. (2019). Adolescents and Pets. *Clinician's Guide to Treating Companion Animal Issues*, 47–75. https://doi.org/10.1016/B978-0-12-812962-3.00004-6

Polheber, J. P., & Matchock, R. L. (2014). The presence of a dog attenuates cortisol and heart rate in the Trier Social Stress Test compared to human friends. *Journal of behavioral medicine*, 37(5), 860-867.

Purewal, R., Christley, R., Kordas, K., Joinson, C., Meints, K., Gee, N., & Westgarth, C. (2017). Companion animals and child/adolescent development: A systematic review of the evidence. *International Journal of Environmental Research and Public Health,* 14(3), 234. https://doi.org10.3390%2Fijerph14030234

Robino, A. E., Corrigan, V. K., Anderson, B., Werre, S., Farley, J. P., Marmagas, S. W., & Buechner-Maxwell, V. (2021). College student mental health in an animal- assisted intervention program: A preliminary study. *Journal of Creativity in Mental Health*, 16(1), 49-58. https://doi.org/10.1080/15401383.2020.1757002

Robinson, R. (2004). Counterbalancing misrepresentations of critical incident stress debriefing and critical incident stress management. *Australian Psychologist*, 39(1), 29–34.

Rodriguez, K. E., Bryce, C. I., Granger, D. A., & O'Haire, M. E. (2018). The effect of a service dog on salivary cortisol awakening response in a military population with posttraumatic stress disorder (PTSD). *Psychoneuroendocrinology*, 98, 202-210.

Shiloh, S., Sorek, G., & Terkel, J. (2003). Reduction of state-anxiety by petting animals in a controlled laboratory experiment. *Anxiety, Stress and Coping*, 16(4), 387–395. https://doi.org/10.1080/1061580031000091582

Substance Abuse and Mental Health Services Administration. (2021). *Warning signs and risk factors for emotional distress*. https://www.samhsa.gov/find-help/disaster-distress-helpline/warning-signs-risk-factors.

Suzuki, A., Poon, L., Papadopoulos, A. S., Kumari, V., & Cleare, A. J. (2014). Long term effects of childhood trauma on cortisol stress reactivity in adulthood and relationship to the occurrence of depression. *Psychoneuroendocrinology*, 50, 289-299.

Taylor, M., Edwards, M., & Pooley, J. (2013). Nudging them back to reality: Toward a growing public acceptance of the role dogs fulfill in ameliorating contemporary veterans' PTSD symptoms. *Anthrozoös*, 26(4), 593–611.

Uver, T. (2020). Validity and reliability testing of the transitional impact scale. *Stress and Health,* 36(4), 278-486. https://doi.org/10.1002/smi.2944

VandenBos, G. R. (Ed.). (2007). *APA dictionary of psychology.* American Psychological Association.

Vincent, A. (2019). *Feasibility of canine support in pediatric dentistry* [Doctoral dissertation, Case Western Reserve University]. OhioLINK Electronic Theses and Dissertations Center. http://rave.ohiolink.edu/etdc/view?acc_num=case1554476390381119

Weiss, D.S., & Marmar, C.R. The impact of event scale – revised. In: Wilson JP, Keane TM, editors. *Assessing psychological trauma and PTSD*. New York: Guilford Press; 1997. pp. 399–411.

Yount, R. A., Olmert, M. D., & Lee, M. R. (2012). Service dog training program for treatment of posttraumatic stress in service members. *U.S. Army Medical Department Journal*, 63–69.

4 Psychophysiological Effects of Human–Dog Interaction in University Students Exposed to a Stress-Induced Situation Using the Trier Social Stress Test (TSST)

Rafael Martos-Montes[1]*, David Ordóñez-Pérez[2], Jesús Ruiz-Maatallah[2] and Miriam Martínez-Cobos[1]

[1]University of Jaén, Spain; [2]Perruneando, Spain

Abstract

Enjoying the company of a good-natured dog can lend support to a person in a stressful situation. This presence brings benefits across different areas of human well-being and leads to a decrease in levels of sympathetic activation and subjective distress which are triggered in social anxiety situations. This study seeks to provide evidence of these benefits relative to physiological variables—heart rate and blood pressure—as well as a subjective variable, namely anxiety. Thirty-six university students (80% female, M = 22.4, SD = 4.32) exposed to a stress-induced situation using the Trier Social Stress Test (TSST) participated in the study. This type of scenario produces an increase in heart rate, blood pressure, and subjective anxiety levels. The decline in these variable levels was assessed based on whether the participants were alone or accompanied by a friendly dog. Through random selection, half of the students could pet the animal during the stress-induced phase (experimental group), whereas the other half had a toy dog to hold (control group). The levels of all three dependent variables were recorded at three different stages: the pretest relaxation phase, the stress- and anxiety-induced test phase, and the relaxation or return-to-calm post-test phase. The results revealed that the dog's presence during the test phase considerably reduced the levels of anxiety and heart rate experienced by the experimental group participants compared to the control group. No significant differences in blood pressure were observed between both groups during this phase. The results of this research coincide with earlier studies that report on the beneficial effects of human–animal interaction, while highlighting the importance of analyzing this interaction in the field of psychology.

Keywords: Dog, Human–animal interaction, Social anxiety, Stress, TSST

Scientific evidence compiled in recent decades suggests that people and dogs have shared an ecological niche for 15,000 years across three different environments: Europe, Southeast Asia, and the Midwest region of the North American subcontinent (Yilmaz, 2017). Yet this does not rule out socialization that is simultaneous and subject to processes independent of one another. In 1941, fossil remains from a canine burial were found in Bonn-Oberkassel (Germany). It is estimated

*Corresponding author: rmartos@ujaen.es

that these remains date back 14,000 years and reflect the importance of the human–pet bond in the funerary act (Janssens et al., 2016).

Attempts have been made to explain why people form bonds with non-human animals and vice versa through various theoretical proposals. Attachment theory (Bowlby, 1982) emphasizes the importance of attachment and caregiving behavioral systems. Attachment is an innate system that involves early bonding between the offspring and their caregiver(s), and serves an adaptive function in fearful or dangerous situations. This system is characterized by a lasting attraction toward the attachment figure. The caregiving system is a complementary system which sees the caregiver direct their behavior toward providing care and protection. Both systems clearly show the natural need for affiliation that people seek with other human beings and animals via behavioral patterns aimed at building cohesion with others. For its part, the biophilia hypothesis (Wilson, 1984) argues that people have an innate interest in other forms of life, which drives us to connect with other living organisms. As people we pay selective attention to—and interactive with—other types of life, actions which can impact significantly on our knowledge, health, and well-being. The presence of some animals represents a sense of security in people, and this is frequently accompanied by a sense of calm. It is apparent that this bond is the fruit of learning (Brickel, 1979), yet cruelty to animals can also fall under this description.

According to the above author, the basic learning processes that initially take place at the heart of the family teach us how to connect with non-human animals. Principally, these are classical conditioning, operant conditioning, and observational learning processes. Lastly, social support theory (Beck & Katcher, 2003) maintains that social support is a set of human and material resources that people and groups have at their disposal to carry out their life project and which help them to overcome the difficulties and problems that life entails. Contact with a dog provides emotional support, love, acceptance, physical contact, and company to humans, which contributes to their physical and psychological well-being. It is proven that animals are also a source of social support, as demonstrated by the number of Americans who consider their pet "a member of the family", talking to their pet as if they were a person and treating them like a trusted confidant (Cain, 1983). Pets also increase the frequency of human social support (Eddy, Hart, & Boltz, 1988). More recently, and from a psychobiological point of view, research has opted to address the human–animal bond as a result of a neurobiological process (Nagasawa et al., 2015). However, it is widely agreed that we as humans gain numerous benefits from interaction with animals and their company (Beetz, Julius, Turner, & Kotrschal, 2011, 2012; Julius, Beetz, Kotrschal, Turner, & Uvnäs-Moberg, 2012; Silcox & Reed, 2014). These gains can be grouped into three categories: physiological, psychosocial, and psychophysiological.

In terms of physiological gains, pet companionship is related to a lower risk of cardiovascular disease, including obesity and high blood pressure (Levine et al., 2013). People with household animals exhibit lower blood pressure and heart rate levels (Virués-Ortega & Buela-Casal, 2006). In one study, Friedman, Katcher, Thomas, Lynch, and Messent (1983) reported a fall in blood pressure among children accompanied by a dog when taking a stressful test (reading out loud) compared with the control group. Similarly, Jenkins (1986) observed how systolic and diastolic blood pressure in dog owners dropped when joined by their pets during a reading out-loud task.

As for psychosocial gains, pets act as social catalysts, promoting social cohesion, cooperation, and contact among people (Gutiérrez, Granados, & Piar, 2007). According to González-Ramírez and Hernández (2011), owners who perceived their pets as members of the family showed significantly lower perceived stress levels compared with those who viewed their pets as guardians of the home.

Psychophysiologically, animals trigger an immediate state of relaxation just by merely capturing our attention. It is believed that they calm and reduce human stress in the short-term (O'Haire, 2010). People report feeling less alone around their pets, more useful, and with enhanced self- esteem (Wheeler & Faulkner, 2015).

Research on human-animal interaction has shown that a brief contact with a dog, especially when dealing with a pet, relaxes people and brings down their stress levels (Allen, Blascovich, Tomaka, & Kelsey, 1991). Regarding the concept of stress, Selye (1936) defined it as a reaction that gives us the necessary energy to successfully respond to environmental demands. Decades later, Lazarus and Folkman (1984) explained how events do not affect us directly. Rather, our interpretation of them is what has an impact. Ursin and Eriksen (2010) hold a similar view. They claim that the expectations we form about these events will determine the perceived stress. More modern definitions, including that provided by Echeburúa (2016), view stress as a question of environmental demands and the resources that a person has to face up to these challenges.

The present study focuses on the emotional stress that arises in situations where conflictive social interaction comes into play. This can trigger various pathologies depending on the individual's genetic predisposition, their own experiences, and the environment in which they interact with other individuals (Molina-Jiménez, Gutiérrez-García, Hernández-Domínguez, & Contreras, 2008). Speaking in public is an example of a social interaction situation that has seen a sharp increase in a person's stress level. When performing this task, increased heart rate, breathing rate, electrodermal activity, muscle tension, and cortisol levels—among other psychophysiological variables—can be observed (Moya-Albiol & Salvador, 2001).

The resident–intruder paradigm is frequently used in the field of animal research to measure psychosocial stress. It involves exposing an individual to high demands up against their peers. The social defeat inflicted on the person who fails to complete the tasks successfully is a severe stressor. Availing of social support under these circumstances has a positive effect on health (Zarghani et al., 2016). Furthermore, this support is one of the most effective methods for tackling stress as it lessens the stressful experience (Sandín, 2008).

Today, scientific evidence points to a friendly dog as a figure capable of providing support in the previously mentioned situations (Nagasawa, Kikusui, Onaka, & Ohta, 2009). It is for this reason that its presence in therapy-based interventions has increased (for a review of the situation in Spain, see Martos-Montes, Ordóñez-Pérez, De la Fuente-Hidalgo, Martos-Luque, & García-Viedma, 2015). The beneficial role of a friendly dog in stressful situations has been demonstrated in research studies that use the Trier Social Stress Test (TSST) protocol designed by Kirschbaum, Pirke, and Hellhammer (1993). The TSST is an experimental stress-inducing protocol that enables psychophysiological variables to be measured in a controlled manner. In this case, it allows us to empirically study how we as people can harness the benefits that human–animal interaction offers when up against a stressful social situation. This protocol may be modified depending on the aim and resources of each research study.

Various research studies have demonstrated the social support that dogs provide using the TSST protocol. According to Allen (2003), family dogs reduce the physiological indicators of stress, which is widely known as the "pet effect". This was proven in a study involving 45 women who experienced work-related stress. Performing a task similar to the TSST protocol, participants accompanied by their pet perceived the task as less stressful than participants joined by their closest friend (Allen et al., 1991).

In a similar study, 294 university students were administered the TSST protocol. They were randomly assigned to three experimental conditions: performing the task in the company of a dog they did not know, in the company of a friend, and alone. The results showed lower levels in the cortisol and heart rate variables for the group that had contact with the dog, but not in anxiety levels (Polheber & Matchock, 2013). Wheeler and Faulkner (2015) applied this protocol to a similar sample of 223 university students with or without the presence of a dog. In this case, the experimental group exhibited a significant reduction in state anxiety, heart rate, and blood pressure level.

Another noteworthy example is a study involving children with separation anxiety. An adapted version of the TSST protocol was used, namely the Trier Social Stress Test for Children (TSST-C). Forty-seven children were randomly assigned to three conditions: in the presence of a therapy-dog, a toy dog, or a friendly human. According to the results, a dog's companionship was interpreted as the most beneficial (Beetz, Julius, Turner, & Kotrschal, 2012).

A more recent study (Fiocco & Hunse, 2017) also suggests that interacting with a therapy dog may buffer the stress response in university students exposed to a stressful situation through the "Paced Auditory Serial-Addition Test" (PASAT) protocol (Tombaugh, 2006). In this study, the exposure to a brief dog-assisted therapy significantly reduced the participants' electrodermal activity compared to a control group without such exposure. Similarly, Wood, Ohlsen, Thompson, Hulin, and Knowles (2018) exposed 131 university students to a single 15-minutes interaction with a dog, showing a significant reduction in state anxiety levels and blood pressure immediately after the intervention.

In reference to Wheeler and Faulkner's (2015) study, those participants who presented high trait-anxiety levels experienced a significant decrease in the previously mentioned variables following interaction with a dog by applying the TSST protocol. The present study seeks to analyze the potential beneficial effects that human–animal interaction has on three variables: state anxiety, heart rate, and blood pressure (systolic and diastolic). In this case, participants are classified according to their state-anxiety levels and not their trait-anxiety ones. In fact, the focus is on establishing the one-off effect that a brief animal interaction can exercise in a stressful situation. To this end, a social stress-induced situation was created using the TSST protocol. Participants were divided into two groups: an experimental group (dog) and a control group (toy dog). The working hypothesis is as follows: The experimental group's interaction with the dog should mitigate any social stress increases in the dependent measures. Confirming this hypothesis, the results would contribute new evidence to the scientific field with regards to the benefits that human–animal interaction can bring people as a buffer against stress to improve well-being and quality of life.

Method

Participants

Thirty-six students (n = 36) studying a Degree in Psychology at the University of Jaén, Spain, participated in the study. Thirty were women and their ages ranged from 19 to 44 years (M = 22.4, SD = 4.32). Participants were rewarded with course credit for their participation and had no experience with the task before starting the experiment. Theirparticipation was voluntary and an informed consent was sought from all the participants. This experimental study was approved by the ethics committee of the University of Jaén.

Prior to study commencement, an email was sent to all possible participants requesting that they answer an online questionnaire designed to assess personal aspects that could influence the study. These aspects included hours of sleep, lifestyle habits (sedentary/physically active), tobacco use or drug treatment, as well as attitudes toward animals and, especially, toward dogs. The goal was to make sure that no participants had any heart-related illnesses or a dog allergy or phobia. The resulting sample was randomly selected for two conditions. In the first scenario, the control group would complete the test holding a toy dog (n = 18, 14 women and 4 men). In the second scenario, the experimental group would complete the test accompanied by a real friendly dog that they could interact with (n = 18, 16 women and 2 men).

Apparatus

Heart rate was recorded using a CMS-50F wristband pulse oximeter (CONTEC™). The different pulse variations were collected wirelessly and the data were downloaded onto a computer for subsequent analysis. It has a measuring range of 30–250 bpm (beats per minute), a resolution of 1 bpm, and a heart-rate accuracy of ± 2 bpm or ± 2%. The use of portable devices helps to measure the variables of interest reliably and without needing to connect to any equipment.

Blood pressure was measured using the Omron M3-HEM-7051-E automatic digital blood pressure monitor. Readings were taken at the end of each phase by wrapping the monitor around the participant's arm and writing down the different values obtained at each phase onto a record sheet. It has a reliability range of 0-299 mmHG for measuring blood pressure and a pulse frequency range of 40-80 beats per minute. It has been clinically validated in accordance with the European Society of Hypertension International Protocol (Asmar, Khabouth, Topouchian, El Feghali, & Mattar, 2010). Data on systolic and diastolic blood pressure were obtained using this device.

The State-Trait Anxiety Inventory (STAI; Spielberger, Gorsuch, & Lushene, 1982; adapted version to a Spanish sample) was used to measure subjective anxiety. The instrument's reliability (alpha de Cronbach) reports an internal consistency of 0.90–0.93 (State subscale) and of 0.84–0.87 (Trait subscale). The State subscale (STAI-S) was used in this study. This subscale determines the actual intensity levels of anxiety induced by stress-loaded experimental procedures.

A Fujifilm FinePix S4500 professional digital camera and a standard tripod were used to create an experimental space to simulate the recording and evaluation of the participants' performance in the social anxiety tasks.

Procedure

Sessions were spread over two weeks. They were held at the University of Jaén's psychophysiology labs. Animals were allowed to enter the labs with the established protocol in place.

The experimental procedure was an adaptation of the standard TSST protocol (Kirschbaum, Pirke, & Hellhammer, 1993), in which the participants' performance was video recorded. Participants were informed that faculty staff would later assess them, thus lending more credibility to the tasks (Birkett, 2011). This procedure achieves results comparable to those obtained with people actually present in the room (Kelly, Matheson, Martinez, Merali, & Anisman, 2007).

The total duration of each session was 50 minutes. Each session was distributed over three phases: pretest (15 min), test (20 min), and posttest or recovery period (15 min). Both the control group and the experimental group underwent the entire procedure following the same phases and the same cognitive tasks.

Pretest phase (Relaxation period). On the day of their appointment, the participants arrived individually to the laboratory where they were met by the experimenter. This individual handed out the informed consent form which included authorization for taking photos and videos for the purpose of lending credibility to the experimental scenario. Once this was done, the participants sat comfortably in front of the computer screen and watched a relaxing 10-min video designed to lower their activation state (Helland, 2016). On completion of this phase, the participants filled in the STAI-S questionnaire and their heart rate and blood pressure were recorded. These readings were used to establish the baseline of each individual for reference.

Test phase (Experimental phase). For this phase the participants moved to an adjacent room. Inside was a chair where they would take a seat and a camera in front of them which would record their performance on both tasks: a spoken task and a mental arithmetic task. The instructions provided were as follows:

"The first task you have to complete is a short speech for a job interview. Before starting your presentation, you have five minutes to mentally prepare a speech in which you describe in detail why you would be the best candidate for your ideal job. You have some blank pieces of paper and a pen should you wish to take some notes or draw diagrams to help organize your speech. However, you will not be able to use these notes later".

The experimenter left the room and this 5-min interval served as a pre-stress phase, a key step according to the first version of the TSST protocol (Kirschbaum, Pirke, & Hellhammer, 1993). Once this interval had elapsed, the experimenter entered the room again and relayed the following information:

"We're going to begin the task. Your responses will be recorded using the camera in front of you and you must talk in its direction. The recording of your intervention will be analyzed by faculty staff heading this research. Your time starts now".

The experimenter left the room again. Once the first task was completed (10-min speech), the participants moved immediately onto the second task with no rest period. The experimenter entered the room and gave the following instructions:

"The second task requires you to mentally continue a sequence of numbers. Starting from the number 1022, you must subtract 13 each time. You must give your answers out loud and if you make a mistake you must go back to the beginning, to the first number. Your time starts now."

The researcher remained in the room. If the participants made a mistake, the researcher stopped them and they would go back to the start. It was important that the experimenter have a sheet of paper at hand with the correct series of numbers written down in order to correct the mistakes as they happened. Nobody managed to complete the task within the allocated time.

Once both tasks were over, participants were asked to repeat the STAI-S questionnaire and their heart rate and blood pressure were recorded.

During this phase, the experimental group performed each task in the presence of a friendly dog and their carer (handler). The participants were informed that they could freely interact with the dog, stroking and petting it. The dog was positioned close to the participants' lap to facilitate interaction during the tasks. In the case of the control group, the participants were given a toy dog which they could hold during the tasks.

The participating dog was an eight-year-old friendly and trustworthy Golden Retriever, in order to promote a more fluid social interaction with it. The animal was up to date on its vaccinations and had undergone a thorough veterinary checkup, adhering to a complete animal health protocol in order to ensure the dog's and the participants' health. An animal welfare protocol was drawn up to safeguard the dog's comfort. Several aspects were taken into account, including fatigue. The sessions were spread across two weeks (Week 1 = 7 sessions, Week 2 = 11 sessions), with a minimum rest period of 40 minutes and a maximum rest period of 60 minutes between sessions. The dog was always assisted by its handler (owner) who closely monitored the dog's well-being and behavior adapted to the requirements of the interaction protocol.

Post-test phase (Return to calm). Next, the pulse oximeter was removed and the participants were accompanied to the starting room. They were told that the tasks were over and that they would now watch the relaxation video again. Once that was done they were given the STAI-S questionnaire to complete for the last time. Their heart rate and blood pressure were recorded.

Data analysis and dependent measures

A mixed factorial experimental design was used. The experiment conditions (experimental group and control group) and the time points that make up the study's experimental protocol (pretest, test, and post-test) were the factors identified. The first factor had two levels with between-group manipulation. The second factor had three levels with within-subject manipulation. The study's dependent variables were anxiety level, heart rate, and blood pressure levels (systolic and diastolic). These dependent variables were evaluated at the three time points: pretest, test, and post-test. The SPSS (version 22) statistical software was used for data analysis with a significance level set at 0.05.

Results

Table 4.1 shows the means and standard deviations of both groups (control and experimental) at each study phase (pretest, test, and post-test) for each dependent variable.

State anxiety: The mixed factorial Group × Phases analysis of variance (ANOVA) performed on the dependent variable State anxiety showed a significant main effect for the variable Phases, $F(2,68) = 43.236$, $p < 0.000$. The same occurred in the interaction Group × Phases, $F(2,68) = 3.951$, $p < 0.024$. The Group factor was not significant, $F(1,34) = 2.803$, $p < 0.103$. An analysis of the Group × Phases interaction in this study prompted the testing of the Group effect at each phase. To achieve this, the independent-samples t-test was used and the analyses revealed no between-group differences at pretest, $t(34) = -0.65$, $p<0.543$, $d = 0.21$ (Cohen's d for effect size). Nor were there differences at post-test, $t(34) = 1.528$, $p<0.136$, $d = 0.51$. The between differences were observed at the test phase, $t(34) = 2.161$, $p<0.038$, $d = 0.72$. State-anxiety levels were lower in the experimental group compared to the control group (see Fig. 4.1).

The Phases variable was significant for each group. Both groups' anxiety levels were higher at test compared to the other phases. Specifically, the control group yielded a significant effect for the Phases variable, $F(2,34) = 34.139$, $p<0.000$. These data revealed a significant quadratic trend component, $F(1,17) = 40.020$, $p<0.000$. A significant effect was also observed in the experimental group for the Phases variable, $F(2,34) = 12.260$, $p<0.000$; the quadratic trend component was also significant, $F(1,17) = 20.365$, $p<0.000$.

Heart rate: The analysis of variance (ANOVA) performed on the dependent variable Heart rate showed a significant main effect for the variable Phases, $F(2,68) = 109.299$, $p < 0.000$. The same occurred with the Group × Phases interaction, $F(2,68) = 3.158$, $p < 0.049$. The Group factor was not significant, $F(1,34) = 2.354$, $p<0.134$. An analysis of the Group × Phases interaction, which used the independent-samples t-test, revealed no significant differences at pretest,

Table 4.1. Descriptive statistics.

	Group	M	SD
STAI-S_Pretest	C	11.89	5.476
	E	13.06	5.896
STAI-S_Test	C	28.83	9.593
	E	21.56	10.590
STAI-S_Posttest	C	15.44	5.913
	E	12.22	6.717
Heart rate_Pretest	C	75.722	10.4758
	E	74.778	10.0268
Heart rate_Test	C	96.944	12.4195
	E	89.044	11.2445
Heart rate_Posttest	C	77.500	10.6177
	E	72.000	7.9410
Systolic BP_Pretest	C	107.17	8.645
	E	109.39	6.260
Systolic BP_Test	C	109.32	26.867
	E	111.39	8.008
Systolic BP_Posttest	C	105.83	8.082
	E	105.11	5.860
Diastolic BP_Pretest	C	64.44	7.188
	E	64.44	6.233
Diastolic BP_Test	C	67.11	12.03
	E	66.89	6.738
Diastolic BP_Posttest	C	63.83	10.428
	E	63.94	6.384

Note: Descriptive statistics (Mean [M] and Standard deviation [SD]) for each group (Control [C] and Experimental [E]) across the different study phases (Pretest, Test, and Posttest) for each dependent variable (State anxiety [STAI-S], Heart rate, Systolic blood pressure, and Diastolic blood pressure.

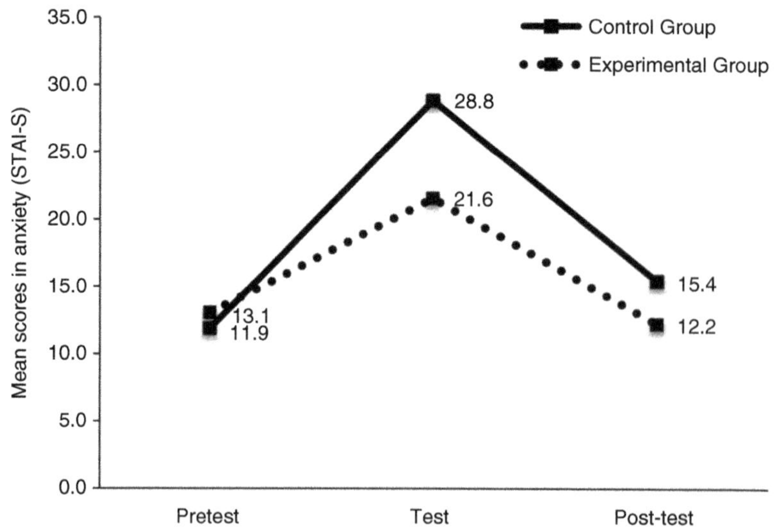

Fig. 4.1. Mean values of state anxiety across the three phases (pretest, test, and posttest) for each group.

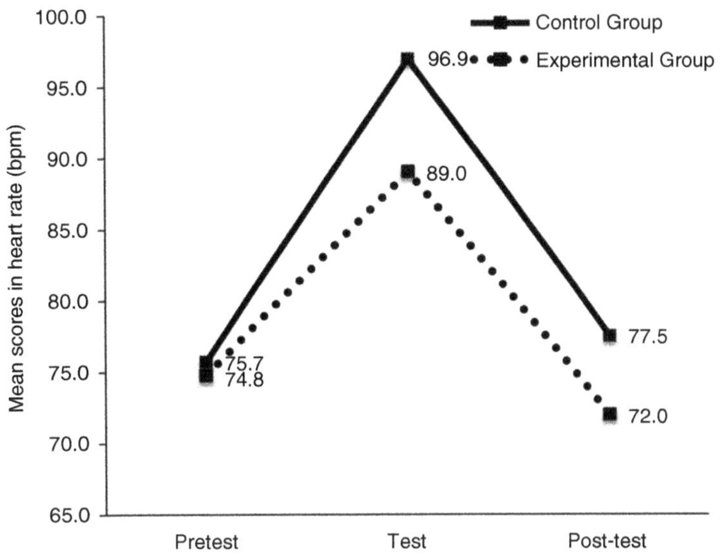

Fig. 4.2. Mean values of heart rate (beats/min) across the three phases (pretest, test, and post-test) for each group.

t(34) = 0.276, p<0.784, d = 0.09, or post-test, t(34) = 1.760, p<0.087, d = 0.59. Differences were found at the test phase, t(34) = 2.041, p<0.050, d = 0.67. The average heart rate in the experimental group was lower compared to the control group (see Fig. 4.2).

The Phases variable was significant for each group in the effects analysis. Both groups' heart rate was higher at test compared to the other phases. The control group yielded a significant effect, F(2,34) = 63.217, p<0.000. These data revealed a significant quadratic trend component, F(1,17) = 100.766, p<0.000. A significant effect was also observed in the experimental group for the variable Phases, F(2,34) = 47.522, p<0.000, with a significant quadratic trend component, F(1,17) = 75.708, p<0.000.

Systolic blood pressure: The corresponding analysis of variance (ANOVA) for this variable showed no significant effect in the Group variable, F(1,34) = 0.244, p <0.625, nor in Phases, F(2,68) = 1.260, p <0.290, or in the interaction between both variables, F(2,68) = 0.144, p<0.866.

Diastolic blood pressure. The corresponding analysis of variance (ANOVA) for this variable showed no significant effect in the Group variable, F(1,34) = 0.000, p <0.987, nor in Phases, F(2,68) = 2.565, p <0.084, or in the interaction between both variables, F(2,68) = 0.007, p<0.993.

Discussion and Conclusions

The results of this study partially support the posed hypothesis. The experimental group's interaction with the dog would mitigate the participants' stress levels compared to the control group's interaction with the toy dog. Indeed, the participants in contact with the real dog showed lower levels of perceived anxiety and heart rate. In fact, the experimental group participants reported feeling less worried and nervous compared with their control group peers. The effect sizes were considerable in both dependent measures (state anxiety and heart rate; Cohen's *d* was 0.72 and 0.67, respectively), what encourages us to continue with this promising research project. However, no significant differences were found between the groups in terms of systolic and diastolic blood pressure.

These results are similar to those obtained by Wheeler and Faulkner (2015). Interacting with a dog while undertaking the TSST protocol significantly reduced the participants' degree of subjective anxiety compared to the group that did not avail of the dog's company. They also coincide with the results reported by Beetz et al. (2012). In this study, children with insecure attachment toward their parents largely benefited from a dog's company compared to the other groups when they took the adapted TSST test. This lends support to the idea that a dog can be a figure capable of providing psychophysiological benefits in stressful situations. In turn, and compared to the classical study proposed by Allen et al. (1991), no equivalent results were found for systolic and diastolic blood pressure. In this research, the experimental group showed significantly lower values than those of the other groups. Women who interacted with a dog exhibited lower stress levels compared to the group that remained alone or interacted with a friend. A possible explanation behind this difference could lie in the participants' degree of closeness with the dog. In their study, the participants completed the test joined by their own pet. However, the dog in the current study was unknown to the participants.

The results of this study also show differences and similarities to Polheber and Matchock's (2013) study, in which 294 university students engaged in the TSST protocol. The presence of a dog was compared to that of a friend or being alone. This research focused on identifying which type of company reports greater perceived (state anxiety) and psychophysiological (heart rate and cortisol level reduction) benefits. In this case, the presence of a dog reduced heart rate levels but not anxiety levels. This reaffirms that an animal's company can exert a positive effect on heart rate. Similar results were reported by Fiocco and Hunse (2017), who found that the presence of a dog significantly reduced the strength of the physiological stress response (electrodermal activity) when exposed to a subsequent stressor. Additionally, the results of the current study do show also significant differences between both groups for perceived anxiety. The group that had the opportunity to interact with the dog reported lower state-anxiety levels. Grajfoner, Harte, Potter, and McGuigan (2017) demonstrated similar results. These authors confirmed that human–dog interaction reduces perceived anxiety levels. This positively impacts on a person's well-being and mood.

In short, the results partially support the hypotheses put forward. The animal's presence mitigated perceived anxiety and heart rate in a social stress situation (TSST). However, it did not have a significant effect on the measures of systolic and diastolic blood pressure. This allows us to suggest that the presence of a friendly dog has calming and dampening effects on social stress. Comparing these results with those of other studies which have introduced dogs that habitually live with the participants (pets) suggests that the effects can be strengthened further (Odendaal, 2000). Moreover, it would be interesting to allow the dog and participant more time to interact before entering the stressful situation. In line with Lass-Hennemann, Peyk, Streb, Holz, and Michael (2014), it is crucial to consider the type of contact that must be established between the participants and the dog to lessen the psychophysiological variables. As the present study used a friendly dog, and not the participant's pet, more research will be necessary to analyse whether present results could be modulated by the type or the intensity of the human–animal bond.

Conneely and Hughes (2010) argue that the participation of university students in research studies is extremely useful when it comes to studying stress and anxiety. However, it would be desirable to use a wider sample that guarantees the confidentiality of the tasks included in the study. Another limitation to consider when interpreting these results could be sample size. If the number of participants per group is not very large, this can represent a limitation (Ato, López, & Banevente, 2013). This could explain why in the study of Wood et al. (2018) with 131 university students, both the reduction of state anxiety and blood pressure were statistically significant. Similar results were found by Wheeler and Faulkner (2015) with 223 university students with respect to measurements of anxiety, heart rate, and blood pressure level. However, differences in the intensity of the stressful situation could not explain the lack of stress effects on blood pressure obtained in the present experiment, since an effect of dog interaction on this measure has been shown in previous studies with similar samples and experimental conditions (Wheeler & Faulkner, 2015; Wood et al., 2018).

In order to make improvements to the design of research studies that implement the TSST protocol, it would be interesting to add a group in which the participants were alone (no dog or toy dog). It would also be desirable to include other variables that might be related to human–animal interaction and the manifestations of stress; for example, cortisol levels (Barker, Knisely, McCain, & Best, 2005; Beetz et al., 2011) and oxytocin levels (Handlin, Nilsson, Ejdebäck, Hydbring-Sandberg, & Uvnäs-Moberg, 2012; Miller et al., 2009; Nagasawa et al., 2009).

To summarize, the results obtained are partially comparable to those achieved in previously conducted research (Beetz et al., 2012; Polheber & Matchock, 2013; Wheeler & Faulkner, 2015). A decrease in state anxiety and heart rate was observed in people who had the opportunity to interact with the friendly dog during the TSST protocol. Yet the results of this study are not comparable to earlier ones in which the animal's presence also had a significant effect on blood pressure (Allen et al., 1991). This could be due to the previously highlighted limitations. However, we can conclude that the results observed point to dogs being a source of social support when faced with conflict situations regardless of the person's age. For this reason, we are seeing more studies attempt to demonstrate their benefits on people's health from a psychological, physiological, and social perspective.

Acknowledgments

We are grateful to the students who gave their time to participate in this study, and specially to Mico, the friendly dog, and his handler.

References

Allen, K. (2003). Are Pets a Healthy Pleasure? The Influence of Pets on Blood Pressure. *Current Directions in Psychological Science,* 12(6), 236–239. doi: 10.1046/j.0963-7214.2003.01269.x

Allen, K. M., Blascovich, J., Tomaka, J., & Kelsey, R. M. (1991). Presence of human friends and pet dogs as moderators of autonomic responses to stress in women. *Journal of Personality and Social Psychology,* 61(4), 582–589. doi: 10.1037/0022-3514.61.4.582

Asmar, R., Khabouth, J., Topouchian, J., El Feghali, R., & Mattar, J. (2010). Validation of three automatic devices for self-measurement of blood pressure according to the International Protocol: The Omron M3 Intellisense (HEM-7051-E), the Omron M2 Compact (HEM 7102- E), and the Omron R3-I Plus (HEM6022-E). *Blood Pressure Monitoring,* 15*(1)*, 49–54. doi: 10.1097/MBP.0b013e3283354b11

Ato, M., López, J. J., & Benavente, A. (2013). Un sistema de clasificación de los diseños de investigación en psicología [A classification system for research designs in psychology]. *Anales de Psicología*, 29(3), 1038-1059. doi: 10.6018/analesps.29.3.178511

Barker, S. B., Knisely, J. S., McCain, N. L., & Best, A. M. (2005). Measuring stress and immune response in healthcare professionals following interaction with a therapy dog: A pilot study. *Psychological Reports*, 96(3), 713–729. doi: 10.2466/pr0.96.3.713-729

Beck, A. M., & Katcher, A. H. (2003). Future Directions in Human-Animal Bond Research. *American Behavioral Scientist*, 47(1), 79–93. doi: 10.1177/0002764203255214

Beetz, A., Julius, H., Turner, D., & Kotrschal, K. (2012). Effects of social support by a dog on stress modulation in male children with insecure attachment. *Frontiers in Psychology*, 3(352), 1–9. doi: 10.3389/fpsyg.2012.00352

Beetz, A., Kotrschal, K., Turner, D. C., Hediger, K., Uvnäs-Moberg, K., & Julius, H. (2011). The effect of a real dog, toy dog and friendly person on insecurely attached children during a stressful task: An exploratory study. *Anthrozoös*, 24(4), 349-368. doi: 10.2752/175303711X13159027359746

Birkett, M. A. (2011). The Trier Social Stress Test protocol for inducing psychological stress. *Journal of Visualized Experiments,* 56(e3238). doi:10.3791/3238

Bowlby, J. (1982). Attachment and loss: Retrospect and prospect. *American Journal of Orthopsychiatry,* 52(4), 664-678. doi: 10.1111/j.1939-0025.1982.tb01456.x

Brickel, C. M. (1979). The Therapeutic Roles of Cat Mascots with a Hospital-based Geriatric Population: A Staff Survey. *The Gerontologist,* 19(4), 368-372. doi: 10.1093/geront/19.4.368

Cain, A. O. (1983). A study of pets in the family system. In A. H. Katcher, & A. M. Beck (Eds.), *New perspectives on our lives with companion animals* (pp. 351-359). Philadelphia: University of Pennsylvania Press.

Conneely, S., & Hughes, B. M. (2010). Test anxiety and sensitivity to social support among college students: effects on salivary cortisol. *Cognition, Brain, Behavior: An Interdisciplinary Journal,* 14(4), 295–310.

Echeburúa, E. (2016). Estrés y recursos de afrontamiento en la sociedad contemporánea [Stress and coping resources in contemporary society]. *Avances en salud mental relacional,* 15(1), 1–10.

Eddy, J., Hart, L. A., & Boltz, R. P. (1988). The effects of service dogs on social acknowledgements of people in wheelchairs. *Journal of Psychology,* 122(1), 39–45. doi: 10.1080/00223980.1988.10542941

Fiocco, A., & Hunse, A. (2017). The buffer effect of therapy dog exposure on stress reactivity in undergraduate students. *International Journal of Environmental Research and Public Health,* 14(7), 707. doi: 10.3390/ijerph14070707

Friedmann, E., Katcher, A. H., Thomas, S. A., Lynch, J. J., & Messent, P. R. (1983). Social interaction and blood pressure: Influence of animal companions. *Journal of Nervous and Mental Disease,* 171(8), 461-465. doi: 10.1097/00005053-198308000-00002

González-Ramírez, M. T., & Hernández, R. L. (2011). Diferencias en Estrés Percibido, Salud Mental y Física de acuerdo al Tipo de Relación Humano-Perro [Differences in Perceived Stress, Mental Health and Physics according to the Type of Human-Dog Relationship]. *Revista Colombiana de Psicologia*, 20(1), 75–86.

Grajfoner, D., Harte, E., Potter, L. M., & McGuigan, N. (2017). The effect of dog-assisted intervention on student well-being, mood, and anxiety. *International Journal of Environmental Research and Public Health*, 14(5), 483–492. doi: 10.3390/ijerph14050483

Gutiérrez, G., Granados, D. R., & Piar, N. (2007). Interacciones humano- animal: características e implicaciones para el bienestar de los humanos [Human-animal interactions: characteristics and implications for the well-being of humans]. *Revista Colombiana de Psicología*, 16, 163–184.

Handlin, L., Hydbring-Sandberg, E., Nilsson, A., Ejdebäck, M., Jansson, A., & Uvnäs-Moberg, K. (2011). Short-term interaction between dogs and their owners: effects on oxytocin, cortisol, insulin and heart rate—an exploratory study. *Anthrozoös*, 24(3), 301-315. doi: 10.2752/175303711X13045914865385

Helland, P. B. (2016, july 15). *Feelings* [video]. Retrieved from https://youtu.be/I80tjkXhZes

Janssens, L. A. A., Street, M., Miller, R., Hazewinkel, H. A. W., Giemsch, L., & Schmitz, R. (2016). The oldest case yet reported of osteoarthritis in a dog: an archaeological and radiological evaluation. *Journal of Small Animal Practice*, 57(10), 568–574. doi: 10.1111/jsap.12548

Jenkins, J. L. (1986). Physiological Effects of Petting a Companion Animal. *Psychological Reports,* 58, 21–22.

Julius, H., Beetz, A., Kotrschal, K., Turner, D., and Uvnäs-Moberg, K. (2012). *Attachment to Pets.* New York: Hogrefe.

Kelly, O., Mathenson, K., Martínez, A., Merali, Z., & Anisman, H. (2007). Psychosocial Stress Evoked by a Virtual Audience: Relation to Neuroendocrine Activity. *CyberPsychology & Behavior,* 10(5), 655-662. doi: 10.1089/cpb.2007.9973

Kirschbaum, C., Pirke, K. M., & Hellhammer, D. H. (1993). The "Trier Social Stress Test"—a tool for investigating psychobiological stress responses in a laboratory setting. *Neuropsychobiology*, 28, 76–81. doi: 10.1159/000119004

Lass-Hennemann, J., Peyk, P., Streb, M., Holz, E., & Michael, T. (2014). Presence of a dog reduces subjective but not physiological stress responses to an analog trauma. *Frontiers in Psychology*, 5(1010), 1–7. doi: 10.3389/fpsyg.2014.01010

Lazarus, R. S., & Folkman, S. (1984). *Stress, appraisal, and coping*. New York: Springer.

Levine, G. N., Allen, K., Braun, L. T., Christian, H. E., Friedmann, E., Taubert, K. A., ... Lange, R. A. (2013). Pet ownership and cardiovascular risk: A scientific statement from the American Heart Association. *Circulation*, 127(23), 2353–2363. doi: 10.1161/CIR.0b013e31829201e1

Martos-Montes, R., Ordóñez-Pérez, D., De la Fuente-Hidalgo, I., Martos-Luque, R., & García-Viedma, M. R. (2015). Intervención asistida con animales (IAA): Análisis de la situación en España [Animal-assisted intervention (AAI): The current situation in Spain]. *Escritos de Psicología,* 8(3), 1-10. doi: 10.5231/psy.writ.2015.2004

Miller, S. C., Kennedy, C. C., DeVoe, D. C., Hickey, M., Nelson, T., & Kogan, L. (2009). An examination of changes in oxytocin levels in men and women before and after interaction with a bonded dog. *Anthrozoös*, 22(1), 31-42. doi: 10.2752/175303708X390455

Molina-Jiménez, T., Gutiérrez-García, A. G., Hernández-Domíngueza, L., & Contreras, C. M. (2008). Estrés psicosocial: Algunos aspectos clínicos y experimentales [Psychosocial stress: Some clinical and experimental aspects]. *Anales de Psicología*, 24(2), 353–360.

Moya-Albiol, L., & Salvador, A. (2001). Empleo de estresores psicológicos de laboratorio en el estudio de la respuesta psicofisiológica al estrés [Use of psychological laboratory stressors in the study of the psychophysiological response to stress]. *Anales de Psicología,* 17(1), 69–81.

Nagasawa, M., Kikusui, T., Onaka, T., & Ohta, M. (2009). Dog's gaze at its owner increases owner's urinary oxytocin during social interaction. *Hormones and Behavior*, 55(3), 434–441. doi: 10.1016/j.yhbeh.2008.12.002

Nagasawa, M., Mitsui, S., En, S., Ohtani, N., Ohta, M., Sakuma, Y., ... Kikusui, T. (2015). Oxytocin-gaze positive loop and the coevolution of human-dog bonds. *Science*, 348, 333–336. doi: 10.1126/science.1261022

O'Haire, M. (2010). Companion animals and human health: Benefits, challenges, and the road ahead. *Journal of Veterinary Behavior: Clinical Applications and Research*, 5(5), 226–234. doi: 10.1016/j.jveb.2010.02.002

Odendaal, J. S. (2000). Animal-assisted therapy—magic or medicine? *Journal of Psychosomatic Research*, 49(4), 275–280. doi: 10.1016/s0022-3999(00)00183-5

Polheber, J. P., & Matchock, R. L. (2013). The presence of a dog attenuates cortisol and heart rate in the Trier Social Stress Test compared to human friends. *Journal of Behavioral Medicine,* 37(5), 860–867. doi: 10.1007/s10865-013-9546-1

Sandín, B. (2008). *El Estrés psicosocial: Conceptos y Consecuencias Clínicas* [Psychosocial stress: Concepts and clinical consequences] (2nd ed.). Madrid: Klinik.

Selye, H. (1936). A syndrome produced by diverse nocuous agents. *Nature, July* 4: 32.

Silcox, D., & Reed, B. J. (2014). The Human Animal Bond: Applications for Rehabilitation Professionals. *Journal of Applied Rehabilitation Counselling*, 45(3), 27–38.

Spielberger, C. D., Gorsuch, R. L., & Lushene, R. (1982). *Manual del Cuestionario de Ansiedad Estado/ Rasgo* [State / Trait Anxiety Inventory] (STAI). Madrid, España: TEA Ediciones.

Tombaugh, T. N. (2006). A comprehensive review of the paced auditory serial addition test (PASAT). *Archives of Clinical Neuropsychology,* 21(1), 53–76. doi: 10.1016/j.acn.2005.07.006

Ursin, H., & Eriksen, H. R. (2010). Cognitive activation theory of stress (CATS). *Neuroscience and Biobehavioral Reviews*, 34(6), 877–881. doi: 10.1016/j.neubiorev.2009.03.001

Virués-Ortega, J. & Buela-Casal, G. (2006). Psychophysiological Effects of Human-Animal Interaction: Theoretical Issues and Long-Term Interaction Effects. *The Journal of Nervous and Mental Disease*. 194(1), 52–57. doi: 10.1097/01.nmd.0000195354.03653.63

Wheeler E. A. & Faulkner, M. E. (2015). The "Pet Effect". *Society & Animals*, 23(5), 425–438. doi: 10.1163/15685306-12341374

Wilson, E. O. (1984). *Biophilia.* Massachusetts: Harvard University Press.

Wood, E., Ohlsen, S., Thompson, J., Hulin, J., & Knowles, L. (2018). The feasibility of brief dog-assisted therapy on university students stress levels: the PAwS study. *Journal of Mental Health*, 27(3), 263–268. doi: 10.1080/09638237.2017.1385737

Yilmaz, O. (2017). Controversies of Origin of Domestic Dog - III - References of Modern Dogs until 2006. *Journal of Agriculture and Veterinary Sciences* 4(11), 484–490. doi: 10.21276/sjavs.2017.4.11.8

Zarghani, N. H., Nazari, M., Shayeghian, Z., y Shahmohammadi, S. (2016). Social support in the pregnant and non-pregnant women and its associated dimensions. *Journal of Nursing and Midwifery Sciences,* 3(2), 11–18. doi: 10.18869/acadpub.jnms.3.2.11

5 Effects of Human–Animal Interactions on Affect and Cognition

Elise R. Thayer and Jeffrey R. Stevens*
University of Nebraska-Lincoln Department of Psychology, Center for Brain, Biology & Behavior, University of Nebraska

Abstract
Human-animal interaction has clear positive effects on people's affect and stress. But less is known about how animal interactions influence cognition. We draw parallels between animal interactions and exposure to natural environments, a research area that shows clear improvements in cognitive performance. The aim of this study is to investigate whether interacting with animals similarly enhances cognitive performance, specifically executive functioning. To test this, we conducted two experiments in which we had participants self-report their affect and complete a series of cognitive tasks (long-term memory, attentional control, and working memory) before and after either a brief interaction with a dog or a control activity. We found that interacting with a dog improved positive affect and decreased negative affect (in one of the two experiments), stress, and anxiety compared to the control condition. However, we did not find effects of animal interaction on long-term memory, attentional control, or working memory. Thus, we replicated existing findings providing evidence that interacting with animals can improve affect, but we did not find similar improvements in cognitive performance. These results suggest that either our interaction was not of sufficient dose or timed appropriately to elicit effects on cognition or the mechanisms underlying effects of human-animal interaction on cognition differ from effects generated by other cognition-enhancing interventions such as exposure to nature. Future research should continue to increase knowledge of the connection between nature exposure and human-animal interaction studies to build our understanding of cognition in response to animal interactions.

Keywords: affect, animal-assisted interventions, cognitive performance, executive function, human-animal interaction

Acknowledgments

We thank Megan Bosworth, Kendall Kelly, and Maggie Kempf for assistance in collecting the data and Francine Goh and London Wolff for comments on a previous draft. We dedicate this work to the memory of Koda, who made the project possible and a joy at every turn.

Conflict of interest

The authors declare no conflicts of interest.

Imagine that you have an hour-long lunch break to take your dog for a walk. Would you rather take Fido down a city street or down a tree-shrouded trail? If you chose the leafy trail, it's not by chance—there is a mountain of evidence to suggest

Corresponding author email: jeffrey.r.stevens@gmail.com

that exposure to natural landscapes is psychologically restorative. Specifically, nature exposure has been shown to increase positive mood (e.g., Mayer et al., 2008), decrease feelings of anxiety (e.g., Bratman et al., 2015), decrease psychological and physiological responses to stress (e.g., Gidlow et al., 2016), and improve cognitive functioning (e.g., Berman et al., 2008; Bratman et al., 2012). The aim of this study is to investigate whether interacting with animals has a similar effect on well-being and cognition as exposure to nature.

At the core of the scientific endeavor to quantify the influence of natural landscapes on human health and well-being is the *biophilia* hypothesis, which postulates that humans have an innate tendency toward and affinity for life and life-like processes (Wilson, 2009). Two relevant theories based on the biophilia hypothesis have been proposed to account for effects of exposure to nature on well-being and cognition. First, *Stress Reduction Theory* proposes that aesthetic features of nature reduce autonomic responses to stress captured by decreases in physiological and experiential indicators of stress (Ulrich, 1981). Second, *Attention Restoration Theory* postulates that experiences in nature restore cognition by replenishing attentional capacities (Kaplan & Kaplan, 1989; Kaplan, 1995). In this view, an individual requires a finite and exhaustible mental resource to maintain focus on a particular task without distraction (i.e., to maintain directed attention). In turn, this resource can be restored while engaging in tasks or activities that do not require marked cognitive demand, such as interacting with nature.

Though directed attention itself is not clearly defined or quantifiable, it is a key component of executive functions (i.e., those related to complex, goal-directed behaviors) and can be tested with well-established paradigms (Miyake et al., 2000). For example, researchers have investigated the effects of experiences in nature on executive functions such as *attentional control* (i.e., the ability to simultaneously attend to relevant information and ignore distracting information) and *working memory* (i.e., the ability to mentally hold and manipulate information in the short-term). The improvement in cognitive performance often observed following nature exposure thereby provides evidence for the restorative effects of nature (for a review, see Stevenson et al., 2018). Though some researchers posit that decreases in stress facilitate attention restoration, evidence indicates that autonomic and cognitive effects of exposure to natural landscapes are distinguishable (Li & Sullivan, 2016). As such, the quantification of nature's influence on cognition is concentrated in research working through the Attention Restoration framework.

The study of human-animal interactions—the mutual and dynamic exchanges between humans and non-human animals (Griffin et al., 2019)—also rests on the same foundational principle of biophilia, though it is minimally integrated with the nature exposure literature (but see Franco et al., 2017). Yet human-animal interactions (HAIs) elicit strikingly similar effects on human health and well-being as nature exposure. Human-animal interactions encompass the interactions between owners and pets, handlers and trained service dogs, and individuals and unfamiliar dogs (Thayer & Stevens, 2019b). This is of particular public interest in light of the rapidly increasing presence of dogs in hospitals, schools, and therapeutic contexts (Barker & Wolen, 2008; Friedmann & Son, 2009; Hosey & Melfi, 2014). Here, we focus on animal-assisted interventions or facilitated interactions between an unfamiliar animal and a person to improve individual health or well-being (Thayer & Stevens, 2019a). These interactions between individuals and unfamiliar dogs can evoke positive mood (Beetz et al., 2012; Crossman et al., 2020) and mitigate behavioral and physiological responses to stress (Odendaal & Meintjes, 2003; Lass-Hennemann et al., 2014; Barker et al., 2016; Fiocco & Hunse, 2017; Ein et al., 2018). However, these effects are not always present. For example, Johnson et al. (2008) found no effect of canine- assisted activities on mood, and Barker et al. (2003) found no effect on anxiety.

Akin to the understanding that human preferences for natural views are evolved, HAI practitioners believe the stress- and anxiety-reducing effects of animal interactions to be largely a function of humans' evolutionary need to attend to environmental cues for survival, animals being key indicators of environmental safety (Serpell, 1996; Kruger & Serpell, 2010). In turn, it is assumed that there are subconscious feelings of safety elicited by these benign interactions that induce a calming effect that reduces stress (Beetz, 2017). Since animal interactions and natural experiences elicit similar stress-reducing effects, do human-animal interactions possess the same cognitive restorative potential as experiences in nature?

There is a gap in the human-animal interaction literature with regard to the place of HAIs in relation to cognitive performance. HAIs and cognitive performance in adults are disproportionately understudied compared to the presence of HAIs in educational contexts (Gee et al., 2017). There have been few direct tests of HAIs and cognitive performance in adults (Gee et al., 2014, 2015; Trammell, 2019) or children (Gee et al., 2010, 2012; Hediger & Turner, 2014). Most of these studies approached cognition from a bio-psycho-social model of stress reduction, analogous to Stress Reduction Theory. Trammell (2019) replicated effects of human-dog interactions on self-reported affect but found no differences between control and HAI groups' performance in a long-term memory paradigm. Long-term memory, however, is not a part of the executive function system, so it is perhaps unsurprising that it is not influenced by HAI. Working memory and attentional control, on the other hand, are components of executive function (McCabe et al., 2010). Yet interacting with a dog does not seem to influence working memory in adults (Gee et al., 2014, 2015) or attentional control in children (Hediger & Turner, 2014). With so few studies, we need to quantify the influence of HAIs on cognition.

Our aim in the present study was to examine the influence of human-animal interactions on affect and cognitive performance in adults using established methods from the adjacent exposure to nature literature. In Experiment 1, we sought to replicate positive affective effects of HAIs observed in previous research (Beetz et al., 2012; Thelwell, 2019; Crossman et al., 2020) and test whether HAI induces restorative effects on cognition using tasks implemented in the experience in nature literature (e.g., Berman et al., 2008). We selected tests of cognitive performance used in the nature exposure literature to capture the attentional control and working memory components of directed attention. We also included a long-term memory task to assess cognitive performance outside of directed attention to investigate if HAI effects might influence cognition generally or executive functioning specifically. We hypothesized that HAI would evoke greater improvements in mood and directed attention but not long-term memory compared to a control condition. We tested these hypotheses using a between-groups pre-post intervention design where we administered affective and cognitive tasks both before and after either a three-minute human- animal interaction or control activity. Further, due to potential moderating effects of affect and pet attitudes on interaction efficacy (Barker et al., 2010), we conducted exploratory moderation analyses of positive and negative affect change and pet attitudes on the effect of animal interaction on cognition. In Experiment 2, we sought to replicate our findings and also replicate self-reported stress- and anxiety-reducing effects of HAI observed in previous research (e.g., Grajfoner et al., 2017) to better characterize the influence of animal interaction on cognition.

Experiment 1

Methods

Participants

We recruited participants who did not have a physical or emotional aversion to dogs (i.e., allergy, fear) from the University of Nebraska-Lincoln (UNL) Department of Psychology subject pool between Sep to Nov 2018. When recruiting participants, we did not include any information about dogs in the study description to avoid introducing self-selection bias into our sample. We also did not include references to dogs in the consent procedure to avoid building expectations about interacting with dogs. We collected data from 73 undergraduate students of whom 60 (82.2%) identified as female, 13 (17.8%) identified as male, and 0 (0.0%) identified as neither female nor male (race/ethnicity and parental income information available in Table S1). Participants were on average 19.2 (SD = 1.4) years of age. There were 39 individuals (53.40%) who currently lived with at least one pet in their primary residence and 62 (84.90%) who lived with at least one pet as a child. All participants received one hour of research credit in exchange for their participation.

Measures

Unless otherwise indicated, all stimuli were presented and all responses were collected with

Psychopy version 1.90.2 (Peirce et al., 2019) on a computer with a 16-inch monitor in a private room with only the participant and experimenter present.

Affect. We assessed participants' affect with the Positive and Negative Affect Schedule [PANAS; Watson et al. (1988)]. Participants viewed 10 positive and 10 negative adjectives (e.g., "excited," "disinterested") and rated each from one (*very slightly or not at all*) to five (*extremely*) as they pertained to how they felt. Higher values for positive adjectives represent more positive affect, and higher values for negative adjectives represent more negative affect. We calculated Revelle's omega total (ω) as our measure of internal consistency reliability of scales (Revelle & Zinbarg, 2008; McNeish, 2018): $\omega_{positive} = 0.90$, $\omega_{negative} = 0.92$).

Cognitive tasks. We administered four separate cognitive tasks: Deese-Roedinger-McDermott (long-term memory), Necker cube pattern control (attentional control), backwards digit span (working memory), and n-back (working memory).

Deese-Roedinger-McDermott. We used the Deese-Roedinger-McDermott long-term memory (DRM) paradigm to examine participants' capacity for long-term memory retention (Roediger & McDermott, 1995; McEvoy et al., 1999). While this task is primarily used for studying false memory, it can be used as a general memory distortion task as well (MacDuffie et al., 2012; Cadavid & Beato, 2016). During the presentation phase of this task, participants passively viewed two sets of ten words associated with a not-presented critical word (e.g., child) presented one at a time. In the recall phase at the end of the experiment, participants were told that they would view some of the words they were instructed to remember at the beginning of the experiment. They viewed 6 of the 20 previously presented words, the two critical words, and four unrelated words in random order and responded via key press whether they recalled seeing the words previously in the experiment (Table S2). We analyzed mean accuracy as the proportion of items correctly recognized, with 1 representing perfect recognition and 0 representing complete lack of recognition. We also calculated d' as $z(P(\text{recall} \mid \text{presented word})) - z(P(\text{recall} \mid \text{not presented word}))$ (Tajika, 2001), but the outcomes are identical to accuracy, so we only report the accuracy results.

Necker Cube Pattern Control. We used the Necker Cube Pattern Control Test to measure participants' attentional control (Orbach et al., 1963; Cimprich, 1993; Sahlin et al., 2016). The Necker cube is an optical illusion that consists of a cube outline that lacks visual cues to indicate its orientation (Figure S1a); with continued viewing, the viewer observes shifts in perspective between back-in-focus and front-in-focus. In this task, participants were prompted to observe the cube and record perceived perspective shifts for 30 s. After this initial trial, they were prompted to observe the cube in a second trial while purposefully holding each focus for as long as possible and minimizing shifts. We calculated the difference in the number of shifts reported between the first and second trials as a measure of participants' attentional control. Positive values represent more shifts in the first trial, which can be interpreted as exerting more attentional control in the second trial.

Backwards digit span. We presented participants with a backwards digit span task to measure their working memory capacity (Berman et al., 2008). In this task, participants viewed sequences of numbers presented individually for one second each, then wrote the sequence down on a sheet of paper in the reverse order from which it was presented (Figure S1b). Following a practice sequence of numbers, participants responded to a total of 14 unique sequences that increased in span (number of digits), starting with three digits and ending with nine digits. We pseudo-randomly generated each sequence such that no digit was repeated within a given sequence. If the participant correctly recorded an entire sequence in reverse order, that response was coded as correct. We measured performance by identifying participants' digit span index, or the greatest span they reversed correctly before failing two consecutive sequences of the same length (Schutte et al., 2017). Spans ranged from 3-9 digits, so higher values represent greater spans, which indicates better working memory.

N-back. We administered an n-back task as an additional measure of working memory capacity (Cohen et al., 1994; Rich, 2007). In this task, participants observed a stream of phonologically distinct letters [B, F, K, H, M, Q, R, X; Kane et al. (2007)] and responded when the current stimulus was presented *n* (two) trials prior

(Figure S1c). Each letter was presented for 0.5 seconds and followed by a 2.5 second interstimulus interval (fixation cross). Participants completed a brief practice before viewing a total of 96 letters, of which 16-19 were targets (i.e., matching the stimulus from two trials prior). We assessed participants' working memory performance on the n-back task by calculating d' as $z(P(\text{hit} \mid \text{target}) - z(P(\text{hit} \mid \text{not target}))$ to capture both correct recognition and false alarm rates (Tajika, 2001). A value of 0 indicates that a participant was not able to discriminate between previously presented and not presented words and larger values indicate greater propensities to discriminate between presented and not-presented words (Haatveit et al., 2010). Higher values can be interpreted as better working memory.

Animal-related measures. In addition to standard demographic metrics (e.g., age and sex), at the end of the experiment, we asked participants whether they owned pets as a child and whether they currently owned pets. We also assessed participants' attitudes towards pets with the Pet Attitude Scale [PAS; Templer et al. (1981); Templer et al. (2004)]. Participants rated the extent to which they agreed with 18 statements (e.g., "House pets add happiness to my life, or would if I had one") on a scale from one (strongly disagree) to seven (strongly agree) ($\omega = 0.93$). Higher values represent more positive attitudes toward pets.

For those assigned to the HAI condition, we administered an additional questionnaire used by Gee et al. (2015) to assess participants' evaluation of the quality of the dog interaction. Participants rated on a scale from one (strongly disagree) to four (strongly agree) the extent to which they agreed with 11 statements (e.g., "I felt more relaxed when the dog was present") pertaining to their comfort, discomfort, ambivalence, and desire to interact with the dog ($\omega = 0.88$). Higher values represent more positive experiences with the interaction.

Cardiovascular activity. Participants wore an Empatica E4 wristband on their left wrist for the duration of the experiment to provide a continuous measure of cardiovascular activity, specifically heart rate variability (McCarthy et al., 2016; Empatica, 2018). The E4 wristband uses a photoplethysmogram (PPG) sensor located on the backside of the device face seated atop the wearer's wrist that samples heart beats at 64 Hertz. We do not provide analyses of cardiovascular data because the device did not sample at a sufficient frequency to detect fine changes in heart rate variability (Shaffer & Ginsberg, 2017).

Procedures

Participants were pseudo-randomly assigned to either an animal interaction (*human–animal interaction* or *HAI*) or control condition before arrival. After participants arrived to the experimental session, they completed informed consent and sat calmly for three minutes to attain a resting state. Then, the researcher instructed the participant to begin the experiment on the computer at their desk. The researcher remained seated in the room throughout the duration of the experiment. The experiment was partitioned into three components, pre-condition, condition, and post-condition, which correspond to the time before, during, and after the animal interaction or control activity, respectively. Participants took about 45 minutes to complete the study.

Pre-condition. Participants experienced the task set in the following order: PANAS, DRM (presentation phase), Necker cube, digit span, and n-back. We administered the affect task first to capture affect upon arrival, the DRM second to allow time to elapse between presentation and recall phases, then followed these with the remaining cognitive tasks in a fixed order for the sake of simplicity.

Condition. Participants experienced three minutes of either the HAI or control condition. We based this timing on changes observed in cortisol, oxytocin, and heart rate after a three-minute dog interaction in Handlin et al. (2011). Participants were not informed which of the three-minute conditions they were assigned to experience until the pre-condition phase was completed.

HAI. We employed JRS's pet dog for every animal-interaction session. The dog used for the HAI condition was a 65-pound, neutered, male Catahoula leopard mix that was Canine Good Citizen certified. Prior to this study, he had completed approximately 35 similar sessions in a previous study. When not interacting with participants, the dog was housed in JRS's office or adjacent experiment room that were both equipped with a large kennel and access to water. The dog participated in 1-5 sessions spread throughout the day with at least 40 minutes between sessions. JRS was not involved in the actual behavioral testing or human-animal interaction to minimize potential bias. Researchers monitored the dog for signs of stress (e.g., excessive panting or licking, avoidance of interacting with participants, barking, aggression, fatigue) and stopped the interaction if he showed signs of stress. Signs of stress were never observed during a session, but when they occurred prior to a session, we reassigned the subsequent participant from the HAI to the control condition.

Before introducing participants to the dog, the researcher asked participants if they had a physical or emotional aversion to dogs; no participants reported any dog aversions. The researcher then brought in the dog, inviting the participant to pet and verbally interact with the dog calmly: "Feel free to pet [dog name] and talk with him all you want. Please try not to rile him up. Other than that, we'll get back to it in a few minutes." Participants were not required to interact with the dog for the whole three minutes.

Participants remained seated for the duration of the interaction. If participants asked questions of or made conversation with the researcher, the researcher briefly informed participants that they would be able to discuss more at the end of the experiment. The dog remained in the experiment room within visual contact after the animal interaction period to rest next to the researcher.

After the experiment ended, researchers debriefed participants who experienced the HAI condition. The researcher explained that participants were not made aware of the dog in recruitment or consent materials to avoid biasing the sample and the results. Researchers requested that participants not discuss the presence of the dog in the experiment with other individuals to help maintain an unbiased sample. Then, researchers invited participants to ask any questions about the nature of the study.

Control. Researchers provided participants with a sheet of paper with a full page of Latin text printed on it and instructed them to circle every 'e' and 'f' for "the next few minutes." Researchers emphasized that the task would not be graded and incorrect answers would incur no penalty. The researcher collected the sheet after the three minutes passed; no data were extracted from the activity.

Post-condition. Participants completed the tasks again in the following order: PANAS, Necker cube, digit span, n-back, and DRM (recall phase). They then completed the Pet Attitude Scale, and those assigned to the HAI condition also completed the animal experience questionnaire. All participants answered standard and animal-related demographic questions (e.g., age, number of pets owned) to conclude the experiment.

Ethics. All procedures were conducted in an ethical and responsible manner, in full compliance with all relevant codes of experimentation and legislation and were approved by the UNL Internal Review Board (protocol # 19552) and Institutional Animal Care and Use Committee (protocol # 1599). All participants gave written consent to participate, and they acknowledged that de-identified data could be published publicly.

Analysis

We analyzed data from 73 participants, with 36 participants experiencing the animal-interaction condition and 37 experiencing the control condition. The sample size was based on previous studies showing effects of HAI on stress responses (Lass-Hennemann et al., 2014; Crossman et al., 2015) with some additional participants added to enhance our ability to detect any potential effects.

Participant characteristics. We compared pre-condition scores for affective measures, cognitive tasks, and animal-related measures (PAS, pet history) between animal interaction and control groups using independent samples t-tests (or Wilcoxon rank sum test in the case of test violations) to ensure that any experimental differences could not be attributed to participant characteristics. There were no significant between-group differences in any measure (Table 5.1).

Data analysis. We used R [Version 4.0.4; R Core Team (2020)] and the R-packages *BayesFactor* [Version 0.9.12.4.2; Morey and Rouder (2018)], *ggbeeswarm* [Version 0.6.0; Clarke and Sherrill-Mix (2017)], *ggcorrplot* [Version 0.1.3; Kassambara (2019)], *here* [Version 1.0.1; Müller (2017)], *Hmisc* [Version 4.4.2; Harrell Jr et al. (2020)], *papaja* [Version 0.1.0.9997; Aust and Barth (2020)], *patchwork* [Version 1.1.1; Pedersen (2020)], *psych* [Version 2.0.12; Revelle (2019)], *rcompanion* [Version 2.3.26; Mangiafico (2020)], and *tidyverse* [Version 1.3.0; Wickham et al. (2019)] for all our analyses. We prepared the manuscript using *rmarkdown* [Version 2.6; Xie et al. (2018)] and *papaja* [Version 0.1.0.9997; Aust and Barth (2020)]. Data, analysis scripts, supplementary methods, tables, and figures, and the reproducible research materials are available in Supplementary Materials at the Open Science Framework (https://osf.io/v7wxt/).

In addition to frequentist analyses, we calculated and drew inferences based on Bayes factors, that is, the strength of evidence for the alternative over the null hypothesis. For example, BF_{10} = 15 suggests that there is 15 times more evidence for the alternative than the null hypothesis. Bayes factors between 3-10 provide moderate evidence for the alternative hypothesis, those between 10-30 provide strong evidence, those between 30-100 provide very strong evidence, and those above 100 provide extreme evidence; reciprocal values (1/3, 1/10, 1/30, 1/100) provide comparable evidence for the null hypothesis (Wagenmakers et al., 2018). We used the *BayesFactor* package to calculate most Bayes factors (using default priors and settings), except for the Wilcoxon rank sum tests, which we calculated from code provided by van Doorn et al. (2020).

Condition effects. To assess potential condition differences pre-condition, we conducted independent samples t-tests or Wilcoxon rank sum tests in the case of test violations. For condition effects, we used analysis of covariance to examine the effects of condition on post-scores controlling for pre-scores. We report predicted marginal means and 95% confidence intervals and calculated effect sizes with generalized eta squared ($\hat{\eta}_G^2$). We used both visual and test-based methods to check analysis of covariance test assumptions: linearity between covariate and outcome variable, homogeneity of regression slopes, normally distributed residuals on outcome variable, and homogeneity of variance (Johnson, 2016). Since we recorded responses only at post-condition for the long-term memory task, we compared between-groups differences with a Wilcoxon rank sum test, as it violated assumptions of an independent samples t-test. For these, we calculated effect sizes with *r*, the z-score of the test statistic divided by the total number of observations.

The analyses of covariance for negative affect and Necker cube significantly violated model assumptions, so we log-transformed negative affect pre- and post-scores and removed outliers (standard deviation × 3; 2 observations) from Necker post-scores to conform to model assumptions. We excluded one observation from DRM (participant expressed comprehension issues after task), three from Necker cube (participants expressed comprehension issues after task), and three from digit span (participants did not request response sheet) when running respective analyses, inserting missing data for these subjects.

Moderation analyses. We conducted follow-up exploratory analyses to identify potential moderators of the relationship between animal interaction and cognitive performance. Because we have three cognitive measures and several potential moderators, combining all of these would result in a large number of statistical tests. To reduce the number of statistical tests run, we aggregated all of the cognition scores into a single composite measure, as used in the nature exposure literature. Following Van Hedger et al. (2019), we constructed the cognitive composite measure by averaging the z-scores for the Necker cube, digit span, and n-back post - pre difference scores. We tested whether positive and negative affect change (i.e., post - pre difference scores; PANAS) and pet attitude (PAS) explained the relationship between experimental condition and composite cognitive performance change. For each moderation analysis, we used multiple linear regression with predictors *condition*, *moderator*, and *condition×moderator* and outcome *post - pre cognitive composite*. We report model fit results alone, as no moderation model accounted for more than a negligible amount of the variance in the data.

Animal experience correlations. We also conducted follow-up exploratory analyses to identify correlations between the animal-related measures, affect, and cognitive performance composite.

Results

Affect

To test the effect of animal interaction on affect, we compared positive and negative PANAS scores following the control and HAI condition. Figure 5.1 shows the effect of condition on positive and negative affect (Table 5.1; Figure S2). Analyses of covariance indicate very strong evidence that positive affect is greater post-condition for those who experienced HAI than those who did not, controlling for pre-interaction scores ($F(1,70) = 30.21$, $MSE = 0.15$, $p<0.001$, $\hat{\eta}_G^2 = 0.30$, $BF_{10} >100$). For negative affect, on the other hand, there is not sufficient evidence to determine whetherthe log post-condition scores differed between control and HAI groups ($F(1,70) = 4.32$, $MSE = 0.03$, $p = 0.041$, $\hat{\eta}_G^2 = 0.06$, $BF_{10} = 1.39$).

Cognitive tasks

To test the effect of animal interaction on cognition, we compared scores on four cognitive tasks following control and HAI conditions. There is evidence to suggest that animal interaction and control groups did not differ on any cognitive task post-condition (Table 5.1; Fig. 5.2 and S3). Specifically, there is moderate evidence that there is no difference between control and HAI groups for accuracy in the long-term memory task post-condition scores ($W = 681$, $p = 0.696$, $r = 0.05$, $BF_{10} = 0.19$). Similarly, the analyses of covariance provide evidence of no difference between groups—controlling for pre-condition scores—for the number of switches in the Necker cube attentional control task ($F(1,67) = 0.76$, $MSE = 12.85$, $p = 0.385$, $\hat{\eta}_G^2 = 0.01$, $BF_{10} = 0.34$), the backwards digit span index for working memory ($F(1,67) = 0.31$, $MSE = 1.98$, $p = 0.578$, $\hat{\eta}_G^2 =0.01$, $BF_{10} = 0.28$), and the n-back d' for working memory ($F(1,70) = 0.12$, $MSE = 1.09$, $p = 0.726$, $\hat{\eta}_G^2 = 0.01$, $BF_{10} = 0.25$).

Exploratory analyses

We tested affect and pet attitude as potential moderators of the effect of HAI on cognition.

There is substantial evidence to suggest that there were no observable moderators on the effect of experimental condition on composite cognitive performance. Specifically, the moderation model did not outperform an intercept-only model for positive affect change ($R^2 = 0.01$, $F(3,36) = 0.30$, $p = 0.828$, $BF_{10} = 0.04$), negative affect change ($R^2 = 0.02$,

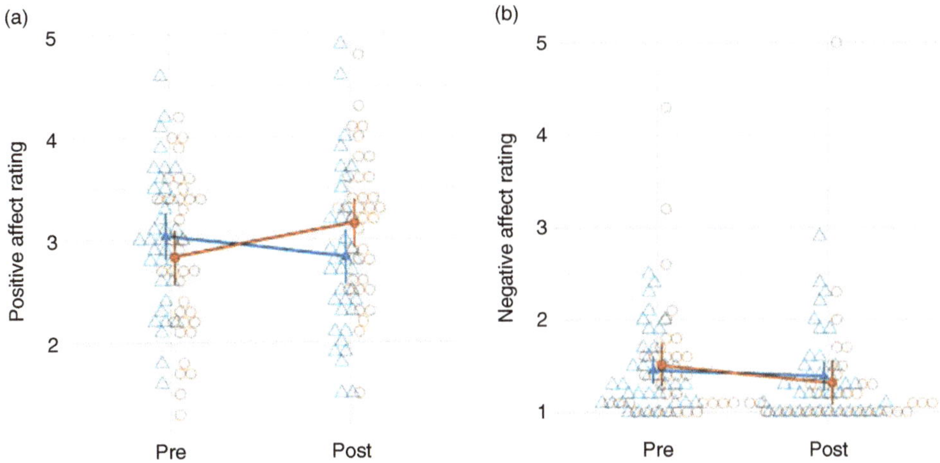

Fig. 5.1. Affect scores pre- and post-condition for control and HAI (human–animal interaction) groups in Experiment 1. Scores show (a) positive PANAS ratings and (b) negative PANAS ratings. Open triangles (blue) represent individual control participant scores, open circles (orange) represent individual HAI participant scores, closed triangles and circles represent condition group means (with lines connecting condition means), error bars represent 95% confidence intervals. Figure used with permission under a CC- BY4.0 license: Thayer & Stevens, 2020; available at https://doi.org/10.31234/osf.io/7v5nq.

Table 5.1. Experiment 1 scores

Measure	Pre-condition					Post-condition				
		Control	HAI				Control	HAI		
	n	*M*	*M*	*p*	BF_{10}	*n*	*M*	*M*	*p*	BF_{10}
Animal measures	73	72.97	33.33	–	–	–	–	–	–	–
Pets now (%)										
Pets as a child (%)	73	91.89	77.78	–	–	–	–	–	–	–
Pet attitude (PAS)	73	5.74	5.63	0.84	0.18	–	–	–	–	–
Affective measures										
Positive affect (PANAS)	73	3.04	2.83	0.24	0.44	73	2.74	3.25	<0.001	>100
Negative affect (PANAS)	73	1.45	1.51	0.79	0.17	73	0.29	0.21	0.04	1.43
Cognitive measures										
Accuracy (DRM)	–	–	–	–	–	72	0.76	0.77	0.70	0.19
Average shifts (NCPC)	70	–0.76	–1.12	0.63	0.27	70	–2.41	–1.66	0.39	0.34
Index (Digit span)	70	6.69	6.12	0.25	0.31	70	7.11	7.30	0.58	0.28
d' (N-back)	73	0.08	–0.08	0.74	0.20	73	0.04	–0.04	0.73	0.28

Note: Post-condition scores control for pre-condition scores. Table used with permission under a CC-BY4.0 license: Thayer & Stevens, 2020; available at https://doi.org/10.31234/osf.io/7v5nq.

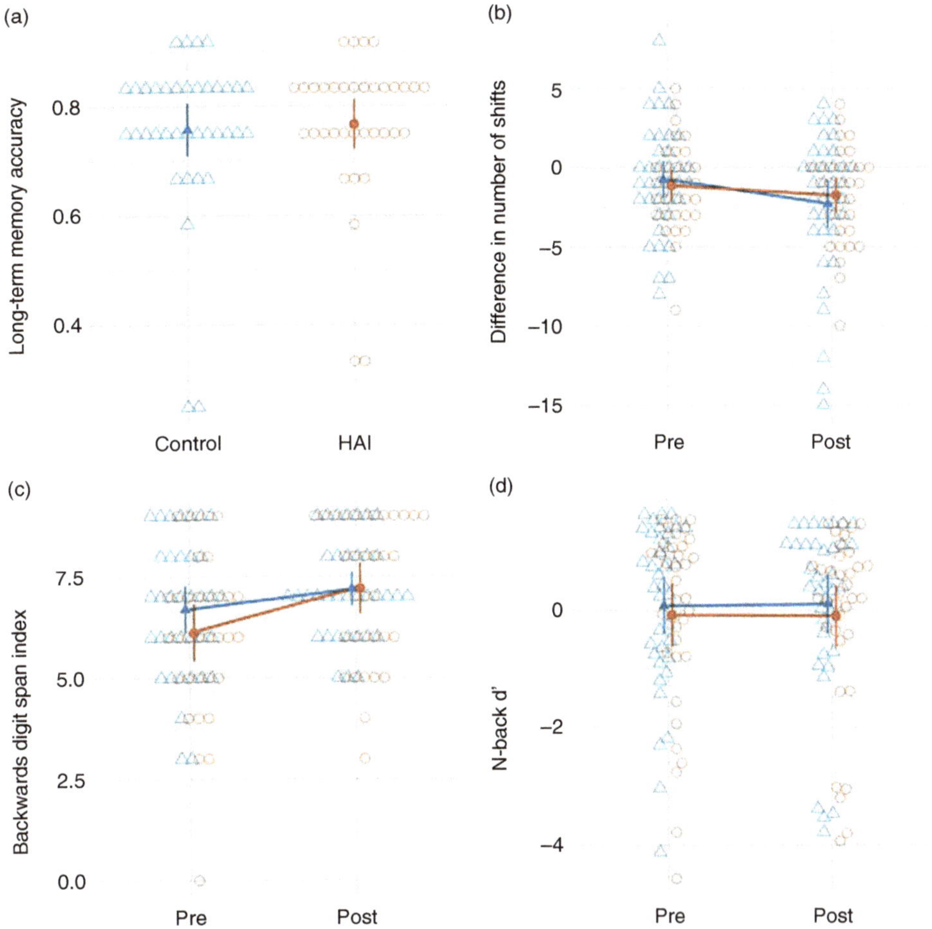

Fig. 5.2. Cognitive performance for control and HAI (human–animal interaction) groups in Experiment 1. (a) Long-term memory accuracy from the Deese-Roedinger-McDermott task was calculated only post-condition. Pre- (Pre) and post-condition (Post) performance was calculated for (b) the difference in number of attentional shifts between the two Necker cube trials, (c) the index for the backwards digit span task, and (d) *d′* for the n-back task. Open triangles (blue) represent individual control participant scores, open circles (orange) represent individual HAI participant scores, closed triangles and circles represent condition group means (with lines connecting condition means), error bars represent 95% confidence intervals. Figure used with permission under a CC-BY4.0 license: Thayer & Stevens, 2020; available at https://doi.org/10.31234/osf.io/7v5nq.

$F(3,63) = 0.41$, $p = 0.746$, $BF_{10} = 0.04$), or pet attitude ($R^2 = 0.04$, $F(3,63) = 0.86$, $p = 0.468$, $BF_{10} = 0.07$).

We found that pet attitude positively correlated with the positive interaction quality measures from Gee et al. (2015) (comfort and desire to interact with the dog) and the change in positive PANAS between pre- and post-condition (Figure S4a), while negatively correlating with discomfort and ambivalence with the dog. The cognitive performance composite score did not correlate with any animal-related measures.

Summary of results

Our first investigation of the effects of HAI on affect and cognition replicated effects of HAI on affect but did not evoke predicted improvements in cognitive performance. Specifically, a three-minute animal interaction bolstered positive affect more so than a control activity. But we did not observe improvements in attentional control or working memory. Our follow-up moderation analyses indicated that affect and pet attitude did not moderate a relationship between experimental condition and cognitive performance.

Experiment 2

Our aim with Experiment 2 was to replicate Experiment 1 and extend the investigation to the influence of HAI on anxiety and stress. We assessed self-reports of anxiety and stress throughout the experiment using visual analogue scales. We again conducted follow-up exploratory analyses to identify potential moderators of the relationship between experimental condition and cognitive performance.

Methods

Participants

We recruited a new sample of participants between Nov 2018 to Apr 2019 from the University of Nebraska-Lincoln psychology subject pool who did not have a physical or emotional aversion to dogs (i.e., allergy, fear), again without providing information about dogs in the study description or consent materials. We analyzed data from 83 of 84 participants, excluding one person who progressed through the study without completing the experimental manipulation. Of the 83 eligible participants, 66 (79.5%) identified as female, 17 (20.5%) identified as male, and 0 (0.0%) identified as neither male nor female (race/ethnicity and parental income information available in Table S1). Participants were on average 19.9 (*SD* = 1.8) years of age (Table S1). There were 47 individuals (56.6%) who currently live with at least one pet in their primary residence and 67 (80.7%) who lived with at least one pet as a child. All participants received one hour of research credit in exchange for their participation.

Measures

In addition to the measures used in Experiment 1, we also explored the influence of human–animal interaction on affect through measures of anxiety and stress.

Affect. We assessed participants' present and general feelings of anxiety with the State and Trait Anxiety Inventory [STAI; Spielberger et al. (1999)]. Participants were presented with 20 statements (e.g., "I feel calm") and rated each from one (*not at all*) to four (*very much so*) to describe their feelings in the moment (*state*; ω = 0.93), then rated another set of 20 to describe their feelings in general (*trait*; $\omega = 0.95$). We also measured present feelings of anxiety with the single-item Anxiety Visual Analogue Scale [AVAS; Cella and Perry (1986)]. Participants indicated how anxious they felt in the moment via mouse-click between poles *not at all anxious* and *extremely anxious* on a 100-tick horizontal line. Participants also indicated how stressed they felt in the moment with the similar Stress Visual Analogue Scale [SVAS; Cella and Perry (1986)]. Higher values represent stronger feelings of anxiety and stress.

Animal-related measures. Participants responded to the same animal-related measures used in Experiment 1, including the pet attitude scale (ω = 0.93) and the HAI experience questions (ω = 0.86). In addition, the researcher logged the amount of time the participant spent physically interacting with the dog, which ranged from 30 sec to the full 3 min.

Procedures

All procedures from Experiment 1 carried over to Experiment 2. However, instead of beginning with the Positive and Negative Affect Schedule, participants first completed Anxiety and Stress Visual Analogue Scales (*baseline*), then STAI prior to PANAS. Participants also completed Visual Analogue Scales immediately preceding the 3-minute animal interaction/control condition (*pre-condition* or *pre*), immediately following the condition (*post-condition* or *post*), and following completion of the experiment (*post+20*).

Analysis

Of the 83 eligible participants, 42 participants experienced the animal-interaction condition and 41 experienced the control condition. We increased our sample size slightly from Experiment 1 to enhance our ability to detect any potential effects in negative affect.

Participant characteristics. There were no between-group differences in pre-condition scores for any affective measures, cognitive tasks, or animal-related measures (Table 5.2).

Data analysis. We utilized the same data analysis approach as Experiment 1 and also used this approach to analyze AVAS and SVAS (immediately before and after intervention). For moderation analyses, we tested all Experiment 1 moderators in addition to state and trait anxiety (from STAI), anxiety change from immediately pre- to post-condition (from AVAS), and stress change from immediately pre- to post-condition (from SVAS). We also included these additional measures in exploratory correlations between pet experience, affect, and cognition for those who experienced the animal interaction.

We log-transformed negative affect pre- and post-scores and removed a single outlier (standard deviation × 3) to conform to analysis of covariance model assumptions. We excluded one observation from DRM (participant expressed comprehension issues after task), three from Necker cube (participants expressed comprehension issues after task), six from digit span (participants did not request response sheet or did not complete more than half of task), and three from n-back (two participants did not record any responses and one participant expressed comprehension issues after task).

The effect of condition on anxiety and stress ratings is demonstrated by Fig. 5.3c&d and S5c&d and Table 5.2. There is strong evidence that anxiety was lower post-condition for HAI compared to control ($F(1,80) = 9.50$, $MSE = 172.0$, $p = 0.003$, $\hat{\eta}^2_G = 0.11$, $BF_{10} = 11.22$) and moderate evidence that stress was lower for those who experienced HAI than control ($F(1,80) = 6.20$, $MSE = 228.7$, $p = 0.015$, $\hat{\eta}^2_G = 0.07$, $BF_{10} = 2.96$) when controlling for pre-condition scores.

Cognitive

There is no evidence to suggest that human–animal interaction and control groups differed on any measure of cognition (Table 5.2; Figs. 5.4 and S6). Specifically, there is moderate evidence that there is no difference between control and HAI groups for the long-term memory task at post-condition ($W = 767$, $p = 0.485$, $r = 0.08$, $BF_{10} = 0.20$), the average switches in the Necker cube controlled attention task ($F(1,77) = 0.43$, $MSE = 8.19$, $p = 0.516$, $\hat{\eta}^2_G = 0.01$, $BF_{10} = 0.29$), the n-back working memory task ($F(1,77) = 0.26$, $MSE = 0.92$, $p = 0.610$, $\hat{\eta}^2_G = 0.01$, $BF_{10} = 0.25$), and the digit span working memory task ($F(1,74) = 0.76$, $MSE = 2.42$, $p = 0.385$, $\hat{\eta}^2_G = 0.01$, $BF_{10} = 0.32$).

Exploratory analyses

In line with Experiment 1, there is no evidence that the same variables nor the anxiety- and stress-related variables moderated the relationship between experimental condition and composite cognitive performance. Specifically, there is evidence that condition-cognition moderation models did not outperform intercept-only models for pet attitude ($R^2 = 0.01$, $F(3,68) = 0.07$, $p = 0.973$, $BF_{10} = 0.02$), positive affect change ($R^2 = 0.05$, $F(3,68) = 1.15$, $p = 0.336$, $BF_{10} = 0.08$), negative affect change ($R^2 = 0.03$, $F(3,68) = 0.64$, $p = 0.589$, $BF_{10} = 0.05$), stress change from pre- to post- condition ($R^2 = 0.02$, $F(3,68) = 0.36$, $p = 0.781$, $BF_{10} = 0.03$), anxiety change from pre- to post- condition ($R^2 = 0.01$, $F(3,68) = 0.06$, $p = 0.979$, $BF_{10} = 0.02$), STAI-State anxiety ($R^2 = 0.04$, $F(3,68) = 1.02$, $p = 0.390$, $BF_{10} = 0.07$), and STAI-Trait anxiety ($R^2 = 0.04$, $F(3,68) = 1.00$, $p = 0.400$, $BF_{10} = 0.07$).

We replicated finding (1) positive relationships between pet attitude and comfort with the dog, desire to interact with the dog, and the change in positive PANAS, (2) negative relationships with discomfort and ambivalence with the dog, and (3) no relationships with cognitive performance composite (Figure S4b). Pet attitude also positively correlated with trait anxiety and negatively correlated with change in negative PANAS, feelings of stress, and feelings of anxiety.

Summary of results

Our findings from Experiment 2 provided nearly identical results to those we observed in Experiment 1. We observed once more that a three-minute HAI bolstered positive affect more so than a control; however, unlike in Experiment 1, HAI reduced negative affect. Further, human–animal interaction evoked lower stress

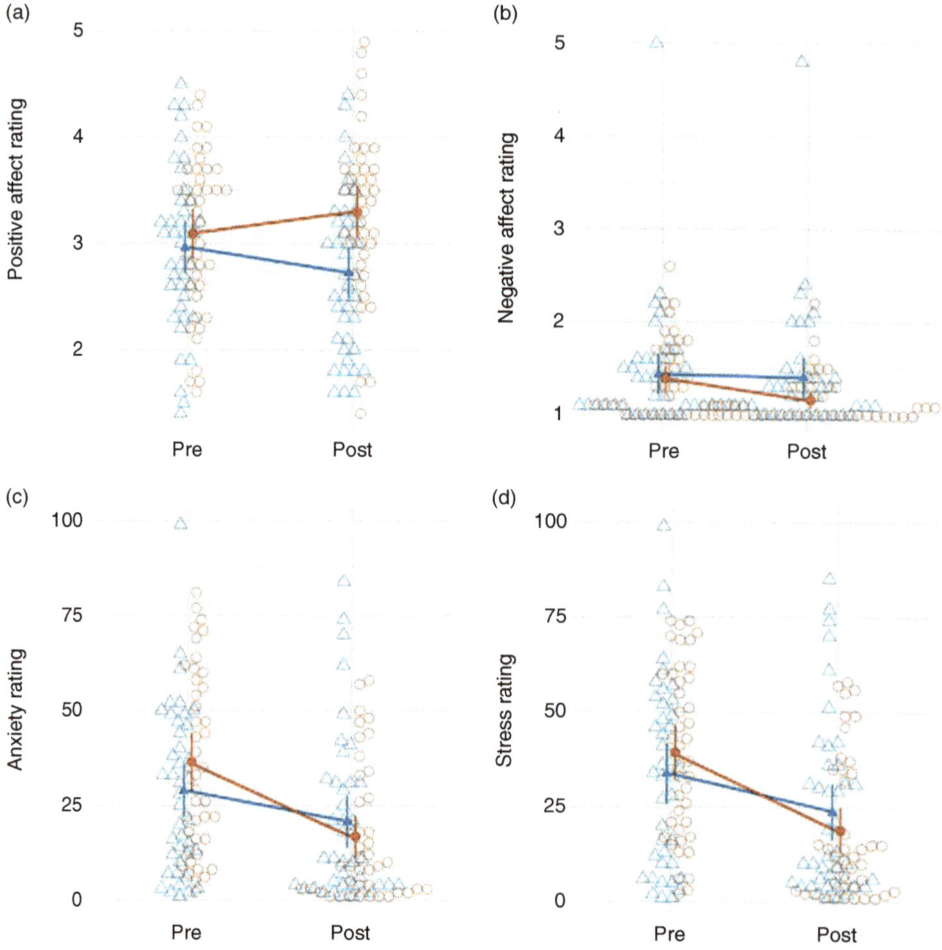

Fig. 5.3. Affect scores pre- and post-condition for control and HAI (human–animal interaction) groups in Experiment 2. Scores show (a) positive PANAS ratings, (b) negative PANAS ratings, (c) anxiety ratings, and (d) stress ratings. Open triangles (blue) represent individual control participant scores, open circles (orange) represent individual HAI participant scores, closed triangles and circles represent condition group means (with lines connecting condition means), error bars represent 95% confidence intervals. Figure used with permission under a CC-BY4.0 license: Thayer & Stevens, 2020; available at https://doi.org/10.31234/osf.io/7v5nq.

and anxiety than the control. We did not observe differential improvements in attentional control or working memory between control and HAI groups. All follow-up moderation analyses mirrored those conducted in Experiment 1 such that affect change, ratings of anxiety and stress change, pet attitude, and state and trait anxiety did not influence the relationship between experimental condition and cognitive performance.

Discussion

Taken together, our findings provide support for the efficacy of animal interaction on affect but no evidence to suggest that animal interaction influences executive function. Specifically, there was greater positive affect improvement in HAI compared to control groups in both Experiments 1 and 2. Though we did not have evidence of

Table 5.2. Experiment 2 scores

Measure	Pre-condition					Post-condition				
	n	Control M	HAI M	p	BF_{10}	n	Control M	HAI M	p	BF_{10}
Animal measures	–	60.98	52.38	–	–	–	–	–	–	–
Pets now (%)										
Pets as a child (%)	–	82.93	78.57	–	–	–	–	–	–	–
Pet attitude (PAS)	83	5.84	5.90	0.67	0.19	–	–	–	–	–
Affective measures										
Positive affect	83	2.96	3.09	0.45	0.30	83	2.77	3.25	<0.001	>100
(PANAS)										
Negative affect	83	1.44	1.40	0.96	0.17	82	0.25	0.13	<0.001	9.31
(PANAS)										
Anxiety (AVAS)	83	28.83	36.45	0.11	0.59	83	23.28	14.28	<0.001	11.08
Stress (SVAS)	83	33.73	39.36	0.18	0.34	83	25.44	17.12	0.01	3.00
State anxiety (STAI)	83	36.22	34.00	0.25	0.31	–	–	–	–	–
Trait anxiety (STAI)	83	40.88	38.55	0.37	0.26	–	–	–	–	–
Cognitive measures	–	–	–	–	–	82	0.74	0.71	0.48	0.21
Accuracy (DRM)										
Average shifts	80	0.15	–1.15	0.19	0.36	80	–1.51	–1.93	0.52	0.28
(NCPC)	77	5.84	6.13	0.43	0.21	77	6.83	6.52	0.39	0.32
Index (Digit span)										
d' (N-back)	80	–0.09	0.30	0.19	0.49	80	0.00	0.11	0.61	0.26

Note: Post-condition scores control for pre-condition scores. Table used with permission under a CC-BY4.0 license: Thayer & Stevens, 2020; available at https://doi.org/10.31234/osf.io/7v5nq.

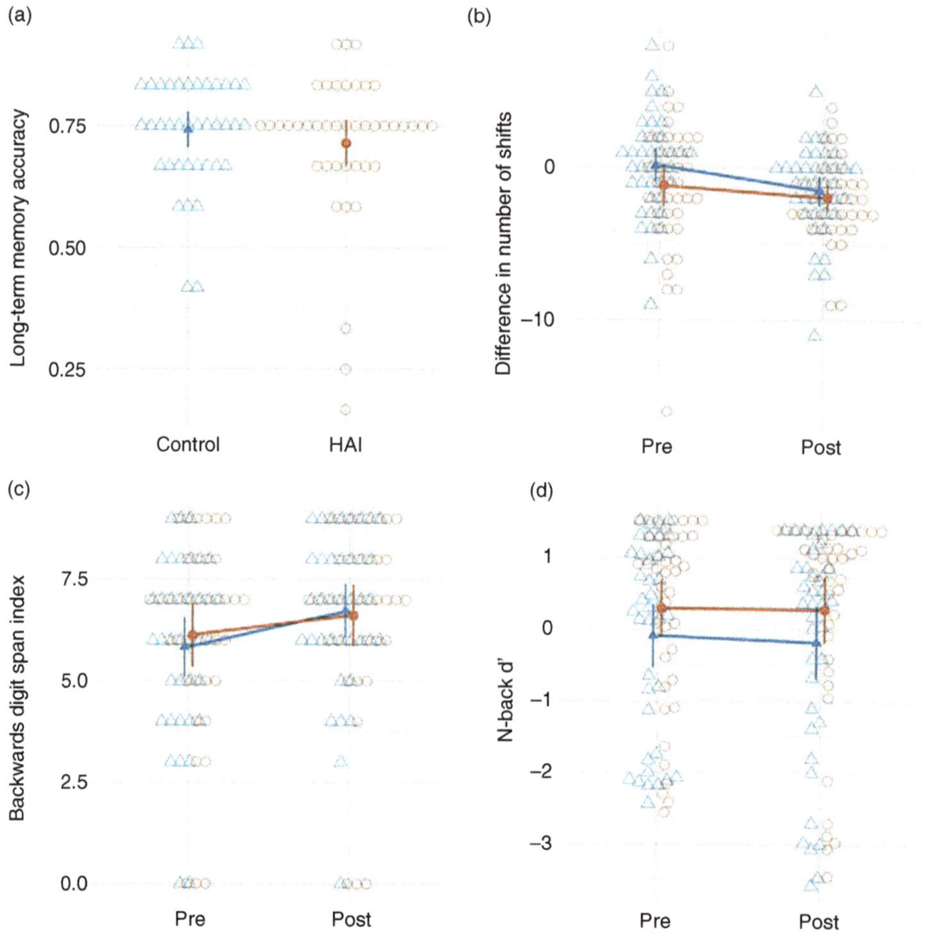

Fig. 5.4. Cognitive performance for control and HAI (human–animal interaction) groups in Experiment 2. (a) Long-term memory accuracy from the Deese-Roedinger-McDermott task was calculated only post-condition. Pre- (Pre) and post-condition (Post) performance was calculated for (b) the difference in number of attentional shifts between the two Necker cube trials, (c) the index for the backwards digit span task, and (d) *d′* for the n-back task. Open triangles (blue) represent individual control participant scores, open circles (orange) represent individual HAI participant scores, closed triangles and circles represent condition group means (with lines connecting condition means), error bars represent 95% confidence intervals. Figure used with permission under a CC-BY4.0 license: Thayer & Stevens, 2020; available at https://doi.org/10.31234/osf.io/7v5nq.

effects of HAI on negative affect in Experiment 1, this likely resulted from a slightly smaller sample size. With the larger sample size of Experiment 2, we found that negative affect was reduced more in human–animal interaction than control groups. Anxiety and stress measures included in Experiment 2 captured more pronounced decreases in anxiety and stress for HAI compared to control groups. Nevertheless, measures of cognitive performance (long-term memory, working memory, and attentional control) did not differ between control and HAI groups in Experiments 1 or 2.

Improvements in affect following brief interactions with an unfamiliar animal are commonly observed in experimental HAI manipulations

(Beetz et al., 2012; Lass-Hennemann et al., 2014; Crossman et al., 2015; Grajfoner et al., 2017), although future research should explore how long these effects last. Our evidence of a positive affect-boosting effect of animal interaction in both experiments validates our experimental design. We observed similar improvements in negative affect, anxiety, and stress in Experiment 2. Given the modest effect sizes observed here, three minutes may be a *minimally* effective interaction period. In fact, a recent dose-response investigation found that low doses of HAI (i.e., three minutes) elicited stress improvement in a majority of participants but that *maximal* improvement relative to time spent was reached with 15 minute doses (Fournier, 2019). Thus, longer interaction durations could induce changes in cognition not observed here. Note that this work focuses on the short-term interactions used in animal-assisted interventions. It is not clear whether they carry over into longer-term interactions associated with pet ownership.

Given the evidence that HAI influences affect and stress, which in turn can influence cognition, we expected HAI to influence cognition. In particular, we expected HAI to influence executive functioning because HAI shares characteristics with another literature—exposure to natural landscapes—that does influence attentional control and working memory. Because animals are an inherent part of nature, and HAI has been tied to biophilia as well, the nature exposure literature created a conceptual framework for predicting that HAI could influence executive functioning. However, our results—and the results of others (Gee et al., 2014, 2015; Hediger & Turner, 2014; Trammell, 2019)—run counter to the findings in the exposure to nature literature.

There are at least two possible reasons why our results do not follow the findings in the nature exposure literature. First, there may just be a fundamental difference between exposure to nature and interacting with animals. Perhaps biophilia may elicit strong affective effects in both nature and animal interactions because they share a similar experiential component. However, the improvement in affect triggers downstream effects on cognition differently with animals and nature. Similarly, cognitive restoration observed following experiences in nature may not be attributable to biophilia alone because these effects are dependent on aesthetic features unique to natural environments, whereby cognitive improvement is facilitated by a more complex mechanism. Also, using biophilia as the framework connecting the nature exposure literature with human–animal interaction may not be as clear-cut as would be expected. While early work suggested that animal interactions should fit within the biophilia framework (Lawrence, 1993), more recent critiques suggests a more nuanced approach (Joye & De Block, 2011). For example, observed HAI effects on well-being may be due to the calming and supernormal stimulus properties of animals or social/cultural effects rather than them being historically important in our evolution (Serpell, 2004; Kruger & Serpell, 2010). Even within an evolutionary framework, animals typically fall into categories of predator or prey, and we may have evolved specific cognition to avoid predators and capture prey (Barrett, 2015). From this perspective, some species are functional in terms of consuming their meat, whereas others are to be feared and avoided. This view would predict differences between species, with predator species probably not enhancing well-being to the degree that less threatening species might. Thus, human–animal relationships are not as straightforward as proposed in the original biophilia hypothesis, and this hypothesis may not have strong predictions about how interacting with animals should influence human well-being.

An alternative possibility is that our experimental paradigm did not trigger latent cognitive effects of HAI. Perhaps exposure to nature can reach the threshold for triggering these effects easily, but the threshold is higher or harder to reach for animal interactions. Or the time lag for these effects may be delayed (e.g., Handlin et al., 2011). Thus, experimental design could be critical for studying HAI effects on cognition. Decisions about durations of exposure, number and timing of cognitive tasks, and the presence of stress induction could be important in eliciting effects of animal interactions (Fournier, 2019; Griffin et al., 2019), as has been demonstrated in the exposure to nature literature (Shanahan et al., 2016; Cox et al., 2017; Stevenson et al., 2018; Stenfors et al., 2019).

Alternatively, other factors could moderate potential HAI effects on cognition. Individual and cultural differences in interactions with animals can moderate effects on well-being (Barker et al., 2010) and could potentially moderate effects on cognition. This possibility necessitates inclusion of individual difference measures, such as pet attitudes, to better understand the factors influencing potential HAI effects on cognition. Though we found no moderating effect of pet attitudes or ownership in our analysis, these types of factors are important to help profile individuals and groups best suited for animal interventions (Melson, 2011; McCune et al., 2014, 2020).

Thus far in the field, the experimental design attributes of human–animal interaction delivery, duration, and features have been a function of convenience and guesswork as opposed to driven by theory. The field is in need of a grounding framework to systematically grow this understanding. The neighboring domain of exposure to nature literature may provide a suitable, rigorously studied foundation (Kaplan & Berman, 2010; Bratman et al., 2012; Schertz & Berman, 2019). By taking advantage of the affective and cognitive frameworks embedded within the exposure to nature literature, HAI practitioners provide themselves with the chance to standardize investigations of cognitive performance and draw theoretically sound inferences from their findings. Evidence of this sort is well-positioned to inform decisions regarding the implementation of HAIs in schools and other performance-dependent contexts for healthy and clinical populations. A deeper understanding of the influence of HAIs on cognition can also provide necessary footing to investigate whether observations are moderated by life experiences, such as growing up in an urban or rural community, race/ethnicity, socio-economic status, or personal history with animals. With affiliative animals like dogs so accessible in daily life, it is crucial to profile the restorative potential of these therapeutic agents by furthering research into the influence of animal interactions on cognition.

Our study investigated HAI in student participants and replicated effects on affect (Stewart et al., 2014; Crossman et al., 2015; Crump & Derting, 2015) and lack of effects on cognition (Gee et al., 2014, 2015; Trammell, 2019) observed in similar populations. Undergraduate students are a unique and unrepresentative population, potentially limiting the application of these findings to other populations. Nevertheless, the high levels of stress and anxiety experienced by students— and the pressure for high levels of cognitive performance—underscore the importance of understanding these effects in this population. Furthermore, the effect of HAI on affect (Crossman et al., 2020) and and the lack of an effect on cognition (Hediger & Turner, 2014) has also been documented in children, suggesting that our findings may generalize beyond undergraduate students. Yet even the sample of undergraduates that we tested is not representative, with a bias toward female, white, affluent participants who owned pets as children. Further research must assess if these findings generalize to other populations.

In addition to a potentially unrepresentative sample of participants, the experimental design may have imposed limitations on the ecological validity of the study. The controlled nature of the experimental setting may have inhibited participants from engaging with the dog in a natural way. Participants may have found having the experimenter in the room or the admonition to avoiding ‘riling up’ the dog to be awkward for engaging in a natural interaction. Thus, differently structured interactions (e.g., in less prescribed or group settings) could result in different outcomes.

Experimental outcomes could also depend on how familiar participants are with the dogs. People interacting with their own dog or a familiar dog may have a more enjoyable experience, which may put them in a different state of mind for completing the cognitive tasks. Not knowing the dog may have made the participants more inhibited, precluding them from fully experiencing any possible benefits in cognitive performance.

Conclusion

In the present study, we addressed a need to strengthen theory-driven tests of the influence of human–animal interaction on cognition. We observed positive effects of HAI in affective measures—including positive affect, negative affect, anxiety, and stress—but did not observe improvement in cognitive performance. Future research should continue to enhance the connection between nature exposure and human–animal interaction studies to build our understanding of cognition in response to animal interactions.

References

Aust, F., & Barth, M. (2020). papaja: Create APA manuscripts with R Markdown. [Version 0.1.0.9997] https://github.com/crsh/papaja

Barker, S. B., Barker, R. T., McCain, N. L., & Schubert, C. M. (2016). A randomized cross-over exploratory study of the effect of visiting therapy dogs on college student stress before final exams. *Anthrozoös*, 29(1), 35–46. https://doi.org/10.1080/08927936.2015.1069988

Barker, S. B., Knisely, J. S., McCain, N. L., Schubert, C. M., & Pandurangi, A. K. (2010). Exploratory study of stress-buffering response patterns from interaction with a therapy dog. *Anthrozoös*, 23(1), 79–91. https://doi.org/10.2752/175303710X12627079939341

Barker, S. B., Pandurangi, A. K., & Best, A. M. (2003). Effects of animal-assisted therapy on patients' anxiety, fear, and depression before ECT. *The Journal of ECT*, 19(1), 38. https://doi.org/10.1097/00124509-200303000-00008

Barker, S. B., & Wolen, A. R. (2008). The benefits of human-companion animal interaction: A review. *Journal of Veterinary Medical Education*, 35(4), 487–495. https://doi.org/10.3138/jvme.35.4.487

Barrett, H. C. (2015). Adaptations to predators and prey. In *The Handbook of Evolutionary Psychology* (pp. 200–223). John Wiley & Sons, Ltd. https://doi.org/10.1002/9780470939376.ch7

Beetz, A. M. (2017). Theories and possible processes of action in animal assisted interventions. *Applied Developmental Science*, 21(2), 139–149. https://doi.org/10.1080/10888691.2016.1262263

Beetz, A., Uvnäs-Moberg, K., Julius, H., & Kotrschal, K. (2012). Psychosocial and psychophysiological effects of human-animal interactions: The possible role of oxytocin. *Frontiers in Psychology*, 3, 234. https://doi.org/10.3389/fpsyg.2012.00234

Berman, M. G., Jonides, J., & Kaplan, S. (2008). The cognitive benefits of interacting with nature. *Psychological Science*, 19(12), 1207–1212. https://doi.org/10.1111/j.1467-9280.2008.02225.x

Bratman, G. N., Daily, G. C., Levy, B. J., & Gross, J. J. (2015). The benefits of nature experience: Improved affect and cognition. *Landscape and Urban Planning*, 138, 41–50. https://doi.org/10.1016/j.landurbplan.2015.02.005

Bratman, G. N., Hamilton, J. P., & Daily, G. C. (2012). The impacts of nature experience on human cognitive function and mental health. *Annals of the New York Academy of Sciences*, 1249(1), 118–136. https://doi.org/10.1111/j.1749-6632.2011.06400.x

Cadavid, S., & Beato, M. S. (2016). Memory distortion and its avoidance: An event-related potentials study on false recognition and correct rejection. *PLOS ONE*, 11(10), e0164024. https://doi.org/10.1371/journal.pone.0164024

Cella, D. F., & Perry, S. W. (1986). Reliability and concurrent validity of three visual-analogue mood scales. *Psychological Reports*, 59(2), 827–833. https://doi.org/10.2466/pr0.1986.59.2.827

Cimprich, B. (1993). Development of an intervention to restore attention in cancer patients. *Cancer Nursing*, 16(2), 83–92.

Clarke, E., & Sherrill-Mix, S. (2017). ggbeeswarm: Categorical scatter (violin point) plots. [Version 0.6.0] https://CRAN.R-project.org/package=ggbeeswarm

Cohen, J. D., Forman, S. D., Braver, T. S., Casey, B. J., Servan-Schreiber, D., & Noll, D. C. (1994). Activation of the prefrontal cortex in a nonspatial working memory task with functional MRI. *Human Brain Mapping*, 1(4), 293–304. https://doi.org/10.1002/hbm.460010407

Cox, D. T. C., Shanahan, D. F., Hudson, H. L., Fuller, R. A., Anderson, K., Hancock, S., & Gaston, K. J. (2017). Doses of nearby nature simultaneously associated with multiple health benefits. *International Journal of Environmental Research and Public Health*, 14(2), 172. https://doi.org/10.3390/ijerph14020172

Crossman, M. K., Kazdin, A. E., & Knudson, K. (2015). Brief unstructured interaction with a dog reduces distress. *Anthrozoös*, 28(4), 649–659. https://doi.org/10.1080/08927936.2015.1070008

Crossman, M. K., Kazdin, A. E., Matijczak, A., Kitt, E. R., & Santos, L. R. (2020). The influence of interactions with dogs on affect, anxiety, and arousal in children. *Journal of Clinical Child & Adolescent Psychology*, 49(4), 535–548. https://doi.org/10.1080/15374416.2018.1520119

Crump, C., & Derting, T. L. (2015). Effects of pet therapy on the psychological and physiological stress levels of first-year female undergraduates. *North American Journal of Psychology*, 17(3), 575.

Ein, N., Li, L., & Vickers, K. (2018). The effect of pet therapy on the physiological and subjective stress response: A meta-analysis. *Stress and Health*, 34(4), 477–489. https://doi.org/10.1002/smi.2812

Empatica. (2018). E4 Wristband User's Manual. https://empatica.app.box.com/E4-User-Manual

Fiocco, A. J., & Hunse, A. M. (2017). The buffer effect of therapy dog exposure on stress reactivity in undergraduate students. *International Journal of Environmental Research and Public Health*, 14(7), 707. https://doi.org/10.3390/ijerph14070707

Fournier, A. K. (2019). HAI dose in animal-assisted intervention. In A. K. Fournier (Ed.), *Animal- Assisted Intervention: Thinking Empirically* (pp. 31–51). Springer International Publishing. https://doi.org/10.1007/978-3-030-32972-3_3

Franco, L. S., Shanahan, D. F., & Fuller, R. A. (2017). A review of the benefits of nature experiences: More than meets the eye. *International Journal of Environmental Research and Public Health*, 14(8), 864. https://doi.org/10.3390/ijerph14080864

Friedmann, E., & Son, H. (2009). The human-companion animal bond: How humans benefit. *Veterinary Clinics of North America: Small Animal Practice*, 39(2), 293–326. https://doi.org/10.1016/j.cvsm.2008.10.015

Gee, N. R., Belcher, J. M., Grabski, J. L., DeJesus, M., & Riley, W. (2012). The presence of a therapy dog results in improved object recognition performance in preschool children. *Anthrozoös*, 25(3), 289–300. https://doi.org/10.2752/175303712X13403555186172

Gee, N. R., Church, M. T., & Altobelli, C. L. (2010). Preschoolers make fewer errors on an object categorization task in the presence of a dog. *Anthrozoös*, 23(3), 223–230. https://doi.org/10.2752/175303710X12750451258896

Gee, N. R., Fine, A. H., & McCardle, P. (2017). Companion animals as moderators of stress responses: Implications for academic performance, testing, and achievement. In N. R. Gee & E. Friedmann (Eds.), *How Animals Help Students Learn: Research and Practice for Educators and Mental-Health Professionals* (pp. 120–132). Taylor & Francis.

Gee, N. R., Fine, A. H., & Schuck, S. (2015). Animals in educational settings: Research and practice. In A. H. Fine (Ed.), *Handbook on Animal-Assisted Therapy* (Fourth, pp. 195–210). Academic Press. https://doi.org/10.1016/B978-0-12-801292-5.00014-6

Gee, N. R., Friedmann, E., Stendahl, M., Fisk, A., & Coglitore, V. (2014). Heart rate variability during a working memory task: Does touching a dog or person affect the response? *Anthrozoös*, 27(4), 513–528. https://doi.org/10.2752/089279314X14072268687763

Gidlow, C. J., Jones, M. V., Hurst, G., Masterson, D., Clark-Carter, D., Tarvainen, M. P., Smith, G., & Nieuwenhuijsen, M. (2016). Where to put your best foot forward: Psycho- physiological responses to walking in natural and urban environments. *Journal of Environmental Psychology*, 45, 22–29. https://doi.org/10.1016/j.jenvp.2015.11.003

Grajfoner, D., Harte, E., Potter, L. M., & McGuigan, N. (2017). The effect of dog-assisted intervention on student well-being, mood, and anxiety. *International Journal of Environmental Research and Public Health*, 14(5), 483. https://doi.org/10.3390/ijerph14050483

Griffin, J. A., Hurley, K., & McCune, S. (2019). Human-animal interaction research: Progress and possibilities. *Frontiers in Psychology*, 10, 2803. https://doi.org/10.3389/fpsyg.2019.02803

Haatveit, B. C., Sundet, K., Hugdahl, K., Ueland, T., Melle, I., & Andreassen, O. A. (2010). The validity of d prime as a working memory index: Results from the "Bergen n-back task." *Journal of Clinical and Experimental Neuropsychology*, 32(8), 871–880. https://doi.org/10.1080/13803391003596421

Handlin, L., Hydbring-Sandberg, E., Nilsson, A., Ejdebäck, M., Jansson, A., & Uvnäs-Moberg, K. (2011). Short-term interaction between dogs and their owners: Effects on oxytocin, cortisol, insulin and heart rate—an exploratory study. *Anthrozoös*, 24(3), 301–315. https://doi.org/10.2752/175303711X13045914865385

Harrell Jr, F. E., Charles Dupont, with contributions from, & others., many. (2020). Hmisc: Harrell miscellaneous. [Version 4.4.2] https://CRAN.R-project.org/package=Hmisc

Hediger, K., & Turner, D. C. (2014). Can dogs increase children's attention and concentration performance? A randomised controlled trial. *Human Animal Interaction Bulletin*, 2, 21–39.

Hosey, G., & Melfi, V. (2014). Human-animal interactions, relationships and bonds: A review and analysis of the literature. *International Journal of Comparative Psychology*, 27(1).

Johnson, R. A., Meadows, R. L., Haubner, J. S., & Sevedge, K. (2008). Animal-assisted activity among patients with cancer: Effects on mood, fatigue, self-perceived health, and sense of coherence. *Oncology Nursing Forum*, 35(2), 225–232. https://doi.org/10.1188/08.ONF.225-232

Johnson, T. R. (2016). Violation of the homogeneity of regression slopes assumption in ANCOVA for two-group pre-post designs: Tutorial on a modified Johnson-Neyman procedure. *The Quantitative Methods for Psychology*, 12(3), 253–263. https://doi.org/10.20982/tqmp.12.3.p253

Joye, Y., & De Block, A. (2011). 'Nature and I are two': A critical examination of the biophilia hypothesis. *Environmental Values*, 20(2), 189–215.

Kane, M. J., Conway, A. R. A., Miura, T. K., & Colflesh, G. J. H. (2007). Working memory, attention control, and the N-back task: A question of construct validity. *Journal of Experimental Psychology. Learning, Memory, and Cognition*, 33(3), 615–622. https://doi.org/10.1037/0278-7393.33.3.615

Kaplan, R., & Kaplan, S. (1989). *The Experience of Nature: A Psychological Perspective*. Cambridge University Press.

Kaplan, S. (1995). The restorative benefits of nature: Toward an integrative framework. *Journal of Environmental Psychology*, 15(3), 169–182. https://doi.org/10.1016/0272-4944(95)90001-2

Kaplan, S., & Berman, M. G. (2010). Directed attention as a common resource for executive functioning and self-regulation. *Perspectives on Psychological Science*, 5(1), 43–57. https://doi.org/10.1177/1745691609356784

Kassambara, A. (2019). ggcorrplot: Visualization of a correlation matrix using 'ggplot2'. [Version 0.1.3] https://CRAN.R-project.org/package=ggcorrplot

Kruger, K. A., & Serpell, J. A. (2010). Animal-assisted interventions in mental health: Definitions and theoretical foundations. In A. H. Fine (Ed.), *Handbook on Animal-Assisted Therapy* (Third Edition) (pp. 33–48). Academic Press. https://doi.org/10.1016/B978-0-12-381453-1.10003-0

Lass-Hennemann, J., Peyk, P., Streb, M., Holz, E., & Michael, T. (2014). Presence of a dog reduces subjective but not physiological stress responses to an analog trauma. *Frontiers in Psychology*, 5, 1010. https://doi.org/10.3389/fpsyg.2014.01010

Lawrence, E. A. (1993). The sacred bee, the filthy pig, and the bat out of hell: Animal symbolism as cognitive biophilia. In S. R. Kellert & W. E. O. (Eds.), *The Biophilia Hypothesis* (pp. 301–344). Island Press.

Li, D., & Sullivan, W. C. (2016). Impact of views to school landscapes on recovery from stress and mental fatigue. *Landscape and Urban Planning*, 148, 149–158. https://doi.org/10.1016/j.landurbplan.2015.12.015

MacDuffie, K. E., Atkins, A. S., Flegal, K. E., Clark, C. M., & Reuter-Lorenz, P. A. (2012). Memory distortion in Alzheimer's disease: Deficient monitoring of short and long-term memory. *Neuropsychology*, 26(4), 509–516. https://doi.org/10.1037/a0028684

Mangiafico, S. (2020). rcompanion: Functions to support extension education program evaluation. [Version 2.3.26] https://CRAN.R-project.org/package=rcompanion

Mayer, F. S., Frantz, C. M., Bruehlman-Senecal, E., & Dolliver, K. (2008). Why is nature beneficial?: The role of connectedness to nature. *Environment and Behavior.* https://doi.org/10.1177/0013916508319745

McCabe, D. P., Roediger, H. L., McDaniel, M. A., Balota, D. A., & Hambrick, D. Z. (2010). The relationship between working memory capacity and executive functioning: Evidence for a common executive attention construct. *Neuropsychology*, 24(2), 222–243. https://doi.org/10.1037/a0017619

McCarthy, C., Pradhan, N., Redpath, C., & Adler, A. (2016). Validation of the Empatica E4 wristband. 2016 *IEEE EMBS International Student Conference (ISC)*, 1–4. https://doi.org/10.1109/EMBSISC.2016.7508621

McCune, S., Kruger, K. A., Griffin, J. A., Esposito, L., Freund, L. S., Hurley, K. J., & Bures, R. (2014). Evolution of research into the mutual benefits of human-animal interaction. *Animal Frontiers*, 4(3), 49–58. https://doi.org/10.2527/af.2014-0022

McCune, S., McCardle, P., Griffin, J. A., Esposito, L., Hurley, K., Bures, R., & Kruger, K. A. (2020). Human-animal interaction (HAI) research: A decade of progress. *Frontiers in Veterinary Science*, 7. https://doi.org/10.3389/fvets.2020.00044

McEvoy, C. L., Nelson, D. L., & Komatsu, T. (1999). What is the connection between true and false memories? The differential roles of interitem associations in recall and recognition. *Journal of Experimental Psychology. Learning, Memory, and Cognition*, 25(5), 1177–1194. https://doi.org/10.1037//0278-7393.25.5.1177

McNeish, D. (2018). Thanks coefficient alpha, we'll take it from here. *Psychological Methods*, 23(3), 412–433. https://doi.org/10.1037/met0000144

Melson, G. F. (2011). Principles for human-animal interaction research. In P. McCardle, S. McCune, J. A. Griffin, & V. Maholmes (Eds.), *How Animals Affect Us: Examining the Influences of Human-Animal Interaction on Child Development and Human Health* (pp. 13–33). American Psychological Association. https://doi.org/10.1037/12301-001

Miyake, A., Friedman, N. P., Emerson, M. J., Witzki, A. H., Howerter, A., & Wager, T. D. (2000). The unity and diversity of executive functions and their contributions to complex "frontal lobe" tasks: A latent variable analysis. *Cognitive Psychology*, 41(1), 49–100. https://doi.org/10.1006/cogp.1999.0734

Morey, R. D., & Rouder, J. N. (2018). BayesFactor: Computation of Bayes factors for common designs. [Version 0.9.12.4.2] https://CRAN.R-project.org/package=BayesFactor

Müller, K. (2017). here: A simpler way to find your files. [Version 1.0.1] https://CRAN.R- project.org/package=here

Odendaal, J. S. J., & Meintjes, R. A. (2003). Neurophysiological correlates of affiliative behaviour between humans and dogs. *The Veterinary Journal*, 165(3), 296–301. https://doi.org/10.1016/S1090-0233(02)00237-X

Orbach, J., Ehrlich, D., & Heath, H. A. (1963). Reversibility of the Necker cube: I. An examination of the concept of "satiation of orientation." *Perceptual and Motor Skills*, 17(2), 439–458. https://doi.org/10.2466/pms.1963.17.2.439

Pedersen, T. L. (2020). patchwork: The composer of plots. [Version 1.1.1] https://CRAN.R- project.org/package=patchwork

Peirce, J., Gray, J. R., Simpson, S., MacAskill, M., Höchenberger, R., Sogo, H., Kastman, E., & Lindeløv, J. K. (2019). PsychoPy2: Experiments in behavior made easy. *Behavior Research Methods*, 51(1), 195–203. https://doi.org/10.3758/s13428-018-01193-y

R Core Team. (2020). R: A language and environment for statistical computing. [Version 4.0.4] R Foundation for Statistical Computing. https://www.R-project.org/

Revelle, W. (2019). psych: Procedures for psychological, psychometric, and personality research. [Version 2.0.12] Northwestern University. https://CRAN.R-project.org/package=psych

Revelle, W., & Zinbarg, R. E. (2008). Coefficients Alpha, Beta, Omega, and the glb: Comments on Sijtsma. *Psychometrika*, 74(1), 145. https://doi.org/10.1007/s11336-008-9102-z

Rich, D. L. (2007). Effects of exposure to nature and plants on cognition and mood: A cognitive psychology perspective [PhD thesis]. Cornell University.

Roediger, H. L., & McDermott, K. B. (1995). Creating false memories: Remembering words not presented in lists. *Journal of Experimental Psychology: Learning, Memory, and Cognition*, 21(4), 803–814. https://doi.org/10.1037/0278-7393.21.4.803

Sahlin, E., Lindegård, A., Hadzibajramovic, E., Grahn, P., Matuszczyk, J. V., & Jr, G. A. (2016). The influence of the environment on directed attention, blood pressure and heart rate—An experimental study using a relaxation intervention. *Landscape Research*, 41(1), 7–25. https://doi.org/10.1080/01426397.2014.982079

Schertz, K. E., & Berman, M. G. (2019). Understanding nature and its cognitive benefits. *Current Directions in Psychological Science*, 28(5), 496–502. https://doi.org/10.1177/0963721419854100

Schutte, A. R., Torquati, J. C., & Beattie, H. L. (2017). Impact of urban nature on executive functioning in early and middle childhood. *Environment and Behavior*, 49(1), 3–30. https://doi.org/10.1177/0013916515603095

Serpell, J. (1996). *In the Company of Animals: A Study of Human-Animal Relationships*. Cambridge University Press.

Serpell, J. A. (2004). Factors influencing human attitudes to animals and their welfare. *Animal Welfare*, 13(S1), 145–151.

Shaffer, F., & Ginsberg, J. P. (2017). An overview of heart rate variability metrics and norms. *Frontiers in Public Health*, 5, 258. https://doi.org/10.3389/fpubh.2017.00258

Shanahan, D. F., Bush, R., Gaston, K. J., Lin, B. B., Dean, J., Barber, E., & Fuller, R. A. (2016). Health benefits from nature experiences depend on dose. *Scientific Reports*, 6, 28551. https://doi.org/10.1038/srep28551

Spielberger, C. D., Sydeman, S. J., Owen, A. E., & Marsh, B. J. (1999). Measuring anxiety and anger with the State-Trait Anxiety Inventory (STAI) and the State-Trait Anger Expression Inventory (STAXI). In M. E. Maruish (Ed.), *The Use of Psychological Testing for Treatment Planning and Outcomes Assessment* (Second, pp. 993–1021). Lawrence Erlbaum Associates Publishers.

Stenfors, C. U. D., Van Hedger, S. C., Schertz, K. E., Meyer, F. A. C., Smith, K. E. L., Norman, G. J., Bourrier, S. C., Enns, J. T., Kardan, O., Jonides, J., & Berman, M. G. (2019). Positive effects of nature on cognitive performance across multiple experiments: Test order but not affect modulates the cognitive effects. *Frontiers in Psychology*, 10, 1413. https://doi.org/10.3389/fpsyg.2019.01413

Stevenson, M. P., Schilhab, T., & Bentsen, P. (2018). Attention Restoration Theory II: A systematic review to clarify attention processes affected by exposure to natural environments. *Journal of Toxicology and Environmental Health,* Part B, 21(4), 227–268. https://doi.org/10.1080/10937404.2018.1505571

Stewart, L. A., Dispenza, F., Parker, L., Chang, C. Y., & Cunnien, T. (2014). A pilot study assessing the effectiveness of an animal-assisted outreach program. *Journal of Creativity in Mental Health*, 9(3), 332–345. https://doi.org/10.1080/15401383.2014.892862

Tajika, H. (2001). Psychology of recognition memory. In N. J. Smelser & P. B. Baltes (Eds.), *International Encyclopedia of the Social & Behavioral Sciences* (pp. 12832–12835). Pergamon. https://doi.org/10.1016/B0-08-043076-7/01520-5

Templer, D., Arikawa, H., Canfield, M., Munsell, K., & Tangan, K. (2004). Modification of the Pet Attitude Scale. *Society & Animals*, 12(2), 137–142. https://doi.org/10.1163/1568530041446580

Templer, D. I., Salter, C. A., Dickey, S., Baldwin, R., & Veleber, D. M. (1981). The construction of a Pet Attitude Scale. *The Psychological Record*, 31(3), 343–348. https://doi.org/10.1007/BF03394747

Thayer, E. R., & Stevens, J. R. (2019a). Animal-assisted intervention. In J. Vonk & T. Shackelford (Eds.), *Encyclopedia of Animal Cognition and Behavior* (pp. 1–4). Springer. https://doi.org/10.1007/978-3-319-47829-6_2057-1

Thayer, E. R., & Stevens, J. R. (2019b). Human-animal interaction. In J. Vonk & T. Shackelford (Eds.), *Encyclopedia of Animal Cognition and Behavior* (pp. 1–5). Springer. https://doi.org/10.1007/978-3-319-47829-6_2058-1

Thayer, E., & Stevens, J. R. (2020). Effects of human-animal interactions on affect and cognition. *PsyArXiv*. https://doi.org/10.31234/osf.io/7v5nq

Thelwell, E. L. R. (2019). Paws for thought: A controlled study investigating the benefits of interacting with a house-trained dog on university students mood and anxiety. *Animals*, 9(10), 846. https://doi.org/10.3390/ani9100846

Trammell, J. P. (2019). Therapy dogs improve student affect but not memory. *Anthrozoös*, 32(5), 691–699. https://doi.org/10.1080/08927936.2019.1645514

Ulrich, R. S. (1981). Natural versus urban scenes: Some psychophysiological effects. *Environment and Behavior*, 13(5), 523–556. https://doi.org/10.1177/0013916581135001

van Doorn, J., Ly, A., Marsman, M., & Wagenmakers, E.-J. (2020). Bayesian rank-based hypothesis testing for the rank sum test, the signed rank test, and Spearman's ρ. *Journal of Applied Statistics*. https://doi.org/10.1080/02664763.2019.1709053

Van Hedger, S. C., Nusbaum, H. C., Clohisy, L., Jaeggi, S. M., Buschkuehl, M., & Berman, M. G. (2019). Of cricket chirps and car horns: The effect of nature sounds on cognitive performance. *Psychonomic Bulletin & Review*, 26(2), 522–530. https://doi.org/10.3758/s13423-018-1539-1

Wagenmakers, E.-J., Love, J., Marsman, M., Jamil, T., Ly, A., Verhagen, J., Selker, R., Gronau, Q. F., Dropmann, D., Boutin, B., Meerhoff, F., Knight, P., Raj, A., Kesteren, E.-J. van, Doorn, J. van, Šmíra, M., Epskamp, S., Etz, A., Matzke, D., … Morey, R. D. (2018). Bayesian inference for psychology. Part II: Example applications with JASP. *Psychonomic Bulletin & Review*, 25(1), 58–76. https://doi.org/10.3758/s13423-017-1323-7

Watson, D., Clark, L. A., & Tellegen, A. (1988). Development and validation of brief measures of positive and negative affect: The PANAS scales. *Journal of Personality and Social Psychology*, 54(6), 1063–1070.

Wickham, H., Averick, M., Bryan, J., Chang, W., McGowan, L. D., François, R., Grolemund, G., Hayes, A., Henry, L., Hester, J., Kuhn, M., Pedersen, T. L., Miller, E., Bache, S. M., Müller, K., Ooms, J., Robinson, D., Seidel, D. P., Spinu, V., … Yutani, H. (2019). Welcome to the tidyverse. *Journal of Open Source Software*, 4(43), 1686. https://doi.org/10.21105/joss.01686

Wilson, E. O. (2009). *Biophilia*. Harvard University Press.

Xie, Y., Allaire, J. J., & Grolemund, G. (2018). *R markdown: The definitive guide*. Chapman; Hall/CRC. https://bookdown.org/yihui/rmarkdown

6 Examining the Impact of a Brief Human–Canine Interaction on Stress and Attention

Jonathan B. Banks[1]*, Caitlin McCoy[1] and Courtney Trzcinski[2]
[1]*Nova Southeastern University;* [2]*Canine Assisted Therapy, Inc.*

Abstract

The interaction between humans and canines has been linked to a variety of benefits including reductions in ADHD symptoms in children, depression symptoms in nursing home patients, and PTSD symptoms in veterans returning from war. Although the inclusion of therapy dogs on college campuses has increased over the last few years, little evidence exists demonstrating the effect of canine interaction in these settings. The current study examined the effects of college student's interactions with therapy dogs during an exam period. Fifty-six students interacted with therapy dogs before or after completing measures of sustained attention, mind wandering, perceived stress, cognitive test anxiety, and state anxiety. Interacting with the therapy dogs reduced state anxiety and resulted in lower perceived stress but did not alter sustained attention task performance or mind wandering. The results suggest that interaction with therapy dogs may help reduce perception of stress and anxiety but may not alter the cognitive functions measured in the current study. Due to the levels of stress that college students experience during exam periods, on-campus therapy dog programs may provide a low, cost effective intervention that universities could implement to benefit their students.

Keywords: Stress, Sustained attention, Human–canine interaction

Interactions between humans and canines have shaped the evolution of canines in a mutually beneficial manner (Range & Viranyi, 2014). The benefits of the human–canine interaction have been demonstrated across a variety of human outcomes. Interaction with therapy dogs reduces depression symptoms and increases well-being in nursing home patients (Gammonley & Yates, 1991), decreases PTSD, depression, and anxiety symptoms in soldiers returning from war (Beck, Gonzales, Sells, Jones, Reer, & Zhu, 2012), decreases ADHD symptoms in children (Schuck, Emmerson, Fine & Lakes, 2015), reduces physiological arousal but not state anxiety or medical fear in hospitalized children (Tsai, Friedmann, & Thomas, 2010), reduces physiological response to a stressful mental arithmetic task (Allen, Blascovich, Tomaka, & Kelsey, 1991), and increases comfort and stress relief during therapy sessions (Walsh, 2009). Interactions with dogs in long-term settings as pets demonstrate similar benefits including, lower systolic and diastolic blood pressure in older adults with a mildly elevated blood pressure (Friedmann, Thomas, Son, Chapa, & McCune, 2013), increased 1 year survival rate following a cardiac event (Friedmann, Katcher, Lynch, & Thomas, 1980), faster recovery from both psychological and physiological stress

*Corresponding author: email:jonathan.banks@nova.edu

manipulations in married couples, (Allen, Blascovich, & Mendes, 2002) and better cardiovascular health (Friedmann, Thomas, Stein, & Kleiger, 2003). Building on these and other findings, the purpose of the current study is to examine the impact of the interaction between college students and dogs on several measures of cognitive functioning and perceived stress.

It is important to note that not all of the studies examining the impact of interactions with dogs or other pets have shown beneficial effects (see Barker & Wolen, 2008). In fact, some recent studies have shown no difference in the frequency of pet owners and non-pet owners who rate themselves as very happy (Herzog, 2010) and no differences in blood pressure between owners and non-owners (Wright, Kritz-Silverstein, Morton, Wingard, & Barrett-Connor, 2007). In contrast to prior work demonstrating better health in pet owners (Headey, 1999), dog ownership in older adults is associated with poorer physical health and depression (Parslow, Jorm, Christensen, & Rodgers, 2005). Overall, the evidence supporting the benefits of pet ownership and animal interaction on human health and well-being is still mixed (Herzog, 2011).

Of specific interest to the current study, the benefits of interaction with therapy dogs has been examined in a variety of educational settings including preschool, elementary school, and at the collegiate level. The presence of a therapy dog in preschool classes increases speed and accuracy on an object recognition task, possibly due to increased focus or motivation resulting from the canine interaction (Gee, Belcher, Grabski, DeJesus, & Riley, 2012). At the elementary school level, the inclusion of a therapy dog in classroom reading programs results in higher reading scores and increased enthusiasm for reading for kindergarten through fourth graders (Kirnan, Siminerio, & Wong, 2015). College students report high levels of interest in and enjoyment of therapy dog sessions (Adamle, Riley, & Carlson, 2009). However, research examining impact of the canine interaction among college students has resulted in mixed findings.

Among college samples, the impact of canine interaction on stress and cognitive performance is important. Stress has a significant negative impact on college student's academic achievement (Pritchard & Wilson, 2003; Struthers, Perry & Menec, 2000). Interactions with a dog are associated with reductions in subjective but not physiological stress following viewing a traumatic film (Lass-Hennemann, Peyk, Streb, Holz, & Michael, 2014). A brief unstructured interaction with a dog, but not viewing a dog, results in decreases in negative affect, state anxiety, and increases in positive affect in medical school residents and students (Crossman, Kazdin, & Knudson, 2015). Further, college students that interact with a therapy dog during a week prior to final exams report lower levels of stress following the interaction than following a control manipulation (Barker, Barker, McCain, & Schubert, 2016). Canine interaction did not result in changes in salivary alpha amylase, suggesting that interacting with therapy dogs does not alter physiological stress.

Despite the benefits of interaction with a dog on perceived stress, the effects do not appear to extend to physiological or cognitive benefits. The presence of a dog does not buffer the effect of a difficult cognitive task on heart rate variability (Gee, Friedmann, Stendahl, Fisk, & Coglitore, 2014) or reduce arousal while preparing for a delivering a speech (Straatman, Hanson, Endenburg, & Mol, 1997). Further, the presence of a dog during a working memory task does not improve task performance (Gee, Friedmann, Coglitore, Fisk, & Stendahl, 2015). The lack of a clear effect of interaction with a dog on cognitive task performance may be a result of a methodological flaw. In prior studies, participants were required to remain in physical contact with the dog during the tasks. Requiring participants to remain in contact with a dog while completing a cognitive task may be problematic. First, requiring the participants to remain in contact gives the participants a second task to complete (e.g., remain touching the dog) while completing the cognitive task. This second task places an extra load on limited cognitive resources (Kane & Engle, 2000). Second, any movement the dog makes during the task may result in additional distraction for the participant, thereby reducing task performance. Therefore, this methodological flaw may be responsible for the lack of evidence for a benefit of canine interaction on cognitive performance.

The reductions in stress that occur as a result of canine interaction may play a role in possible cognitive changes as a result of the interaction. Stress results in increases in mind wandering, or Task-Unrelated Thoughts (TUTs; Banks & Boals, 2016). Mind wandering is a common experience, occurring in approximately 50% of all waking hours (Killingsworth & Gilbert, 2010). Despite the frequency of these thoughts, when individuals experience mind wandering, their ongoing task performance is impaired (McVay & Kane, 2009; Randall, Oswald, & Beier, 2014). Impaired performance as a result of mind wandering has been demonstrated on a variety of tasks, including working memory (Banks & Boals, 2016; Banks, Tartar, & Tamayo, 2015), sustained attention (Banks, Tartar, & Welhaf, 2014; McVay & Kane, 2009), and academic performance (Wammes, Seli, Cheyne, Boucher, & Smilek, 2016). This is especially problematic for college students during exam periods, as exam periods are stressful (Bosch, Ring, de Geus, & Amerongen, 2004) and require the ability to sustain attention to goal directed tasks, such as taking an exam or studying. Given the benefits of canine interaction on stress reduction, the use of therapy dogs during periods of stress may have a variety of benefits, including reducing mind wandering and increasing sustained attention. Despite prior work demonstrating changes in stress following an interaction with a therapy dog (Barker et al., 2016), no prior work has examined the impact of this interaction on mind wandering. Since mind wandering is a mediator for the impact of stress on cognitive task performance – specifically tasks requiring working memory (Banks & Boals, 2016) – then reductions in stress that result from interacting with therapy dogs may also result in the downstream effects of reducing mind wandering and increasing some cognitive task performance. The current study examined the impact of college students interacting with therapy dogs during an examination week—a period examined as a time of mild chronic stress (Bosch et al., 2004). Increased levels of cortisol, a stress hormone, have been observed during examination periods, providing supporting evidence for the stressful nature of examination periods (Viena, Banks, Barbu, Schulman, & Tartar, 2012). Unlike other studies that have examined the impact of the interaction between people and dogs on cognitive tasks in a laboratory setting (Gee et al., 2014; 2015), the interaction between people and dogs in the current study occurred in a university-wide Canine Therapy event, consistent with events that occur on university campuses across the U.S. Therefore, any effects observed in the current study will mirror effects that might be observed in the real world. It was hypothesized that college students who interact with therapy dogs during examination periods will have lower levels of perceived stress than those who do not interact with the therapy dogs. Secondly, it was hypothesized that college students who interact with therapy dogs during examination periods would experience higher performance on several cognitive tasks, including higher levels of sustained attention, increased speed of processing, and lower levels of mind wandering compared to those who do not interact with the therapy dogs. Finally, based on prior work demonstrating the beneficial effect of owning a dog (Friedmann et al., 1980; 2003; 2013), we controlled for dog ownership in examining the impact of the brief on-campus intervention.

Methods

Participants

Fifty-six students (43 = Females, 13 = Males; *M* age years = 20.05, *SD* = 3.38) from a university in the southeastern United States participated in the current study in exchange for a gift card or course credit. Students were randomly assigned to a control ($n = 27$) or brief on-campus canine interaction condition ($n = 29$). Participants were recruited via flyers posted on campus and online advertisements for the psychology department research pool. Participants that reported a fear of dogs or any allergic reaction to dogs were excluded from participation.

The study was approved by the Nova Southeastern University Institutional Review Board and the Nova Southeastern University Institutional Animal Care and Use Committee. Sample size was determined based on effect sizes reported in prior work examining the impact of canine interaction on reports of perceived stress, which demonstrated large effect of interaction on changes in reported perceived stress (d = 1.63–1.87; Barker et al., 2016; d =1.11–1.48; Crossman et al., 2015). A power analysis suggested a required sample size of 46 to achieve an alpha = 0.05 with an effect size of d = 1.11.

Materials

Cognitive Outcome Measures Letter and Pattern Comparison. The letter and pattern comparison tasks are established measures of speed of information processing (Salthouse & Babcock, 1991). The letter comparison consists of two trials, each with a row of consonants presented on a page of paper, with a line in between each of the rows (i.e., XLD___XLD). Participants are asked to classify whether the letters in the rows are the same or are different for each pair of letters, by writing either an "s" or a "d" on the line between the pairs. The pattern comparison task is analogous to the letter comparison task although in this task the participant is asked to compare two patterns of lines. For both tasks the participant completes two 30-second trials. The score on each task is the combined number of correct responses on the two trials minus the number of incorrect responses. Scores on each task were converted to z-scores and a composite speed of processing score was created by averaging the z-scores for each task.

Sustained Attention to Response Task (SART). The SART is a go/no-go task in which participants must respond rapidly to all frequent non-target stimuli while withholding a respond to infrequent target stimuli (Robertson, Manly, Andrade, Baddeley, & Yiend, 1997). In this version of the SART, the infrequent target stimuli was the number 3 and the frequent non-target stimuli were any number between 1 and 9, excluding 3. The SART consisted of 180 trials, made of 160 non-target trials and 20 target trials. Participants were instructed to complete the task as accurately and quickly as possible. Accuracy on the SART was measured as the number of correctly withheld responses to the target stimuli (TACC).

Thought Probes. Thought probes were inserted into the SART task to measure frequency of mind wandering. Consistent with prior work (McVay & Kane, 2009) with the SART, participants were interrupted at random intervals and asked, "What were you thinking about" just prior to the probe. Participants selected one of the following response options: "a. Task related thought, exclusively", "b. Task performance/ evaluative thoughts", "c. Task-unrelated, neutral content", "d. Task-unrelated, positive content", "e. Task-unrelated, negative content". The percent of task-unrelated thoughts was calculated by summing the number of off-task response choices, options c though e, endorsed and dividing by number of probes presented during the task (12 total probes). Due to the intermediate nature of task-related intrusions being between on- and off- task thoughts, the percentage of task-related intrusions, option b, was not included in any analysis.

Self-report Outcome Measures Perceived Stress Scale (PSS; Cohen, Kamarck, & Mermelstein, 1983). The PSS measures the degree to which an individual perceives a situation as stressful. Participants responded to a series of items examining perceived stress a scale of 0 (*never*) to 4 (*very often*). The PSS was scored by summing the items, such that the higher the PSS score, the greater the level of perceived stress (Cohen et al., 1983). The PSS has been shown to correlate well with other measures of stress (Cohen et al., 1983). Internal consistency in the current data set was high ($\alpha = 0.85$).

Positive and Negative Affect Schedule (PANAS; Watson, Clark, & Tellegen, 1988). The PANAS is a 20-item measure of positive and negative affect. Participants rated their current mood in relation to items on a five-point Likert-type scale, ranging from 1 (*very slight or not at all*) to 5 (*extremely*). The PANAS was scored by summing the positive and negative items for each individual participant to create a positive and negative affect score. The PANAS has been shown to be reasonably related to other measures of depression, anxiety, and stress (r's= 0.30–0.67; Crawford & Henry, 2004). Reasonable internal consistency was found in the current sample at both time points for positive affect (α = 0.82–0.86) and negative affect (α = 0.75–0.81).

Mind Wandering Questionnaire (MWQ). The MWQ is a five-item questionnaire that measures mind wandering (Mrazek, Phillips, Franklin, Broadway, & Schooler, 2013). Participants respond on a 6-point scale from 1 "almost never" to 6 "almost always" to a series of items such as "I have difficulty maintaining focus on simple or repetitive work." Scores on the MWQ are related to other well-known measures of mind wandering including, probe-caught mind wandering during a working memory task ($r = 0.299$) and during a self- report stress scale, the PSS, or perceived stress scale, ($r = 0.303$; Mrazek et al., 2013). Internal consistency in the current sample was reasonable ($\alpha = 0.80$).

Cognitive Test Anxiety Scale (Cassady & Johnson, 2002). The cognitive test anxiety scale is a 27-item questionnaire measuring the amount of anxiety individuals experience in evaluative situations such as exams (Cassady & Johnson, 2002). Participants respond to items on a scale from 1 "Not at all typical of me" to 4 "Very typical of me" in response to questions such as "I lost sleep worrying about examinations". The cognitive test anxiety scale is highly related to other measures of test anxiety (r's = 0.61–0.81; Cassady & Johnson, 2002). Internal consistency in the current sample was high (α = 0.93).

State-Trait Anxiety Inventory (STAI-S; Spielberger, Gorsuch, Lushene, Vagg, & Jacobs, 1983). The STAI-S was used to measure state anxiety. The STAI-S is a 20-item measure that evaluates subjective emotional states like nervousness, restlessness, tension, and worrying. Higher scores indicate higher state anxiety. The STAI-S has demonstrated adequate convergent validity with other measures of state anxiety (Spielberger et al., 1983). Internal consistency was high in the current sample for state (α = 0.89) and trait (α = 0.89) anxiety.

Animal History Questionnaire. Participants were asked a series of questions designed to determine their level of prior interaction with animals and their current number of pets, including "Do the dog(s) currently reside with you (do you see them daily)?", "Do you have an overall positive experience with animals?" and "Do you enjoy interacting with dogs?". Participants responded to these questions with a "yes" or "no" response. This measure was included to control for any effects attributable to owning a dog.

Demographics. Participants completed a demographics form to indicate age, ethnicity, and gender.

Procedure

Data collection occurred as part of a university-wide Canine Therapy event for all students on campus during a midterm exam week. Study participants were recruited prior to the day of the event and reported to a location near the canine therapy event. No participants interacted with the therapy dogs prior to participation in the study. All participants completed an informed consent form, a baseline measure of the PANAS, and an Animal History Questionnaire. Participants were randomly assigned to a control or canine interaction condition. Control condition participants proceeded directly to the laboratory to complete subsequent measures. The control condition was designed to control for the effects of repeated testing and to provide a comparison group experiencing similar amounts of examination period stress. Canine interaction condition participants interacted with a dog for 10 minutes. Prior work has used similar durations for canine interaction, ranging from 7 minutes (Crossman et al., 2015) to 15 minutes (Barker et al., 2016). Participants were allowed to choose the dog they interacted with from several possible dog breeds including Beagles, Golden Retrievers, and German Shepherds. Participants were permitted to interact with as many of the dogs as they wished. Most participants sat on the ground next to one of the dogs and petted the dog for the interaction period. While petting the dogs, participants were also seen talking with the dogs, talking with the handlers, and taking pictures with the dogs. The dog handlers had the dogs on a leash and were asked to behave as they normally would during a campus visitation event, including allowing the college students to pet the dog, having the dogs do tricks, and answering questions about the dogs or the therapy dog program. The dogs were all certified therapy dogs with Canine Assisted Therapy, and all dogs had experience visiting individuals in a variety of settings, including academic settings. The dog handlers were also certified handlers with Canine Assisted Therapy that had been certified independently of their dogs. To ensure minimal fatigue on the dogs, the event was limited to two hours and handlers could remove their dogs during the event for a break if they felt the dogs were fatigued. Following the 10-minute interaction period, canine interaction participants proceeded to the laboratory. Upon arrival at the lab all participants completed the SART on a computer in a semi-private room. Participants completed the Letter and Pattern comparison tasks in a group led by a research assistant and then were given the self-report questionnaires to complete in a room with a trained research assistant. Participants completed the MWQ, PSS, PANAS, and demographics to determine if the canine interaction altered mind wandering, perceived stress, or mood. Completing these measures took approximately 35 minutes. All participants were thanked for their participation, awarded a gift card, and debriefed as to the purpose of the study. Following completing the study, participants in the control condition were then given the option of interacting with the dogs in the same setting as the experimental participants.

Data analysis

A series of independent samples t-tests were conducted to ensure that participants in the brief on-campus canine interaction and control conditions did not differ on baseline levels of positive or negative affect prior to interacting with the canines or on the number of dogs they currently own, have owned in the past, number the currently reside with, or whether they enjoy interacting with dogs. A chi-square analysis was conducted to compare participants in the brief on-campus canine interaction and control conditions in terms of the current presence or absence of a dog at home.

A series of linear regression analyses were conducted predicting the dependent variables of perceived stress, positive and negative affect, state anxiety, cognitive test anxiety, SART performance, speed of processing, and mind wandering. Pet ownership was entered as a covariate in all analyses, with condition entered as the primary predictor of interest. Condition was dummy coded for the purpose of the regression analyses; brief on-campus canine interaction condition dummy coded as 1 and control dummy coded as 0. Pet ownership was also dummy coded for entry into the regression analyses; pet owners dummy coded as 1 and non-pet owners dummy coded as 0.

A series of mixed model ANOVA's were conducted to determine if scores on the PANAS positive or PANAS negative changed over time and if this change was moderated by condition. All analyses were conducted using SAS 9.4 software. Significance threshold was $p = 0.05$.

Results

Descriptive statistics for all dependent variables can be found in Table 6.1. No differences were found between participants in the canine interaction and control conditions on baseline levels of positive or negative affect prior to interacting with the canines. Additionally, no differences were found between participants in either condition in regard to the number of dogs they currently own, have owned in the past, number they currently reside with, or whether they enjoy interacting with dogs, all p's > 0.05. Further, the presence or absence of a dog at home did not differ significantly by condition, $\chi^2 (1) = 2.08, p = 0.15$.

Condition did not serve as a significant predictor for positive and negative affect, cognitive test anxiety, SART performance, speed of processing, or mind wandering, all *p*'s > 0.05. As can be seen in Table 6.2, significant regression models were found for predicting perceived stress and state anxiety. For both models condition served as a significant predictor; participants in the brief on-campus canine interaction condition evidenced lower levels of perceived stress and state anxiety. To determine if the effect of the intervention on perceived stress and state anxiety was altered by pet ownership, an interaction term was added to the two regression models. The interaction terms were not significant in either regression, p's > 0.05, and did not improve model fit. To visualize the effect of the canine interaction condition, perceived stress and state anxiety are plotted in Fig. 6.1, by condition.

A significant effect of time was discovered on the PANAS positive, $F(1, 53) = 10.86, p < 0.01$, *partial* $\eta^2 = 0.17$, such that participants reported lower levels of positive affect at the end of the study than at the beginning of the study (as seen in Table 6.1). Importantly, there was no effect of condition or time × condition interaction, all *p*'s >0.05. No effect of time, condition, or time × condition interaction was observed for scores on the PANAS negative, all *p*'s > 0.05.

Discussion

The current study examined the impact of interaction between dogs and college students during an exam period on perceived stress and cognitive functioning. We hypothesized that a brief ten-minute interaction with a therapy dog would reduce levels of state anxiety, perceived stress, mind wandering, and increase sustained attention. Our results suggest that interacting with a

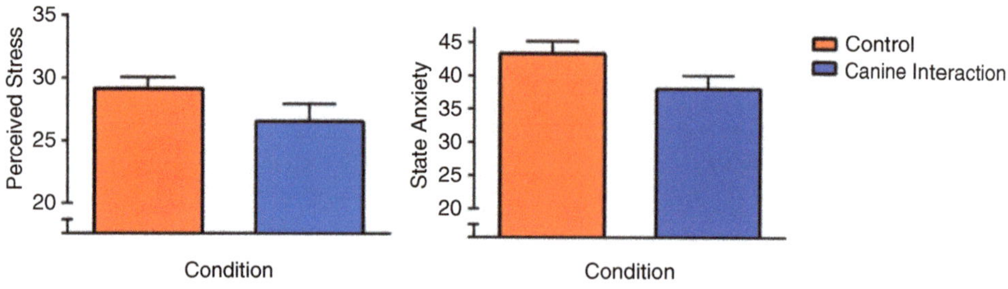

Fig. 6.1. The impact of canine interaction on perceived stress and state anxiety. Note: error bars represent standard error of the mean.

Table 6.1. Descriptive Statistics by Condition.

	Brief Canine Interaction	Condition	Control	Condition
	M	*(SD)*	*M*	*(SD)*
PSS	26.54	(7.44)	29.15	(4.68)
STAI-S	38.04	(10.05)	43.28	(9.28)
STAI-T	42.07	(9.55)	44.21	(8.90)
Cognitive Test Anxiety	66.59	(14.92)	65.31	(17.74)
MWQ	19.41	(4.66)	17.89	(5.56)
SART-TACC	6.79	(3.64)	7.11	(3.36)
Speed of Processing Composite	0.17	(0.84)	–0.18	(0.86)
PANAS Positive T1	30.41	(6.82)	30.15	(6.84)
PANAS Positive T2	25.90	(7.35)	26.67	(7.25)
PANAS Negative T1	13.48	(3.40)	14.56	(4.48)
PANAS Negative T2	13.69	(4.48)	13.74	(4.37)
Percentage of TUTs	33.33	(30.29)	21.30	(23.92)

Note: PSS = Perceived Stress Scale, STAI-S = State Anxiety Inventory-State, STAI-T- State Anxiety Inventory-Trait, MWQ = Mind Wandering Questionnaire, SART-TACC = Target accuracy on the Sustained Attention to Response Task, TUTs- Percentage of Off-Task thoughts.

dog during the intervention was related to lower levels of perceived stress and state anxiety. Decreased perceived stress and state anxiety could have a positive impact on scholastic achievement since higher levels of stress in college students have negative impacts scholastically (Pritchard & Wilson, 2003; Struthers et al., 2000). Although the covariate—presence of a dog at home—was a significant predictor of both perceived stress and state anxiety, the presence of a dog at home was related to lower levels of each measure, the variable was included for the purposes of a covariate and not a main effect. The perceived stress scale asks participants to report their level of perceived stress over the last month, however, the interaction with the canines appears to have been sufficient to alter perception of recent stress.

Interestingly, no benefit of the interaction with dogs was observed on the PANAS. In fact, a main effect of time was found: participants decreased in level of positive affect over the course of the study. This finding may be due to the timing of participants completing the PANAS. Since the second PANAS was completed after the SART and speed of processing tasks, it is possible that any effect of interacting with the dogs on positive affect was counter acted by the cognitive tasks.

Consistent with prior findings in college students (Gee et al., 2015), we did not find any changes on either cognitive measure. One strength of the current study is the inclusion of multiple cognitive measures examining two different cognitive functions; sustained attention and speed of processing. The lack of an effect of the interaction on either sustained attention or

Table 6.2. Regression analysis.

	B	*SE*	β	*t*	*p*	*F*	*df*	*p*	Adjusted R^2
Predicting PSS									
Dog at home	–5.06	1.99	–0.33	–2.54	0.014	4.53	2,51	0.015	0.117
Condition	–3.45	1.66	–0.27	–2.09	0.042				
Predicting STAI									
Dog at home	–6.33	3.16	–0.27	–2.00	0.051	3.98	2,48	0.025	0.107
Condition	–6.29	2.69	–0.32	–2.34	0.023				
Predicting PANAS Positive T2									
Dog at home	4.42	2.37	0.25	1.86	0.07	1.82	2,53	0.17	0.029
Condition	–0.07	1.95	–0.01	–0.04	0.97				
Predicting PANAS Negative T2									
Dog at home	–1.18	1.47	–0.11	–0.80	0.43	0.32	2,53	0.73	–0.025
Condition	–0.24	1.21	–0.03	–0.20	0.84				
Predicting CAT									
Dog at home	5.58	5.44	0.14	1.03	0.31	0.57	2,52	0.57	–0.16
Condition	2.23	4.50	0.07	0.50	0.62				
Predicting SART									
Dog at home	–0.77	1.17	–0.09	–0.67	0.51	0.28	2,53	0.76	–0.027
Condition	–0.44	0.96	–0.06	–0.46	0.65				
Predicting Speed of Processing									
Dog at home	–0.46	0.28	–0.22	–1.67	0.10	2.76	2,53	0.08	0.057
Condition	0.28	0.23	0.17	1.24	0.22				
Predicting TUTs									
Dog at home	0.04	0.06	0.06	0.46	0.64	1.48	2,53	0.24	0.017
Condition	0.13	0.04	0.23	1.71	0.09				
Predicting MWQ									
Dog at home	–1.74	1.70	–0.14	–1.02	0.31	1.15	2,53	0.33	0.005
Condition	1.25	1.40	0.12	0.90	0.37				

Note: PSS = Perceived Stress Scale, STAI = State Anxiety Inventory, MWQ = Mind Wandering Questionnaire, SART = Target accuracy on the Sustained Attention to Response Task, CAT = Cognitive Test Anxiety, TUTs = Percentage of off-task thoughts.

speed of processing is consistent with prior findings demonstrating no effect on cognition (Gee et al., 2015). The current findings do suggest that the methodological flaws in prior studies—requiring participants to touch the dog during the cognitive tasks—may not be responsible for the lack of an improvement in cognitive functioning.

Although prior work has shown cognitive benefits in children as a result of interactions with canines (Gee et al., 2010; 2012; Kirnan et al., 2015), the lack of effect on cognitive functioning in college students may not be surprising. Since college students are approaching peak levels of cognitive functioning (Alloway & Alloway, 2013), interventions such as the one in the current study may have minimal impacts. The changes in levels of perceived stress and state anxiety as a result of canine interaction may have downstream effects on academic performance—one of the main reasons that canine intervention programs are held on college campuses. Consistent with the idea that cognitive changes may occur as a downstream result of changes in state anxiety and perceived stress, the lack of a change in rates of mind wandering may explain the lack of changes in the cognitive tasks. As mind wandering mediates the relationship between stress and cognitive performance (Banks & Boals, 2016), the lack of a change in mind wandering may suggest the intervention was not strong enough to influence mind wandering and cognitive task performance.

There are several limitations in the current study. It is possible that a longer interaction with the dogs would have resulted in a greater effect and possibly changes in cognitive functioning. It is also possible that canine interaction would alter cognitive tasks that require greater attentional demands, such as working memory tasks, as these tasks are more difficult. Further, the setting of the interaction in the current study differed from prior work. Participants in the current study interacted with the dogs in a group setting and then completed the rest of the tasks in the laboratory without the dogs present. In prior studies, the dog was present in the lab as the participants were completing the studies, even to the point of touching the dogs while completing the cognitive tasks (Gee et al., 2015). However, since the methodology in the current study matches the type of interaction that occurs on college campuses across the country, these results may match the effects that are seen in the real world. Additionally, the current study did not examine the impact of the canine interaction on academic performance. It is possible the reduction in perceived stress and state anxiety had downstream consequences on academic performance. Prior work has demonstrated a relationship between state anxiety and academic performance (Pritchard & Wilson, 2003; Struthers et al., 2000). Future work should examine the impact of canine interaction on academic performance in the classroom. Additionally, since the control group used in the current study was a non-treatment control group, it is not possible to determine if the effects seen in the canine interaction condition occurred due to the passage of time. Finally, given the smaller sample used in the current study, it is possible that the current study did not have sufficient power to detect smaller effects that may have occurred on the other constructs examined.

The current study provides evidence for the efficacy of a group canine interaction experience on college student's perceived stress and state anxiety. Caution must be taken in interpreting our results since the benefits seen in the canine interaction group may have been due to them taking a break while they played with the dogs rather than something about the interaction itself. However, despite this possible alternative explanation our results are consistent with prior work demonstrating the beneficial effect of having a dog at home (Allen et al., 2002; Headey, 1999; Siegel, 1990) and of reduced self-reported stress in college students (Barker et al., 2016; Crossman et al., 2015). Importantly, the current results did not provide any evidence for changes on either of the cognitive measures. The lack of changes in rates of mind wandering provide a possible explanation for the lack of changes on the cognitive tasks and a direction for future work. Changes in cognitive task performance may only occur following interaction with a dog when the interaction results in changes in reductions in stress related mind wandering. This is the first study, to the authors' knowledge, to test for an effect of interaction with dogs on measures of sustained attention, speed of processing, and mind wandering. Interaction with dogs, in a group setting on campus, may serve as a beneficial intervention to reduce stress in a college student population. Given the level of stress during examination periods and the importance of strong academic performance during this time, the inclusion of canine interaction periods on college campus may be beneficial for students.

Authors note

We would like to thank Audrey V. B. Hood for her comments on an earlier version of this manuscript and Matthew W. S. Welhaf, Haley Hickey, and Lindsay Craig for their assistance with data collection.

References

Adamle, K., Riley, T., & Carlson, T. (2009). Evaluating college student interest in pet therapy. *Journal of American College Health, 57*(5), 545–548.

Allen, K., Blascovich, J., & Mendes, W. (2002). Cardiovascular reactivity and the presence of pets, friends and spouses: The truth about cats and dogs. *Psychosomatic Medicine, 64*, 727–739.

Allen, K. M., Blascovich, J., Tomaka, J., & Kelsey, R. M. (1991). Presence of human friends and pet dogs as moderators of autonomic responses to stress in women. *Journal of Personality and Social Psychology, 61*, 582–589.

Alloway, T. P., & Alloway, R. G. (2013). Working memory across the lifespan: A cross-sectional approach. *Journal of Cognitive Psychology, 25*, 84–93.

Banks, J. B., & Boals, A. (2016). Don't think about it: Understanding the role of mind wandering in stress related working memory impairments. *Cognition and Emotion,* doi:10.1080/02699931.2016.1179174

Banks, J. B., Tartar, J. L., & Tamayo, B. A. (2015). Examining factors involved in stress related working memory impairments: Independent or conditional effects? *Emotion, 15*(6), 827–836.

Banks, J. B., Tartar, J. L., & Welhaf, M. S. (2014). Where's the Impairment: An Examination of Factors that Impact Sustained Attention Following a Stressor. *Cognition and Emotion, 28*, 856–866.

Barker, S. B., Barker, R. T., McCain, N. L., & Schubert, C. M. (2016). A randomized cross-over exploratory study of the effect of visiting therapy dogs on college students before final exams. *Anthrozoös: A multidisciplinary journal of the interactions of people and animal, 29*(1), 35–46.

Barker, S., & Wolen, A. R. (2008). The benefits of human-companion animal interaction: A review. *Journal of Veterinary Medical Education, 35*(4), 487–495.

Beck, C., Gonzales, F. Jr., Sells, C., Jones, C., Reer, T., & Zhu, Y. (2012). The effects of animal-assisted therapy on wounded warriors in an occupational therapy life skills program. *U.S.Army Medical Department Journal,* 38–45.

Bosch, J. A., Ring, C., de Geus, E. J., & Amerongen, A.V. (2004). Academic examinations and immunity: academic stress or examination stress? *Psychosomatic Medicine 66*, 625–627.

Cassady, J., & Johnson, R. (2002). Cognitive test anxiety and academic performance. *Contemporary Educational Psychology, 27*, 270–295.

Cohen, S., Kamarck, T., & Mermelstein R. (1983). A global measure of perceived stress. *Journal of Health and Social Behavior, 24*, 386–396.

Crawford, J. R., & Henry, J. D. (2004). The Positive and Negative Affect Schedule (PANAS): Construct validity, measurement properties and normative data in a large non-clinical sample. *British Journal of Clinical Psychology, 43*, 245–265.

Crossman, M. K., Kazdin, A. E., & Knudson, K. (2015). Brief unstructured interaction with a dog reduces distress. *Anthrozoös: A multidisciplinary journal of the interactions of people and animals, 28*(4), 649–659.

Friedmann, E., Katcher, A. H., Lynch, J. J., & Thomas, S. A. (1980). Animal companions and one-year survival of patients after discharge from a coronary care unit. *Public Health Reports, 95*(4), 307–312.

Friedmann, E., Thomas, S. A., Son, H., Chapa, D., & McCune, S. (2013). Pet's presence and owner's blood pressure during the daily lives of pet owners with pre- to mild hypertension. *Anthrozoös: A multidisciplinary journal of the interactions of people and animals, 26*(4), 535–550.

Friedmann, E., Thomas, S. A., Stein, P. K., & Kleiger, R. E. (2003). Relation between pet ownership and heart rate variability in patients with healed myocardial infarcts. *The American Journal of Cardiology, 91*(6), 718–721.

Gammonley, J., & Yates, J. (1991). Pet projects: animal assisted therapy in nursing homes. *Journal of Gerontological Nursing, 17*(1), 12–5.

Gee, N. R., Belcher, J., Grabski, J. L., DeJesus, M., & Riley, W. (2012). The presence of a therapy dog results in improved object recognition performance in preschool children. *Anthrozoös: A multidisciplinary journal of the interactions of people and animals, 25*, 289–30.

Gee, N. R., Church, M. R. & Altobelli, C. L. (2010). Preschoolers make fewer errors on an object categorization task in the presence of a dog. *Anthrozoös: A multidisciplinary journal of the interactions of people and animals, 23*(3), 223–230.

Gee, N. R., Friedmann, E., Coglitore, V., Fisk, A., & Stendahl, M. (2015). Does physical contact with a dog or person affect performance of a working memory task? *Anthrozoös: A multidisciplinary journal of the interactions of people and animals, 28*(3), 483–500.

Gee, N. R., Friedmann, E., Stendahl, M., Fisk, A., & Coglitore, V. (2014). Heart rate variability during a working memory task: Does touching a dog or person affect the response? *Anthrozoös: A multidisciplinary journal of the interactions of people and animals, 27*(4), 513–528.

Headey, B. (1999). Health benefits and health cost savings due to pets: Preliminary estimates from an Australian national survey. *Social Indicators Research, 47*, 233–243.

Herzog, H. (2010). *Some we love, some we hate, some we eat: Why it's so hard to think straight about animals.* New York, NY: Harper.

Herzog, H. (2011). The impact of pets on human health and psychological well-being: Fact, Fiction, or Hypothesis? *Current Directions in Psychological Science, 20*(4), 236–239.

Kane, M. J. & Engle, R. W. (2000). Working memory capacity, proactive interference, and divided attention: Limits on long-term memory retrieval, *Journal of Experimental Psychology: Learning, Memory, and Cognition, 26*(2), 336–358.

Killingsworth, M. A., & Gilbert, D. T. (2010). A wandering mind is an unhappy mind. *Science,* 330, 932.

Kirnan, J. P., Siminerio, S., & Wong, Z. (2015). The impact of a therapy dog program on children's reading ability and attitude towards reading. *Early Childhood Education Journal,* 1–15. doi:10.1007/s10643--015-0747--9

Lass-Hennemann, J., Peyk, P., Streb, M., Holz, E., & Michael, T. (2014). Presence of a dog reduces subjective but not physiological stress responses to an analog trauma. *Frontiers in Psychology, 5*, 1–7.

McVay, J. C., & Kane, M. J. (2009). Conducting the train of thought: working memory capacity, goal neglect, and mind wandering in an executive-control task. *Journal of Experimental Psychology, 35*(1), 196–204.

Mrazek, D. M., Phillips, T. D., Franklin, S. M., Broadway, M. J., & Schooler, W. J. (2013). Young and restless: validation of the mind-wandering questionnaire (MWQ) reveals disruptive impact of mind wandering for youth. *Frontiers in Psychology,* 4, 560. doi: 10.3389/fpsyg.2013.00560

Parslow, R. A., Jorm, A. F., Christensen, H., & Rodgers, B. (2005). Pet ownership and health in older adults: Findings from a survey of 2,551 community-based Australians aged 60–64. *Gerontology, 51*, 40–47.

Pritchard, M. E., & Wilson, G. S. (2003). Using emotional and social factors to predict student success. *Journal of College Student Development, 44*(1), 18–28.

Randall, J. G., Oswald, F. L., & Beier, M. E. (2014). Mind-wandering, cognition, and performance: A theory-driven meta-analysis of attention regulation. *Psychological Bulletin,* 140(6), 1411-1431. doi:10.1037/a0037428

Range, F., & Viranyi, Z. (2014). Tracking the evolutionary origins of dog-human cooperation: The "Canine Cooperation Hypothesis". *Frontiers in Psychology, 5*, 1–10.

Robertson, I. H., Manly, T., Andrade, J., Baddeley, B. T., & Yiend, J. (1997). 'Oops!': Performance correlates of everyday attentional failures in traumatic brain injured and normal subjects. *Neuropsychologia, 35*(6), 747–758.

Salthouse T.A., & Babcock R.L. (1991) Decomposing adult age differences in working memory. *Developmental Psychology, 27*, 763–776.

Siegel, J. M. (1990). Stressful life events and use of physician services among the elderly: The moderating role of pet ownership. *Journal of Personality and Social Psychology, 6*, 1081–1086.

Schuck, S. E. B., Emmerson, N., Fine, A., & Lakes, K. (2015). Canine assisted therapy for children with ADHD: preliminary findings from the positive assertive cooperative kids (P.A.C.K.) study. *Journal of Attention Disorders, 19*, 125–137.

Spielberger, C. D., Gorsuch, R. L., Lushene, R., Vagg, P. R., & Jacobs, G. A. (1983). *Manual for the State-Trait Anxiety Inventory.* Palo Alto, CA: Consulting Psychologists Press.

Straatman, I., Hanson, E., Endenburg, N., & Mol, J. (1997). The influence of a dog on male students during a stressor. *Anthrozoös: A multidisciplinary journal of the interactions of people and animals, 10*, 191–197.

Struthers, W. C., Perry, P. R., & Menec, H. V. (2000). An examination of the relationship among academic stress, coping, motivation, and performance in college. *Research in Higher Education, 41*(5), 581–592.

Tsai, C.C., Friedmann, E., & Thomas, S. A. (2010) The Effect of Animal-Assisted Therapy on Stress Responses in Hospitalized Children, *Anthrozoös: A multidisciplinary journal of the interactions of people and animals,* 23(3), 245-258.

Viena, D. T., Banks, J. B., Barbu, M. I., Schulman, H. A., & Tartar, J. L. (2012) Differential effects of mild chronic stress on cortisol and S-IgA responses to an acute stressor. *Biological Psychology, 91*, 307–311.

Walsh, F. (2009). Human-animal bonds II: the role of pets in family systems and family therapy. *Family Process,* 48, 481-499.

Wammes, J. D., Seli, P., Cheyne, J. A., Boucher, P. O., & Smilek, D. (2016). Mind wandering during lectures II: Relation to academic performance. *Scholarship of Teaching and Learning in Psychology, 2*(1), 33–48.

Watson, D., Clark, L. A., & Tellegen, A. (1988). Development and validation of brief measures of positive and negative affect: The PANAS scales. *Journal of Personality and Social Psychology, 54*(6), 1063–1070.

Wright, J. D., Kritz-Silverstein, D., Morton, D. J., Wingard, D. L., & Barrett-Connor, E. (2007). Pet ownership and blood pressure in old age. *Epidemiology, 18*, 613–617.

7 Comparing the Effect of Human–Dog Interactions and Progressive Muscle Relaxation on Self-Report and Physiological Measures of Stress

Nicole L. Beasley, Greg C Elvers*, Roger N. Reeb and Hannah L. Torok
Department of Psychology, University of Dayton

Abstract

This study compares the effects of human–dog interactions and progressive muscle relaxation on stress in college students during the week of their final exams using self-report and physiological measures of stress. Students often cope with stress during the final exams period using various strategies such as spending time with a therapy dog. While students often report that their stress is reduced after visiting with a therapy dog, some studies find physiological evidence for a reduction in stress while others do not. During the first day of finals week, students ($N = 53$) in an introductory psychology or a research methods course were randomly assigned to spend 15 minutes with a therapy dog or to spend 15 minutes doing a progressive muscle relaxation task. Heart rate variability, a physiological measure of stress, and two self-report measures of stress (the PSS-10 which is a 10 item questionnaire on the participants' stress level and the SVAS on which the participants mark a visual scale to indicate their current stress level) were measured both before and after the treatments. Compared to the pre-treatment measures, stress was lower after the treatment. Spending time with a therapy dog can reduce stress associated with final exams. However, the intercorrelations between heart rate variability and the self-report measures were not statistically significant suggesting that the measures might correspond to different dimensions of the stress response, as explained in some theories of stress response and emotion. Future research regarding the effects of therapy dogs on stress should include at least one physiological measure of stress and ideally multiple measures. This inclusion might help clarify the underlying psychological and physiological mechanisms leading to stress reduction.

Keywords: therapy dogs, stress reduction, physiological measurement, self-report measurements

Author Note

The authors attest that there are no conflicts of interest with this research.

We thank the Miami Valley Pet Therapy Association for helping us recruit the therapy dogs (Bailey, Kia, Roger, Sadie, Scout, and Teddy) and their handlers (Gerry Coen, Rene Oyola, Melanie Donbar, Mary Watson, Jack Filia, and Paula Brown) who made this project possible. We also thank Kirah Noble for assisting in the collection of the data.

There are few occurrences during the academic semester that generate as much stress and anxiety among students as exams (Gilbert et al., 1996). In response to stress from final exams, some academic institutions offer stress mitigation

*Corresponding author: email:gelvers1@udayton.edu

strategies such as allowing students to visit with therapy dogs (Trammell, 2017). These students' intuition that interacting with dogs may reduce stress is supported by research that finds such interactions may activate the oxytocin system (Beetz, Unväs-Moberg et al., 2012; Handlin et al., 2012). The impact of therapy dogs on students' stress has been the focus of multiple studies. Some studies fail to find physiological evidence of a reduction in stress after visiting with a therapy dog (Barker et al., 2016; Crump & Derting, 2015; Gee et al., 2014; Grossberg et al., 1988; Lass-Hennemann et al., 2014; Schöberl et al., 2012) while others do find physiological evidence of stress reduction (Barker et al., 2005; Beetz, Julius et al., 2012; Tsai et al. 2010).

Barker et al. (2016) is one study that failed to find a difference in stress reduction when measured physiologically, but which did find a difference in stress reduction using self-report scales. Self-reported stress was measured with the Perceived Stress Scale (PSS) and the Stress Visual Analog Scale (SVAS) while physiological markers of stress included salivary nerve growth factor and alpha amylase. Barker et al. randomly assigned students to either an attention-control condition (no interaction with therapy dogs) or a therapy dog intervention. Afterwards students provided a second set of saliva samples and responded to the PSS and SVAS. Barker et al. found a reduction in self-reported stress, but no reduction in the physiological markers of stress for students who had interacted with the therapy dogs.

At first glance, the studies that fail to find a reduction in stress via physiological measures after interacting with dogs seem to indicate that this is a robust finding, but this may be a premature conclusion as explained later. This finding appears across multiple studies with different physiological measures of stress – salivary alpha amylase (Barker et al., 2016), heart rate and blood pressure (Crump & Derting, 2015; Grossberg et al., 1988; Lass-Hennemann et al., 2016), and heart rate variability (Gee et al., 2014). The null finding appears with different stressors, both acute (stress induced by the study: Gee et al., 2014; Grossberg et al., 1988; Lass-Hennemann et al., 2014) and chronic (stress induced by exams in the following week: Barker et al., 2016; Crump & Derting, 2015). It appears with different populations – students (Barker et al., 2016; Crump & Derting, 2015; Gee et al. 2014), and for some measures, healthcare workers (Barker et al. 2005). It also appears with therapy dogs and with pet dogs (Grossberg et al., 1988). Therapy dogs are trained to remain calm in most situations and are accompanied by their handlers who may be sympathetic, good listeners, and/or calming. These traits may or may not be present in pet dogs and their guardians, and it is possible that these traits contribute to the reduction in stress above and beyond whatever reduction is stress is caused by the therapy dog per se.

There are several possible reasons, ranging from the practical to theoretical, why a study might find a pre- to post-test difference in stress when measured with a self-report and not when measured with a physiological marker. A researcher might have selected an insensitive physiological marker of stress or there might have been some technical difficulty with the measurement per se. This may have been part of the reason that Barker et al. (2016) failed to find a difference with one of their physiological markers – most levels of salivary nerve growth factor were undetectable in their study.

Similarly, the researcher may not have used a sufficiently stressful event. For example, Grossberg et al. (1988) used the Thematic Apperception Test (TAT) (which involves looking at an ambiguous picture and creating a story about it) as one of their stressors. The TAT is not usually considered to be a stressful test. The duration of a laboratory stressor might have been too short (e.g. Lass-Hennemann et al.'s, 2014, stressful event was an 11 minute film clip depicting physical and sexual violence). Weaker manipulations might produce weaker results – results small enough that the researcher's statistical tests might not be powerful enough to detect.

Another possible explanation is that self-reports may be more prone to subject-expectancy effects than are physiological measures. When participating in a study with therapy dogs in which there are pre- and post-test measures of stress, participants may believe that they have figured out the purpose of the study and respond with lower levels of self-reported stress in the post-test, whether the intervention actually reduced stress or not.

A possible theoretical explanation comes from Lang's (1979) tripartite model of emotional responses. This model claims that there are three components to an emotional response –

physiological arousal, cognitive distress, and behavioral avoidance. During strong emotions, such as an intense fear associated with a phobia, these components tend to be concordant – tending to vary together. However, with less strong emotions, such as many students might experience during finals week, these components may be discordant – tending to vary independently (Ollendick et al., 2011). Thus, if the stress is not sufficiently severe, it is not surprising that some researchers find stress reduction with one measure, but not with all measures.

Other studies suggest that therapy dogs can reduce physiological markers of stress. This too seems to be a robust finding which occurs with different measures – cortisol (Barker et al. 2005; Beetz, Julius et al., 2012) and systolic blood pressure (Tsai et al., 2010). This finding occurs in different populations – healthcare workers (at least with some physiological markers, Barker et al., 2005), children with insecure attachment (Beetz, Julius et al., 2012), and hospitalized children (Tsai et al., 2010). For example, Barker et al. (2005) measured serum cortisol, epinephrine, norepinephrine, salivary cortisol, salivary IgA, and lymphocytes in blood both before and after spending 5 or 20 minutes with a therapy dog or 20 minutes of quiet rest. Results indicate that both serum and salivary cortisol were reduced, especially when measured 45 minutes after the interaction with the therapy dog.

One physiological measure of stress is heart rate variability – the variance of the time between heart beats, (technically the variance of the RR intervals). It is thought that heart rate variability is controlled by the interactions of the sympathetic and parasympathetic branches of the autonomic nervous system. The sympathetic nervous system activates the "flight vs. fight" response while the complementary parasympathetic nervous system activates the "rest and digest" responses. During times of stress, the sympathetic nervous system becomes more active and this leads to a decrease in heart rate variability – the period of time between heart beats becomes more regular. In a meta-analysis, Kim et al. (2018) reviewed 37 studies that examined whether heart rate variability is a valid physiological measure of stress or not. The meta-analysis concludes that heart rate variability is a valid measure of stress.

Traditionally, heart rate variability has been measured with an electrocardiogram (ECG or EKG) which involves attaching numerous (often 12) electrodes to a person's limbs and chest. The ECG equipment can be expensive, the electrodes are often discarded after a single use, and placing electrodes on a participant's chest can be intrusive, and perhaps stressful, to some participants. Fortunately, alternatives now exist that are less expensive, less wasteful, and less stressful. Photoplethysmography (PPG), a non-invasive method used in this study to collect heart rate variability, shines a light through a participant's fingertip to a photosensor. The change in volume of blood in the fingertip that naturally occurs during the beating of the heart can be detected and from this, the heart rate variability can be determined. In a review of PPG and its applications in clinical physiological measurement, Allen (2007, p. R27) states that heart rate variability can be "easily extracted from PPG pulse signals."

The present study examines self-report and physiological measures of stress taken from college students on the first day of final exams week both before and after interacting with a therapy dog or participating in a progressive muscle relaxation control condition. It is predicted that stress, measured both with self-reports and physiological markers, will be reduced (heart rate variability will increase) after interacting with therapy dogs or participating in a progressive muscle relaxation control condition.

Method

Sample

The sample consisted of 53 college students (36 female and 17 male) with a mean age of 19.2 years (SD = 1.0 years). Data from one additional participant was discarded due to the loss of the pre-treatment heart rate variability reading. Twenty-six participants (18 females and 8 males) were randomly assigned to the therapy dog with handler condition and the remaining 27 participants (18 females and 9 males) were assigned to the progressive muscle relaxation condition. Human–animal interactions and progressive muscle relaxation are not covered in detail in the courses from which the participants volunteered. The participants were students in an introductory psychology class or a research methods class at a private university in the United States. They participated in partial fulfillment of a research requirement for the introductory psychology class or for extra credit in the research methods class. Students who disliked dogs, were nervous about dogs, were unsure of their ability to interact with dogs, were allergic to dogs, or were very anxious were not allowed to participate. The study was approved by the Institutional Animal Care and Use Committee and a subcommittee of the Institutional Review Board.

The six therapy dogs and handlers were recruited from the Miami Valley Pet Therapy Association (MVPTA). Each dog had passed a seven-week course during which the dogs were trained and verified by MVPTA as appropriate as a therapy animal.

Instruments

Two self-report measures of stress were used – the ten item Perceived Stress Scale (PSS-10) modified to ask about stress during the last week instead of the last month and the Stress Visual Analog Scale (SVAS). The PSS-10 consists of 10 questions (e.g. In the last week, how often have you felt nervous and stressed?) with five point Likert scale responses (0 = never, 4 = very often). The responses to the 10 questions are summed after reverse scaling appropriate responses. Cohen et al. (1983) report that Cronbach's α for the PSS-10 is 0.84 and that the PSS-10 has mild to moderate correlations with negative life events. In the current study, the pre-and post-test PSS-10 Cronbach's α are 0.76 and 0.79.

The SVAS asks participants to indicate their level of stress that they are currently feeling by placing a mark on a 15 cm long line with anchors of "none" on the left end and "most severe imaginable" on the right end of the line. The distance in millimeters of the mark from the left end of the scale is recorded. Barker et al. (2016) report good test-retest reliability (0.79) for the SVAS and good concurrent validity (0.68) between patient ratings and nurse ratings of stress responses in patients.

The physiological measure of stress was heart rate variability. A CorSense PPG sensor from Elite HRV was used. According to the manufacturer's web site, accuracy is comparable to 5-lead ECG/EKG (Elite HRV, 2019). Plews et al. (2017) compared PPG as measured by a smart phone, a heart rate sensor (Polar H7) and ECG and found almost perfect correlations (R = 1.00 with 90% confidence interval of [0.99 to 1.00]) between the PPG and ECG and between the heart rate sensor and ECG. The CorSense PPG sensor has been informally compared to the Polar H7 heart rate sensory used in the previous study by a company (not affiliated with Elite HRV) that writes smart phone software for measuring HRV. The review concludes that the Elite HRV sensor is "very accurate in detecting RR intervals and can therefore be used reliably for HRV analysis." (Altini, 2018).

Participants inserted the index finger of their right hand into the sensor and sat still for two minutes while heart rate variability was measured. The CorSense software captures the equivalent of the R-R intervals, calculates the root mean square of successive differences (RMSSD) of these intervals, takes the natural logarithm of the RMSSD, and normalizes the result to a value between 0 and 100.

Design

Participants were tested in groups of one to six participants depending on how many people signed-up and attended a given session. After getting consent to participate, participants reported their age, sex, the date and time of their next exam, and what, if any, sources of stress they were currently experiencing. Next, they answered the SVAS and PSS-10. Heart rate variability was then measured for two minutes. A randomly selected half of the group was then escorted to a nearby room where a therapy dog and handler were waiting.

Participants in the therapy dog with handler condition were told to initially hold out their hand for the dog to sniff and then they could pet, talk to, or play (but not vigorously) with the dog. All but one of the participants petted the dog and/or talked to the dog. No one played with the dog. Participants spent 15 minutes interacting with the dog and handler. The handlers of the therapy dogs were instructed to behave as they would in any other therapy dog session. All handlers talked to the participants in a friendly way – asking about their finals, if they had pets at home, and answered questions about their therapy dog. Heart rate variability, SVAS, and PSS-10 were then re-administered while the participants remained in the same room as the therapy dog and handler.

The other participants stayed in the original room and did a 15-minute-long progressive muscle relaxation task. Instructions were pre-recorded and told participants to progressively contract, hold, and relax various muscle groups while they sat. Progressive muscle relaxation was first introduced in 1934 and is a commonly used procedure for reducing stress-related anxiety (McCallie et al., 2006). Dolbier and Rush (2012) found reductions in self-reports and physiologically measured stress with 20 minute sessions of progressive muscle relaxation. Heart rate variability, SVAS and PSS-10 were then re-administered.

All participants were debriefed and had their questions answered.

Results

Table 7.1 shows the frequencies of stressors that the participants reported experiencing. Many participants reported more than one stressor. All but three participants reported that they were experiencing stress related to exams or studying for exams.

To help reduce the likelihood of making Type-I errors, univariate tests were only performed if the corresponding multivariate test was statistically significant. Likewise, follow-up tests of simple main effects were only performed if the univariate interaction was statistically significant.

To test if the participants in the therapy dog with handler and progressive muscle relaxation groups were equally stressed initially, a MANOVA with treatment condition as the independent variable and the three stress measures as the dependent variables was performed on the pre-treatment data. The MANOVA failed to find a significant effect of treatment, $F(3, 49) = 1.933$, $p = 0.137$, $\alpha = 0.05$, $\eta_p^2 = 0.106$.

Table 7.1. Participant's Self-Reported Stressors and Their Frequencies.

Stressor	*N*
Finals/studying for finals	50
Moving out/packing	11
Getting work done	5
Jobs	3
Family issues	2
Grades	2
Papers	2
Presentations	2
Friends	1
Future goals	1
Going on a study abroad	1
Graduation	1
Heat	1
Living arrangements	1
Nothing	1
Relationship problems	1
School related topics	1
Switching majors	1
This study	1

To test if the treatments reduced stress, a 2 (treatment: therapy dog with handler vs. progressive muscle relaxation) × 2 (time of measurement: pre- vs. post-treatment) MANOVA was performed with the three stress measures as the dependent variables. The MANOVA revealed effects of treatment, $F(3, 49) = 3.107$, $p = 0.035$, $\eta_p^2 = 0.160$, time of measurement, $F(3, 49) = 33.769$, $p < 0.001$, $\eta_p^2 = 0.674$, and their interaction, $F(3, 49) = 6.847$, $p = 0.001$, $\eta_p^2 = 0.295$.

Shapiro-Wilk tests were used to test ANOVA's assumption of normality. All Shapiro-Wilk tests with the exception of the pre-test SVAS had *p* values that were ≥ 0.077. An inspection of the Q-Q plot for the pre-test SVAS revealed no systematic departure from normality. ANOVA is robust to violations of the assumption of normality when sample sizes are greater than approximately 20. Thus, this assumption is likely sufficiently satisfied. Bartlett's tests for homogeneity of variance were performed for each dependent variable. All *p* values were ≥ 0.233, satisfying this assumption.

Follow-up 2 (treatment: therapy dog with handler vs. progressive muscle relaxation) × 2 (time of measurement: pre- vs. post-treatment) ANOVAs were performed for each dependent variable. Fig. 7.1 shows the means and 95% confidence intervals for the heart rate variability data. The ANOVA for heart rate variability revealed a reliable difference between the pre-treatment (M = 57.0, SE = 1.8) and post-treatment (M = 61.1, SE = 1.4) stress measurements, $F(1, 51) = 5.145$, $MS_{error} = 84.771$, $p = 0.028$, $\eta_p^2 = 0.092$. The ANOVA failed to reveal a reliable difference between the therapy dog with handler (M = 59.6, SE = 1.9) and progressive muscle relaxation (M = 58.5, SE = 1.9) conditions, $F(1, 51) = 0.144$, $MS_{error} = 191.397$, $p = 0.706$, $\eta_p^2 = 0.003$. The ANOVA also failed to reveal a reliable interaction of treatment condition and time of measurement, $F(1, 51) = 2.922$, $MS_{error} = 84.771$, $p = 0.093$, $\eta_p^2 = 0.054$.

Consistent with the philosophy of the *new statistics* (Cumming, 2012), the effect size of visiting with the therapy dog and handler was calculated with a repeated measures t-test and revealed a large effect for the pre- (M = 56.0, SE = 2.6) vs. post-treatment (M = 63.1, SE = 2.0) heart rate variability data, $t(25) = -4.052$, $p < 0.001$, $r^2 = 0.396$. A repeated measures t-test failed to reveal even a small effect for the pre- (M = 58.0, SE = 2.5) vs. post-treatment (M =59.0, SE = 1.9) heart rate variability for participants in the PMR condition, $t(26) = -0.325$, $p = 0.748$, $r^2 = 0.004$.

Fig. 7.2 shows the means and 95% confidence intervals for the SVAS data. The ANOVA for SVAS revealed a reliable difference between the pre-treatment (M = 76.1 mm, SE = 3.5) and post-treatment (M = 54.0 mm, SE = 3.3) stress measurements, $F(1, 51) = 94.967$, $MS_{error} = 135.579$, $p < 0.001$, $\eta_p^2 = 0.651$. The ANOVA failed to reveal a reliable difference between the therapy dog with handler (M = 61.8 mm, SE = 4.6) and progressive muscle relaxation (M = 68.3 mm, SE = 4.5) conditions, $F(1, 51) = 1.034$, $MS_{error} = 1078.618$, $p = 0.314$, $\eta_p^2 = 0.020$. The ANOVA revealed a reliable interaction of treatment condition and pre- to post-test measurements, $F(1, 51) = 13.963$, $MS_{error} = 135.579$, $p < 0.001$, $\eta_p^2 = 0.215$. Repeated measures t-tests were used as follow-up analyses of simple main effects of time of measurement for the therapy dogs with handler ($t(25) = 9.622$, $p < 0.001$, $r^2 = 0.787$) and for progressive muscle relaxation ($t(26) = 4.216$, $p < 0.001$, $r^2 = 0.406$). For SVAS, interacting with therapy dogs and handler reduced perceived stress more than doing a

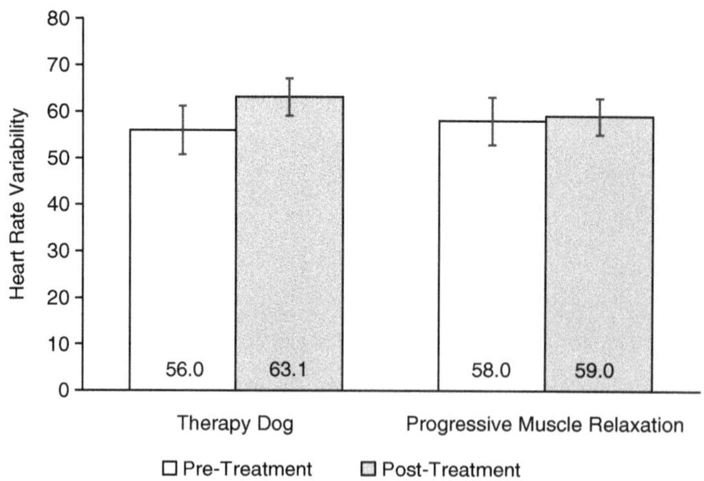

Note. The error bars represent the 95% confidence intervals. Higher values imply *less* stress.

Fig. 7.1. Pre-and Post-Treatment Heart Rate Variabilities for Visiting With Therapy Dogs and Handlers and Progressive Muscle Relaxation.

progressive muscle relaxation task did as indicated by the differences in the effect sizes.

Fig. 7.3 shows the means and 95% confidence intervals for the PSS-10 data. The ANOVA for PSS-10 revealed a reliable difference between the pre-treatment (M = 18.9, SE = 0.7) and post-treatment (M = 17.5, SE = 0.7) stress measurements, $F(1, 51) = 15.860$, $MS_{error} = 3.513$, $p < 0.001$, $\eta_p^2 = 0.237$. The ANOVA revealed a reliable difference between the therapy dog with handler (M = 16.2, SE = 0.9) and progressive muscle relaxation (M = 21.2, SE = 0.9) conditions, $F(1, 51) = 9.403$, $MS_{error} = 44.114$, $p = 0.003$, $\eta_p^2 = 0.156$. The ANOVA revealed a reliable interaction of treatment condition and time of measurement, $F(1, 51) = 7.137$, $MS_{error} = 3.513$, $p = 0.010$, $\eta_p^2 = 0.123$. Repeated measures t-tests were used as follow-up analyses of simple main effects of time of measurement for the therapy dogs with handler ($t(25) = 4.848$, $p < 0.001$, $r^2 = 0.485$) and for progressive muscle relaxation ($t(26) = 0.903$, $p = 0.375$, $r^2 = 0.030$). For PSS-10, interacting with therapy dogs and handler decreased perceived stress while doing a progressive muscle relaxation task did not reliably reduce perceived stress.

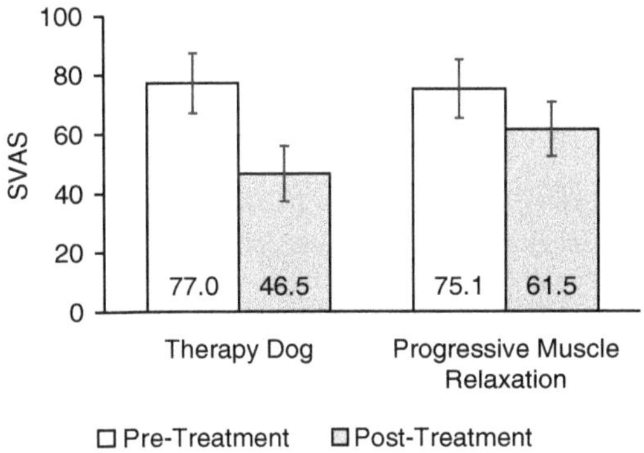

Note. The error bars represent the 95% confidence intervals. Higher values imply more stress.

Fig. 7.2. Pre- and Post-Treatment Stress Visual Analog Scale (SVAS) Ratings for Visiting With Therapy Dogs and Handlers and Progressive Muscle Relaxation.

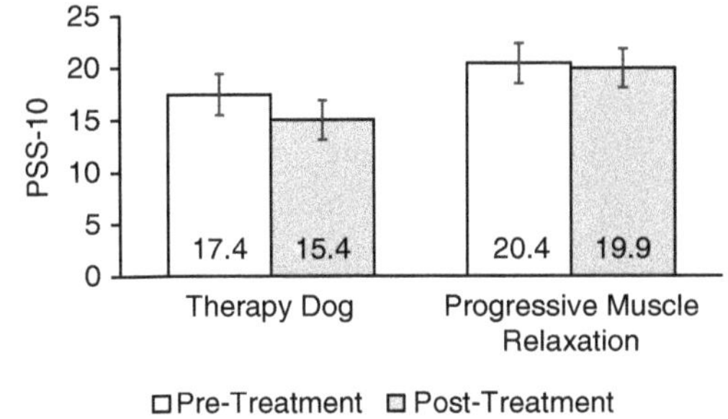

Note. The error bars represent the 95% confidence intervals. Higher values imply more stress.

Fig. 7.3. Pre- and Post-Treatment Perceived Stress Scale (PSS-10) Ratings for Visiting With Therapy Dogs and Handlers and Progressive Muscle Relaxation.

If heart rate variability, SVAS, and PSS-10 measure are at least partially overlapping dimensions of stress, one would expect the three variables to be intercorrelated if the stress level was high according to Lang's (1979) theory. Correlations among the three pre-test measures and the three post-test measures are shown in Table 7.2. None of the correlations are statistically reliable. Variability in heart rate variability explains less than 1% of the variability of the PSS-10 and SVAS. Variability in the SVAS score explains less than 7% of the variability in the PSS-10 score.

Discussion

The results suggest that visiting with therapy dogs and their handlers for 15 minutes reduces stress in college students during final exams week when measured with heart rate variability using a commercially available and relatively inexpensive sensor. Furthermore, interacting with the therapy dog and their handlers yields a relatively large effect size from pre- to post-test, explaining almost 40% of the variability in the heart rate variability data. The PSS-10 and SVAS also had large effect sizes pre- to post-test for interacting with a therapy dog and handler. Making therapy dogs and their handlers available to students during final exams week may be a valuable service that colleges and universities can provide to their students.

Table 7.2. Intercorrelations Among the Three Measures of Stress.

Pre-Test		
	PSS-10	SVAS
Heart rate variability	$r = -0.088$ $p = 0.529$ $r^2 = 0.008$	$r = 0.030$ $p = 0.830$ $r^2 = 0.001$
SVAS	$r = 0.181$ $p = 0.196$ $r^2 = 0.033$	
Post-Test		
	PSS-10	SVAS
Heart rate variability	$r = -0.092$ $p = 0.516$ $r^2 = 0.008$	$r = 0.002$ $p = 0.988$ $r^2 < 0.001$
SVAS	$r = 0.250$ $p = 0.074$ $r^2 = 0.063$	

Students in the progressive muscle relaxation group did not show an increase in heart rate variability with the effect size explaining less than 1% of the variability in the data. The PMR group did have large effect sizes pre- to post-test when measured with the PSS-10 and SVAS. PMR may be an inexpensive and easy way for students to reduce stress as measured with the PSS-10 and SVAS during final exams week. An empirical question is whether students would be at least as likely to engage in PMR as they are in a therapy dog session. Students who are missing their own pets may, or may not, be more willing to attend a therapy dog session than to engage in PMR. If students are not sufficiently interested in PMR as a way to reduce stress, then it would not be a viable option no matter how beneficial and cost effective it is. The relative interest in participating in a PMR session (or other stress-management sessions) versus a therapy dog session during final exam week is an interesting empirical question for future research.

The studies which found reductions in physiological evidence of stress after visiting with a therapy dog and handler (Barker et al., 2005, Beetz, Julius et al., 2012, Tsai et al., 2010) used serum and/or salivary cortisol and/or systolic blood pressure as their measures of stress. Barker et al.'s and Beetz, Julius et al.'s results suggest that cortisol levels might lag changes in stress. Barker et al. found the largest change in cortisol when it was measured 45 minutes after the interaction, and Beetz, Julius et al. found a reliable difference in cortisol levels only between the first of two pre-treatment and the last of two post-treatment measurements. While such delays might be acceptable in a laboratory setting, they are probably less practical in field studies where the participants might be less willing to wait up to 45 minutes after interacting with a therapy dog or undergoing PMR. If other researchers can replicate the finding that heart rate variability is a reliable and valid measure of physiological stress reactivity before and after interacting with therapy dogs or PMR, it might eliminate the delay that appears to be necessary with salivary cortisol measurements. Measuring heart rate variability is likely cheaper and safer than collecting bodily fluids (saliva for salivary cortisol and blood for serum cortisol), storing them appropriately, and having them analyzed.

Because the correlations between heart rate variability and the PSS-10 and SVAS are quite low, the physiological and self-report measures of stress might be assessing different components – Lang's (1979) physiological, cognitive, or behavioral components – of the emotional response associated with stress. During strong emotions, such as an intense fear associated with a phobia, these components tend to be concordant – tending to vary together; with less strong emotions, such as moderate generalized anxiety, these components tend to be discordant – tending to vary independently (Ollendick et al., 2011). The low intercorrelations among the measures are consistent with their exam stress being moderate instead of strong. Future research might study participants who are experiencing higher levels of exam stress, such as those seeking help from the campus counseling center for stress, to see if the physiological and self-report measures from those individuals might be more concordant and more strongly correlated with each other.

Lazarus and Folkman's (1984) transactional model of stress and coping categorizes coping strategies as problem-focused or emotion-focused. Problem-focused coping strategies tend to be more effective when dealing with a stressor that is under one's control, while emotion-focused coping strategies tend to be more effective when dealing with a stressor that is not under one's control. Many stressors, such as exam stress, have some components that are controllable (e.g. how much a student studies and when they start studying) while having other components that are not controllable by the individual (e.g. how difficult the exam will be, how many exams are scheduled in the same day). Therapy dog sessions and PMR are more consistent with emotion-focused coping – the individual is not learning about a particular stressor, but rather is learning pragmatic skills to regulate their emotions as they encounter stressors, which may not be under their control.

In connection with Lazarus and Folkman's (1984) model, researchers have categorized people – including adults (Cohen & Lazarus, 1973; Goldstein, 1973) and children (Peterson & Toler, 1986) – as information-seekers who prefer problem-focused coping strategies or information-avoiders who prefer emotion-focused coping strategies. Thus, therapy dog sessions may be most beneficial for individuals who are information-avoiders, but may also be appropriate for information-seekers if paired with another intervention that is problem-focused. This may also be helpful for information-seekers when forced to face uncontrollable stressors or if paired with another intervention component that is problem-focused in nature. That is, emotion-focused strategies such as visiting with a therapy dog, may allow a person to feel less overwhelmed and more relaxed. Then, a problem-focused strategy, such as teaching a study strategy, could be introduced. Future research might look at the effects of therapy dogs on exam stress for students with various coping dispositions as identified by the aforementioned researchers and whether adding a problem-focused coping strategy, such as a study skill, further reduces stress.

The possibility that part of the reduction in stress is due to "subject-expectancy effects" is worth noting. That is, if a participant successfully perceived the purpose of the study, some may be motivated to respond to self-report measure items in ways that are consistent with their perceptions of the hypothesis, regardless of their physiological reactions, which may or may not be noticeable to them. However, given past research showing decreases in self-reported stress in response to sessions with therapy dogs, accompanied by the evidence of concurrent validity for the self-report measures selected for use in this study, there is reason to believe that participants legitimately experienced a decrease in stress in response to the interventions. In a future study, perhaps the use of a post-experimental inquiry or interview may allow a better understanding of the subjective experience of participants following a therapy dog session.

In order to fully understand the effects of therapy dogs and their handlers on stress, it is recommended that researchers continue to include physiological indicators of stress. According to the concept of individual response stereotypy (Lacey & Lacey, 1958), different people have different autonomic responses to the same stressor and thus no single measure of autonomic response will capture the stress response of all participants. Levenson (1983) recommends a minimum of three measures of the autonomic response – a cardiovascular measure, an electrodermal measure, and a somatic muscle measure. Levenson also recommends, when possible, that a cortical measure be included to measure central nervous system arousal. Individual response-stereotypy accompanied with a failure to measure the three different dimensions of the autonomic response might explain why some of the previous research failed to find an effect of therapy dogs on physiological indicators of stress.

In an ideal experiment, the number of people with the therapy dog and handler in each session should have been controlled. In practice, the number of participants who signed-up for a given session with the therapy dog and handler and the number of participants who came to the session prevented this variable from being controlled. While the number of students with a therapy dog and handler in a session could influence how the students interacted with the dog and therefore influence the results, it would likely influence the results in a way that would work against the hypothesis. That is, if one-on-one is optimal for reducing stress, the larger group sizes would reduce the size of the effect. Likewise, if many-on-one is optimal for reducing stress, the smaller group sizes would reduce the size of the effect. Whatever the optimal group size is, having other group sizes would tend to reduce the size of the effect across the sessions. Variation in group size might also be more similar to what happens in therapy dog sessions outside the laboratory. Future research should systematically vary group size and other factors to see how much, if at all, they contribute to the reduction of stress observed when students interact with therapy dogs.

Future research might attempt to determine the reason that visiting a therapy dog and handler reduces stress. While it may be possible that there is something unique about interacting with a therapy dog that reduces stress, such as the activation of the oxytocin system (Beetz, Uvnäs-Moberg et al., 2012), there are other potential reasons. At least in this study, the therapy dog session was in a calm environment and simply spending time in such an environment might reduce stress. While the interaction between treatment (therapy dog and progressive muscle relaxation) and time of measurement (pre- and post-treatment) was not statistically significant for heart rate variability in this study, progressive muscle relaxation, which was also in a calm environment, had an effect size that was less than the cutoff for a small effect while the therapy dog with handler condition had a large effect size. The handlers of the therapy dogs also interacted with the participants in a friendly manner. Perhaps interacting with another person in a friendly way contributes to the reduction of stress (but see Lass-Hennemann et al., 2014). Future research, for example, could have handlers follow scripts while interacting with the participants. In some scripts, the handler might be friendly while in other scripts the handler might act in a more formal manner.

Interacting with a friendly dog might have reminded some of the participants of pleasant times with their own dog, and this might contribute to the reduction of stress. Future researchers could explore this possible explanation by assessing and statistically controlling for such variables as past experience with dogs or emotional memories of family interactions involving a dog.

References

Allen, J. (2007). Photoplethysmography and its application in clinical physiological measurement. *Physiological Measurement, 28*, R1-R39. https://doi.org/10.1088/0967-3334/28/3/R01

Altini, M. (2018, November 9). *CorSense*. HRV4Training. https://www.hrv4training.com/blog/corsense

Barker, S. B., Barker, R. T., McCain, N. L., & Schubert, C. M. (2016). A randomized cross-over exploratory study of the effect of visiting therapy dogs on college student stress before final exams. *Anthrozoös, 29*(1), 35–46. https://doi.org/10.1080/08927936.2015.1069988

Barker, S. B., Knisely, J. S., McCain, N. L., & Best, A. M. (2005). Measuring stress and immune response in healthcare professionals following interaction with a therapy dog: A pilot study. *Psychological Reports, 96*(3), 713–729. https://doi.org/10.2466/pr0.96.3.713-729

Beetz, A., Julius, H., Turner, D., & Kotrschal, K. (2012). Effects of social support by a dog on stress modulation in male children with insecure attachment. *Frontiers in Psychology, 3*, Article 352. https://doi.org/10.3389/fpsyg.2012.00352

Beetz, A., Uvnäs-Moberg, K., Julius, H., & Kotrschal, K. (2012). Psychosocial and psychophysiological effects of human-animal interactions: The possible role of oxytocin. *Frontiers in Psychology*, *3*, Article 234. https://doi.org/10.3389/fpsyg.2012.00234

Cohen, F., & Lazarus, R. S. (1973). Active coping processes, coping dispositions, and recovery from surgery. *Psychosomatic Medicine*, *35*(5), 375–389. https://doi.org/10.1097/00006842-197309000-00002

Cohen, S., Kamarck, T., & Mermelstein, R. (1983). A global measure of perceived stress. *Journal of Health and Social Behavior*, *24*(4), 385–396. https://doi.org/10.2307/2136404

Crump, C., & Derting, T. L. (2015). Effects of pet therapy on the psychological and physiological stress levels of first-year female undergraduates. *North American Journal of Psychology 17*(3), 575–590.

Cumming, G. (2012). *Understanding the new statistics effect sizes, confidence intervals, and meta-analysis*. Routledge. https://doi.org/10.4324/9780203807002

Dolbier, C. L., & Rush, T. E. (2012). Efficacy of abbreviated progressive muscle relaxation in a high-stress college sample. *International Journal of Stress Management*, *19*(1), 48–68. https://doi.org/10.1037/a0027326

Elite HRV (2019). *CorSense heart rate variability finger sensor by Elite HRV*. https://elitehrv.com/corsense

Gee, N. R., Friedmann, E., Stendahl, M., Fisk, A., & Coglitore, V. (2014). Heart rate variability during a working memory task: Does touching a dog or person affect the response? *Anthrozoös*, *27*(4), 513–528. https://doi.org/10.2752/089279314X14072268687763

Gilbert, D. G., Stunkard, M. E., Jensen, R. A., Detwiler, F. R. J., & Martinko, J. M. (1996). Effects of exam stress on mood, cortisol, and immune functioning: Influences of neuroticism and smoker- non-smoker status. *Personality and Individual Differences*, *21*(2), 235–246. https://doi.org/10.1016/0191-8869(96)00065-7

Goldstein, M. J. (1973). Individual differences in response to stress. *American Journal of Community Psychology*, *1*(2), 113–137. https://doi.org/10.1007/bf00880131

Grossberg, J. M., Alf, E. F., & Vormbrock, J. K. (1988). Does pet dog presence reduce human cardiovascular responses to stress? *Anthrozoös*, *2*(1), 38–44. https://doi.org/10.2752/089279389787058253

Handlin, L., Hydbring-Sandberg, E., Nilsson, A., Ejdebäck, M., Jansson, A., & Uvnäs-Moberg, K. (2011). Short-term interaction between dogs and their owners: Effects on oxytocin, cortisol, insulin and heart rate – an exploratory study. *Anthrozoös*, *24*(3), 301–316. https://doi.org/10.2752/175303711X13045914865385

Kim, H., Cheon, E., Bai, D., Lee, Y. H., & Koo, B. (2018). Stress and heart rate variability: A meta-analysis and review of the literature. *Psychiatry Investigation*, *15*(3), 235–245. https://doi.org/10.30773/pi.2017.08.17

Lacey, J. I., & Lacey, B. C. (1958). Verification and extension of the principle of autonomic response-stereotypy. *The American Journal of Psychology*, *71*(1), 50–73. https://doi.org/10.2307/1419197

Lang, P. J. (1979). A bio-informational theory of emotional imagery. *Psychophysiology*, *16*(6), 495-512. https://doi.org/10.1111/j.1469-8986.1979.tb01511.x

Lazarus, R. S. & Folkman, S. (1984). *Stress, appraisal, and coping*. Springer.

Levenson, R. W. (1983). Personality research and psychophysiology: General considerations. *Journal of Research in Personality*, *17*(1), 1–21. https://doi.org/10.1016/0092-6566(83)90057-0

Lass-Hennemann, J., Peyk, P., Streb, M., Holz, E., & Michael, T. (2014). Presence of a dog reduces subjective but not physiological stress responses to an analog trauma. *Frontiers in Psychology*, *5*, Article 1010. https://doi.org/10.3389/fpsyg.2014.01010

McCallie, M. S., Blum, C. M., & Hood, C. J. (2006). Progressive muscle relaxation. *Journal of Human Behavior in the Social Environment*, *13*(3), 51–66. https://doi.org/10.1300/j137v13n03_04

Ollendick, T., Allen, B., Benoit, K., & Cowart, M. (2011). The tripartite model of fear in children with specific phobias: Assessing concordance and discordance using the behavioral approach test. *Behaviour Research and Therapy*, *49*(8), 459–465. https://doi.org/10.1016/j.brat.2011.04.003

Peterson, L. & Toler, S. M. (1986). An information seeking disposition in child surgery patients. *Health Psychology*, *5*(4), 343–358. https://doi.org/10.1037/0278-6133.5.4.343

Plews, D. J., Scott, B., Altini, M., Wood, M., Kilding, A. E., & Laursen, P. B. (2017). Comparison of heart-rate-variability recording with smartphone photoplethysmography, Polar H7 chest strap, and electrocardiography. *International Journal of Sports Physiology and Performance*, *12*(10), 1324–1328. https://doi.org/10.1123/ijspp.2016-0668

Schöberl, I., Wedl, M., Bauer, B., Day, J., Möstl, E., & Kotrschal, K. (2012). Effects of owner-dog relationship and owner personality on cortisol modulation in human-dog dyads. *Anthrozoös*, *25*(2), 199–214. https://doi.org/10.2752/175303712X13316289505422

Trammell, J. P. (2017). The effect of therapy dogs on exam stress and memory. *Anthrozoös*, *30*(4), 607–621. https://doi.org/10.1080/08927936.2017.1370244

Tsai, C., Friedmann, E., & Thomas, S. A. (2010). The effect of animal-assisted therapy on stress responses in hospitalized children. *Anthrozoös*, *23*(3), 245–258. https://doi.org/10.2752/175303710X12750451258977

8 Experimental Trial Demonstrates Effects of Animal-Assisted Stress Prevention Program on College Students' Positive and Negative Emotion

Patricia Pendry*, Alexa M. Carr, Stephanie M. Roeter and Jaymie L. Vandagriff
Department of Human Development, Washington State University

Abstract

In response to the growing prevalence of mental health issues among college students, campuses across the nation are implementing animal-assisted stress reduction programs, despite a clear lack of evidence supporting their efficacy. Researchers conducted a randomized controlled trial to determine the effects of a universal, campus-based, animal-assisted stress prevention program on college students' moment-to-moment emotion the week preceding final exams. Participants were randomized into three conditions; the experimental group engaged in a 10-minute long interaction with dogs and cats from the local humane society, the control group watched a 10-minute slide show featuring photos of the same animals, while the wait-listed group was assessed in response to waiting for 10 minutes for their turn to participate in the program. Immediately before and after the assigned intervention, participants completed a 25-item checklist assessing how content, irritable, anxious, and depressed they felt in that moment. At post-test, participants who engaged in a 10-minute interaction with live animals reported statistically significant higher levels of contentment, $F(2, 181) = 9.30, p < 0.001$, and lower levels of anxiety, $F(2, 181) = 5.74, p < 0.01$, and irritability, $F(2, 181) = 5.44, p < 0.01$, compared to students in the control and wait-listed groups. This study provides much-needed evidence in support of animal-assisted campus visitation programs, demonstrating that 10 minutes of human–animal interaction increases levels of positive emotion and decreases levels of negative emotion in college students approaching final examinations.

Keywords: animal visitation program, college students, momentary emotion, randomized controlled trial, human–animal interaction

According to several sources, the prevalence of mental health symptoms and disorders in college students is on the rise (Hunt & Eisenberg, 2010). Based on a report by the National College Health Assessment sponsored by the American College Health Association [ACHA] (2014), one in two students reported experiencing 'overwhelming anxiety' in the past year, and one in three reported feeling 'so depressed that it was difficult to function' at some point during the last 12 months (p. 14). Moreover, more than 20% of college students reported being diagnosed or treated by a professional for a mental health condition in the past year, with anxiety (13.2%), depression (11.1%), and panic attacks (6.1%) (p. 15) being the most prevalent disorders.

Although the developmental etiology of these psychopathologies is complex, increasing

Corresponding author email: ppendry@wsu.edu

rates of stress exposure and lack of adaptive coping skills are thought to play a significant role (Grant *et al.*, 2014). The ACHA report (2014) noted that over fifty percent of students reported experiencing 'more than average' (42.3%) or a 'tremendous' amount of stress (10.4%) (p. 16). This is of concern as 28% of students reported that stress was the most significant factor negatively impacting their individual academic performance, including receiving a lower grade on an exam, course or project; receiving an incomplete; dropping the course; or experiencing a significant disruption in daily academic activities (p. 5). Moreover, although college students' stress originated from many different sources, academic stress was quoted by forty-four percent of students to be the 'most traumatic or difficult to handle' (p. 15). In fact, a great majority of students (84.4%) reported having felt 'overwhelmed by all they had to do' at some point during the last 12 months, and 80% reported feeling 'exhausted, not from physical activity' (p. 13).

It is important that we address academic stress, anxiety and depression as they negatively affect academic performance and retention. A summation of epidemiologic and experimental trials found that individuals with early-onset mental health disorders are more likely to terminate their education at the secondary and post-secondary levels (Kessler, 2012); in a nationally representative epidemiologic study of undergraduate students, 2.6% of school terminations prior to college graduation could be attributed to mental disorders (Breslau, Lane, Sampson & Kessler, 2008). Furthermore, in a large-scale longitudinal study, depressive symptomology significantly predicted lower academic performance and drop-out among college students, especially when it co-occurred with anxiety symptoms (Eisenberg, Golberstein & Hunt, 2009). Smaller trials conferred that exam stress in particular is associated with increased symptomology for anxiety and depression (Gilbert, Stunkard, Jensen, Detwiler & Martinko, 1996) and poorer academic performance (Ng, Koh & Chia, 2003). Since academic stress is considered an inevitable part of college life, it is important that we identify and expand evidence-based prevention programs that promote students' ability to cope adaptively with stress, thus reducing the negative implications of stress exposure on mental health and academic achievement.

Prevalence of animal-assisted college-based programs

One type of approach that has been enthusiastically received by college administrators, college-based mental health professionals, and students is to offer animal-assisted activities (AAAs) on college campuses. Different from animal-assisted *therapy*, which is conducted by a licensed healthcare professional as an integrative part of an individualized treatment process reimbursed by health insurance companies, AAAs incorporate interactions with animals (e.g., dogs, cats, horses, guinea pigs) into various program activities in a variety of settings. Over the last decade, AAAs have shown a tremendous increase in use and popularity on college campuses, particularly during the period before final examinations (Daniels, 2010; Devlin, 2011; Gaterud, 2011; Novak, 2010; Palmateer, 2010; Trunnell, 2010). In fact, according to a recent survey (Crossman & Kazdin, 2015), in the US alone close to a thousand college campuses offer AAAs. While some of these programs appear to be ad-hoc in nature, such as university staff bringing their personal pets to campus (Thomson, 2003), other programs utilize a more formal approach, bringing in animals from outside organizations (Riggenbach, 2010; Henry, 2008; Fox, 2010; Trunnell, 2010), including animals from local shelters (Baran, 2003; Cavazos, 2010).

Evidence supporting animal-assisted activities in various populations

In addition to the fact that these types of programs have some intuitive appeal to college administrators and students, their implementation is guided by evidence suggesting that interaction with animals is associated with enhanced stress-related functioning in various populations (Hediger & Beetz, 2015; Kruger, McCune, & Merrill, 2012; Barker & Wolen, 2008 for review). For example, a meta-analysis by Souter and Miller (2007) examining five experimental trials, comprising mainly older adults, concluded that animal-assisted therapy and activity can reduce depressive symptomatology. Additionally, experimental evidence in equine facilitated learning conducted as after-school programs with middle-school children demonstrated that children who participated in an 11-week program showed lower levels of cortisol (Pendry, Smith, & Roeter, 2014b), as well as higher levels of social competence (Pendry, Carr, Smith & Roeter, 2014a), outcomes which are significantly associated with stress-related symptomatology. Additionally, there is ample evidence from therapeutic literatures (Fine, 2015) to suggest that the presence of animals can serve as a "catalyst" for both positive and negative emotional experiences (p. 145).

Several mechanisms have been proposed to explain the potential pathways by which human–animal interaction can assert these effects, including the *biophilia hypothesis* (Wilson, 1984; Wilkes, 2009), which postulates that evolutionary forces leave us innately attuned and wanting to engage with animals and nature. Alongside this framework is the longstanding notion that human–animal interactions elicit feelings of social support and companionship in humans. A landmark study by Friedmann and Katcher (Freidmann, Katcher, Lynch & Thomas, 1980) laid the foundation for this perspective by investigating the effects of pet ownership on one-year survival rates of patients hospitalized in a coronary care unit. Those who owned pets survived at a significantly higher rate than patients who did not own pets after one year, suggesting that pet ownership may provide protective influence similar to that of human companionship.

Interestingly, relatively little nothing is known about the efficacy of college-based, animal-assisted activity programs in preventing or reducing student stress and stress-related mental health problems in naturalistic settings. The handful of studies conducted in these contexts have focused on examining interest of students in pet therapy (Adamle, Riley & Carlson, 2009), characteristics of implementation success (Reynolds & Rabschutz, 2011), and only recently, the effects on the therapy animals involved (Ng *et al.*, 2014). There are only a handful randomized controlled trials that have examined causal effects on college students' functioning in response to exposure to human animal interaction.

Results of these studies suggest that providing students with opportunities to interact with animals appears to have benefits for students' wellbeing. Crossman, Kazdin, and Knudson (2015) randomly assigned a group of Yale medical students to briefly interact with a dog, view a slide presentation of the same dog, or a wait-list condition. Results showed that students who interacted with a dog for less than 10 minutes reported declines in their anxiety and negative mood scores and large increases in their positive mood scores. In addition, Wheeler & Faulkner (2015) found that undergraduate students who were given access to a live dog to pet while engaging in potentially anxiety producing tasks (i.e., an unexpected speech, arithmetic problems) displayed lower levels of state anxiety than their counterparts who were told to pet a stuffed animal. Targeting self-identified homesick students, Binfet & Passmore (2016) found that participation in an 8-week AAT program, during which first year students participated in small-group interactions with therapy dogs, decreased feelings of homesickness. Most recently, a randomized controlled trial by Barker, Barker, McCain & Schubert (2016) found significant differences in college students' perceived stress after a 15 minute-long interaction with a therapy dog prior to final examinations. While important and promising, the aforementioned studies were conducted either with a relatively small or targeted at-risk sample, featured one-on-one or small group interactions, and/or were conducted in the context of a laboratory setting. A logical next step before promoting widespread implementation of AAAs on college campuses is to examine whether these benefits can be obtained in the context of a *universal*, large-scale animal-assisted stress-prevention program in a naturalistic setting.

Rationale and hypotheses

The overall objective of this study was thus to conduct a large-scale, randomized controlled trial to determine the effects of the Pet Your Stress Away (PYSA) program, a universal existing college-based prevention program held in the week before final examinations. The program allows students to engage in a 10-minute long supervised group interaction with suitable cats and dogs from a local animal shelter. The main goal of the study was to examine whether exposure to 10 minutes of human animal interaction affected students' moment-to-moment emotion (e.g., feeling content, anxious, irritable and depressed). We measured changes in student moment-to-moment emotion because they are indicators of individual differences in appraisal and arousal, which are known to play a major role in overall health and well-being (Peterson, Park, & Seligman, 2005). Also, an individual's momentary emotional state is linked to activation of the Hypothalamic Pituitary Adrenal (HPA) axis, the body's physiological stress response system associated with the development of psychopathology in response to chronic or extreme stress. Examining changes in moment-to moment emotional states in response to either a stressor or activity intended to down-regulate emotional and physiological arousal is useful as an indicator of individual differences in stress system activation and development of mental health issues (Adam, 2012). In addition to examining main effects of program participation on students' moment-to-moment indices of emotion, we explored whether treatment effects were moderated by students' reports of stress-related symptomatology including levels of depression, anxiety, worry and perceived stress in the weeks preceding the program.

The central hypotheses of the current study were that 1) Students randomly assigned to participate in the 10-minute PYSA program would report significantly lower levels of negative emotion (i.e., feeling anxious, depressed, irritable) and significantly higher levels of positive emotion (i.e., feeling content) at posttest, compared to students assigned to the control or waitlisted condition and 2) that treatment effects on momentary indices of emotion may be moderated by differences in students' state levels of mental health related symptoms (i.e., depression, perceived stress, worry and anxiety).

Method

Recruitment, design and procedures

All procedures performed in studies involving human participants were in accordance with the ethical standards of the institutional and/or national research committee and with the 1964 Helsinki declaration and its later amendments or comparable ethical standards. All procedures performed in studies involving animals were in accordance with the ethical standards of the University's Institutional Animal Care and Use Committee.

In the week before final exams were to take place, the study team visited a wide variety of general education classes and recruited consenting undergraduate students (N = 233) representing approximately 33 different majors across all student standings. Given the universal orientation of the planned program, students were not approached based on individual characteristics, but rather based on their enrollment in large general education classes, taught by instructors who had given permission to the research team to conduct recruitment presentations during class time. Given that the planned program dates and times had been determined months in advance and were thus unchangeable, we asked interested students to consider these dates and times and confirm that they were indeed available during programming times. At the end of the recruitment presentation, interested and available students were consented and asked to complete a screening survey, which included a participant ID number and a randomized treatment condition identifier meaningless to participants, indicating the treatment condition to which they were randomly assigned ($N_{experimental} = 76$; $N_{control} = 79$; $N_{waitlist} = 78$). The screening survey contained questions pertaining to demographic characteristics (e.g., class standing, gender, age, major), current and prior mental health (e.g., depression, anxiety, worry and perceived stress; see measures) and questions about participation in animal-assisted programming and/or counseling activities. For a flow diagram describing recruitment, condition allocation, reasons for declining participation, and study completion see Fig. 8.1. Participants who completed all study components were mostly female ($N_{female} = 156$, $N_{male} = 25$), upperclassmen ($N_{freshman} = 45$, $N_{sophomore} = 43$, $N_{junior} = 56$, $N_{senior} = 36$; $M_{age} = 20.19$, $SD = 1.69$) with an average GPA of 3.09±0.42.

Description of treatment conditions

Two days after recruitment, participants came to the PYSA program site during a two-hour time frame. Participants were asked to display the provided label containing their condition identifier on the outside of their clothing so research assistants could direct all study participants to check-in rooms specific to each condition. Participants randomly assigned to the *experimental condition* (N = 68) were directed to a curtained off program entry area managed by research as-

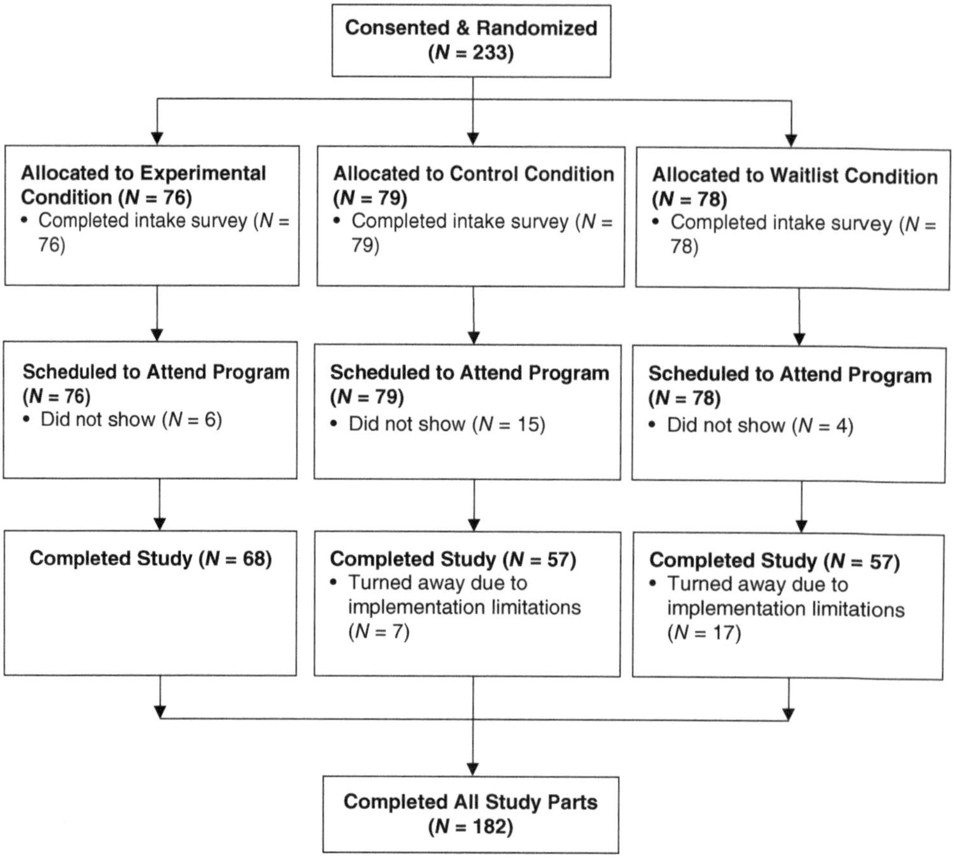

Fig. 8.1. Flow Diagram describing sample recruitment, randomization, program participation and study completion.

sistants who carefully managed and documented students' time of entry and exit into the human animal interaction area, which was located in a large gym. Immediately before entering the program area, students in the experimental condition completed a 2-minute survey reporting on their current emotional state, a measure described in detail in the method section below. Students then entered the animal interaction area, where they engaged with animals of their choosing for exactly 10 minutes. Groups of four to five students engaged with dogs under supervision of an animal handler, while they engaged with cats individually. Dogs (N = 9; N_{female} = 4) were adult, mostly large breed animals (Labrador terrier mix, American Staffordshire Pitbull mix, Labrador Pitbull mix, Boxer Labrador mix, Alaskan malamute, and several dogs with unknown breed mixes) from two local shelters. Dogs were seated on pillows and blankets and kept on their leash, in close proximity of their handler. Cats (N = 12; N_{female} = 9) were housed in large cat condos, which facilitated interaction between individual students and cats. Students were allowed to freely interact with the animals, which most often centered on petting and stroking the animals. After exactly 10 minutes, students were escorted to a curtained- off section where they immediately completed the same 2-minute survey reporting on their emotional state at post-test.

Participants randomly assigned to the *control condition* (N = 57) were told that before entering the program area, they would view a

10-minute slide presentation containing pictures of the program animals so they could indicate their preferences for certain animals using a checklist (i.e., would you pet this animal, which cat do you like best, etc.). Unbeknownst to participants, the only purpose for asking students to complete this checklist was to engage students in viewing of pictures of the program animals to facilitate assessment of momentary emotion in response to the control condition, rather than actually informing with which animals they would later interact. Participants thus completed their pretest and posttest ratings of moment to moment emotional states immediately before and after the 10-minute slide presentation. Upon completion students entered into the program area where they too were allowed to interact with program animals for 10 minutes.

Participants assigned to the *waitlist condition* (N = 57) were directed to a 'waiting' area and instructed to refrain from verbal interaction with others and asked to store their cellphones and reading materials. Immediately after receiving these instructions, they completed their first pretest measure of momentary emotion. They then sat in silence for 10 minutes, after which they were instructed to complete their posttest measure of momentary emotion. They were not informed that they were assessed in response to non-treatment. Following their completion of the research protocol, participants were given entry to engage with the program animals for 10 minutes. All groups were provided extra credit vouchers to be turned into their professors.

Measures

Dependent variable: Moment-to-moment emotion. Immediately before entering the program area, students completed a 25-item scale rating the extent to which they experienced various positive and negative emotions *at that moment* on a 4-point Likert scale ranging from 0 (*not at all*) through 3 (*very much*). The measure used in the present study is based on the experienced sampling method (ESM; Csikszentmihalyi & Larson, 1987) and was utilized in several prior studies by the first author (Papp, Pendry, & Adam, 2009; Papp, Pendry, Simon, & Adam, 2013). The current version of the measure was derived based on data collected during a pilot study conducted by the author with a sample of similar college students during a prior round of PYSA program implementation, during which students completed 45-items measuring the similar moment-to-moment emotions. Researchers conducted a factor analysis using MPlus to reduce the number of variables in the measure, which resulted in four latent constructs including *anxious* (e.g., stressed, overwhelmed, worried, anxious, tense; $\alpha = 0.89$), *content* (e.g., calm, at peace, joyful, positive, at ease; $\alpha = 0.95$), *irritable* (e.g., frustrated, aggravated, agitated, irritable, pissed off; $\alpha = 0.66$), and *depressed* (e.g., depressed, sad, discouraged, unhappy, alone; $\alpha = 0.85$). Further reduction of the measure was then conducted in order to address duplicate items, redundant and/or ambiguous language. After duplicate items and highly correlated items were dropped, a repeated cycle of deletion and testing of remaining items was conducted resulting in each factor retaining 5 items with loadings greater than 0.70. Re-calculation of each of the factors based on current data and sample showed continued high internal reliability ($\alpha_{anxious} = 0.87$, $\alpha_{content} = 0.89$, $\alpha_{irritable} = 0.88$, and $\alpha_{depressed} = 0.86$, respectively).

In order to examine the potential role of state-level indices of emotional functioning as potential moderators of program effects on moment-to-moment indices of emotion, participants were asked to complete various reliable self-report measures at screening examining state-level indices of mental health symptomatology and disorder.

Depressive Symptomology. Depressive symptomology was measured using the Beck Depression Inventory (BDI: Beck, Steer & Brown, 1996), which consists of 21 items (*e.g., I feel sad, I cry all the time*) rated on a 4-point Likert scale, derived from symptoms and attitudes frequently expressed by clinically depressed individuals. There is strong support for the high reliability ($\alpha > 0.83$) of the measure with younger adults (Nezu, Ronan, Meadows, & McClure, 2000), which was echoed in our sample ($\alpha = 0.88$). Based on the guidelines of Beck *et al.* (1996) a composite depression score was calculated for each individual by summing rating scores across the 21 items, which was standardized for analyses.

Composite scores for total depression in our sample ranged from 0 to 46. According to Beck *et al.* (1996), scores were used to categorize participants into one of four levels of depressive symptoms: *minimally depressed* (0–13) (N = 130), *mild depression* (14–19) (N = 37), *moderate depression* (20–28) (N = 12), and *severe depression* (29–63) (N = 3). Moderate depression and above is typically considered clinical in the research setting. Additionally, the overall group mean level of depression (M = 9.7, SD = 6.9) suggests that the sample was experiencing minimal depression at the time of recruitment.

Anxiety. Anxiety was measured using the Beck Anxiety Inventory (BAI: Beck & Steer, 1993), a 21-item scale on a 4-point Likert scale (*0 = not all* to *3 = severely*) describing participants' common symptoms of anxiety (e.g., *numbness and tingling, sweating not due to heat,* and *fear of the worst happening*). The BAI shows excellent internal consistency with average coefficient α values of 0.88 (de Beurs, Wilson, Chambless, Goldstein, & Feske, 1997), which was echoed in our sample (α = 0.93). Scores were summed across the 21 items to create a composite anxiety score, which was standardized for analyses. According to Beck and Steer (1993) our sample contains individuals reporting *very low anxiety* (0–21) (N = 151), *moderate anxiety* (22–35) (N = 25), and individuals reporting *anxiety with potential cause for concern* (> 36) (N = 6). The overall group mean level of anxiety (M = 12.3, SD = 9.98) suggests that the sample was experiencing very low anxiety at the time of recruitment.

Worry. Worry was measured using the Penn State Worry Questionnaire (PSWQ; Meyer, Miller, Metzger, & Borkovec, 1990), a 16-item scale that assesses the frequency and associated ability to control worry, by asking participants to endorse statements (*i.e., I worry all the time, my worries overwhelm me*) on a 5-point Likert scale (*1 = not at all typical* to *5 = very typical*). Among participants with anxiety disorders, college students, and community samples, internal consistency of the PSWQ is excellent (α = 0.83–0.93; Brown, Antony, & Barlow, 1992), which was echoed in our sample (α = 0.93). The scoring procedures of Meyer *et al.* (1990) were followed in order to obtain a composite worry score for analysis. Our sample's mean level of worry was 53.8 (SD = 12.3), with mean levels of worry for females slightly higher than for males (M_{female} = 55.4, SD = 11.7; M_{male} = 44.5, SD = 12.1), echoing work by Meyer *et al.* (1990).

Perceived Stress. Perceived stress was measured with the abbreviated Perceived Stress Scale – 10 (PSS-10; Cohen, Kamarck & Mermelstein, 1983; Cohen & Williamson, 1988), asking participants to endorse 10 statements on a 5-point Likert scale (from 0 = *never* to 4 = *very often*) describing the extent to which events during the previous month were appraised as stressful (*e.g., how often have you felt nervous and stressed*). Internal consistency in our sample was higher than average α =0.70 (Lee, 2012) at α =0.86. Positive items were reverse-coded before summing across all 10 items to create a composite perceived stress score, which was standardized for analyses. Cohen *et al.* (1988) provide norm mean levels of perceived stress for 18–29 year olds in the general population with at least a junior high school education (M = 14.2, SD = 6.2), suggesting that perceived stress in our sample mean is higher at 18.95 (SD = 6.1). The elevated group mean in our sample could potentially be explained by differences in stress due to upcoming final examination week of our participants versus the everyday stresses experienced by the general public.

Analytic strategy

The following analytic strategy was used to demonstrate significant differences in momentary emotion between participants randomly assigned to either the PYSA experimental condition, the control condition or the waitlisted group. The intent-to-treat (ITT) multiple imputation and causal analyses of original and pooled data were conducted using IBM SPSS Statistics 22. The ITT analyses established a representation of group differences due to assigned intervention condition, rather than post-randomization characteristics in the proceeding analyses (Montori & Guyatt, 2001). We used five iterations of the data, and predicted missing ESM values using sample demographics and trait indices of students' emotional functioning including depression, anxiety, worry and perceived stress, which correlated with measures of momentary emotion at pre-test and post-test.

We conducted a set of analyses of variance (ANOVA) by intervention condition with a test of significance at α = 0.05 on pre-test data and post-test data for each emotion factor including feeling content, anxious, irritable and depressed. We included Tukey post-hoc pairwise comparisons to determine specific between-group differences in mean levels of emotion factors, and Cohen's *d* using pooled standard deviations to compare the magnitude of effects between groups. For those scales that main effects were not noted, we examined the effects of interactions between the condition to which participants were assigned and the state-level indices of emotional functioning including clinical levels of depression, anxiety, worry and perceived stress. Paired sample t-tests were also conducted to examine the mean level and significance of within-group differences from pre-test to post-test for each condition along with Cohen's *d* effect sizes, which are presented in the text.

Results

Pre-test group differences

We first conducted a series of t-tests to compare participants' demographic characteristics and state-level indices of emotional functioning across the three experimental conditions and found that there were no significant differences in class standing, $F(2, 180) = 1.88$, $p = 0.16$, gender, $F(2, 180) = 1.07$, $p = 0.34$, age, $F(2, 180) = 1.07$, $p = 0.35$, depression, $F(2, 180) = 0.90$, $p = 0.41$, anxiety, $F(2, 180) = 0.23$, $p = 0.79$, worry, $F(2, 180) = 0.47$, $p = 0.63$, or perceived stress, $F(2, 180) = 1.03$, $p = 0.36$, suggesting random distribution of participant characteristics across conditions was achieved as expected and intended.

To examine whether mean levels of students' moment-to-moment emotion at pretest were similar across treatment conditions, we then conducted an ANOVA by experimental condition on the original data, which indicated no significant differences by group assignment for feeling content, $F(2, 177) = 1.46$, $p = 0.24$; anxious, $F(2, 177) = 2.58$, $p = 0.08$; nor irritable, $F(2, 177) = 1.13$, $p = 0.33$. Unexpectedly, there were significant differences by group in the extent to which students reported feeling depressed, $F(2, 177) = 3.50$, $p = 0.03$. Specifically, a Tukey post-hoc analysis revealed that at pre-test, mean levels of feeling depressed were higher for students randomly assigned to the control group ($M = 0.49$, $SD = 0.56$), than those in the non-treatment group ($M = 0.26$, $SD = 0.72$; $d = 0.49$, $p = 0.02$). However, there were no significant differences in mean levels of feeling depressed between the experimental group ($M = 0.37$, $SD = 0.46$), and the control group ($d = -0.23$, $p = 0.30$), nor between the experimental group and non-treatment group ($d = 0.18$, $p = 0.43$). Given the presence of pre-existing differences at pretest for feeling depressed between the non-treatment and control groups, post-test differences between these groups must thus be interpreted cautiously.

Post-test group differences in moment-to-moment emotion

Feeling content. After students in each group completed their respective assigned treatments, ANOVA results demonstrated that post-test reports of the emotion factor *feeling content* using pooled estimates from the ITT analysis differed significantly by condition (Table 8.1). Tukey post-hoc analyses and effect size calculations indicated that students in the experimental condition reported significantly higher levels of feeling content at post-test, than students in the control group ($d = 0.65$, $p < 0.01$), and those in the non-treatment group ($d = 0.78$, $p < 0.001$). A within-group t-test showed that the mean increase in feeling content for those in the PYSA group was significant ($t = 6.75$, $p < 0.01$), with a moderate within-group effect ($d = 0.67$) indicating that 10 min of HAI increased students' content feelings. Finally, there were no significant or substantial between-group differences of feeling content at post-test between the control group, and the non-treatment group ($d = 0.12$, $p = 0.87$). Thus, we can conclude that participation in the PYSA program had a positive, significant, and substantive effect on the extent to which students felt content as hypothesized.

Feeling anxious. ANOVA results demonstrated that participants reported significant differences in the extent to which they experienced anxious feelings by group at post-test (Table 8.1). Post-hoc analyses and effect size calculations specified that those in the experimental group reported feeling significantly and substantially less anxious than those in the control condition ($d = -0.55$, $p < 0.01$). Similarly, the experimental group reported feeling significantly and

Table 8.1. Momentary Emotion Means and Standard Deviations in 3 groups at post-test with original (N = 167) and pooled estimates (N = 182) from the ITT analysis.

	Total	PYSA	Control	Non-treatment		
Emotion	*M (SD)*	*M (SD)*	*M (SD)*	*M (SD)*	*F*	*p*
Original data					(2, 166)	
Content	1.84 (0.81)	2.14 (0.71)	1.67 (0.87)	1.58 (0.73)	9.00	< 0.01***
Anxious	0.78 (0.72)	0.56 (0.59)	0.95 (0.80)	0.90 (0.75)	5.55	< 0.01**
Irritable	0.30 (0.51)	0.16 (0.31)	0.40 (0.62)	0.40 (0.58)	4.25	0.02*
Depressed	0.25 (0.42)	0.18 (0.35)	0.32 (0.48)	0.30 (0.44)	1.96	0.15
Pooled estimates					(2, 181)	
Content	1.83 (0.80)	2.14 (0.71)	1.67 (0.87)	1.61 (0.71)	9.30	< 0.01***
Anxious	0.78 (0.71)	0.56 (0.59)	0.95 (0.80)	0.88 (0.70)	5.74	< 0.01**
Irritable	0.32 (0.51)	0.16 (0.31)	0.39 (0.62)	0.44 (0.54)	5.44	< 0.01**
Depressed	0.26 (0.41)	0.18 (0.35)	0.32 (0.48)	0.31 (0.40)	2.28	0.11

Note. *p <0.05, **p < 0.01, ***p < 0.001

substantially less anxious at post-test compared to the non-treatment condition (d = –0.49, p = 0.03). The within-group t-test showed that the mean decrease in feeling anxious for those in the PYSA group was significant (t = –10.27, p < 0.01), with a large magnitude within-group effect size (d = 0.99), suggesting that participation in the intervention significantly and substantially decreased feelings of anxiety. Finally, there were no significant post-hoc differences between the control group and non-treatment group (d = 0.09, p =0.87). In sum, these results are consistent with our hypothesis suggesting that students who experienced 10 min of HAI felt significantly and substantially less anxious than those in either the control or non-treatment conditions.

Feeling irritable. Results indicate that groups also differed significantly on how irritable they felt at post-test by treatment condition (Table 8.1). The post-hoc analysis specified that participants in the experimental group felt significantly and moderately less irritable than those in the control group (d = –0.47, p = 0.03) and those in the non-treatment group (d = –0.64 p = 0.02). The within-group t-tests showed that those in the experimental group felt significantly and moderately less irritable (t = –4.21, p <0.01, d = 0.52) after the intervention than they did immediately before interacting with the animals. Levels of irritability of students in the non-treatment group were not significantly or substantially different compared to those experienced by students in the control group (d = –0.09, p = 0.91). These findings are consistent with our hypothesis, suggesting that participation in a 10 min interaction with cats and dogs significantly and substantially reduced feelings of irritability compared to watching a canine-feline themed slide presentation or not receiving any treatment.

Feeling depressed. There were no significant group differences in levels of feeling depressed at post-test (Table 8.1). The effect size comparing feeling depressed in the experimental group and the control group was not significant or substantial (d = –0.33, p = 0.15), nor was the effect size of the experimental and wait-list group comparison (d = –0.35, p =0.22). However, based on within-group comparisons, we found that participants in the experimental group reported significant and moderate decreases in feeling depressed immediately after program participation (t = –4.11, p < 0.01, d = –0.47), compared to before HAI interactions. There were no significant or substantial pre to post-test changes in levels of depressive feelings between students in the control group and non-treatment condition (d = 0.02, p =0.97). Although these results may appear promising, we cannot causally infer that the program caused decreases in feeling depressed.

Given the lack of main effects for depressive states, we explored whether this absence of main effects could be explained by participants' state levels of stress-related symptomatology. A post-hoc multivariate analysis of variance (MANOVA) was conducted to examine the extent to which treatment group and state-levels of clinical depression, perceived stress, worry and anxiety interacted to moderate the effects of the program on moment-to-moment levels of depression. We found no evidence to suggest that clinical levels of mental health symptomatology moderated momentary levels of depression of participants by treatment condition. In sum, we cannot infer that clinical levels of depression, perceived stress, worry or anxiety moderated post-test levels of moment-to-moment levels of depressive feelings by treatment condition.

Discussion

This study adds to an emerging body of literature on randomized controlled trials of college-based animal-assisted stress prevention programs on college students' emotional states and wellbeing. Overall, our results demonstrated support for our hypothesis, suggesting that the PYSA program was effective in positively influencing students' moment-to-moment emotion. Specifically, we found that 10 minutes of interaction time with dogs and/or cats significantly and substantially lowered self-reported feelings of anxiety and irritability in college students compared to either watching a silent slide presentation of animal pictures, or sitting quietly in a room for 10 minutes without socializing. Additionally, 10 minutes of HAI significantly and substantially increased feelings of contentment compared to either of the alternative treatment groups in which students did not engage in direct contact with live animals. These findings provide promising evidence to consider the continued use of universal, animal-assisted campus-based stress prevention programs aiming to reduce student stress. We did not find evidence to suggest that moment-to-moment feelings of sadness and depression were significantly impacted by any of the three treatment conditions nor that state levels of clinical depression, anxiety, and perceived stress moderated these effects. Given that there were preexisting differences in pretest levels of depressive feelings between the PYSA group and control group despite rigorous implementation of randomization, findings on main effects of HAI on depressive states remain inconclusive.

Strengths

This study constitutes a significant contribution by demonstrating significant causal effects of a universal, animal-assisted stress-prevention program on indices of moment-to moment well-being in a large sample of college students. Building on findings by Crossman and colleagues (2015), our findings extend results by Barker, Barker, McCain & Schubert (2016) who found that a 15-minute interaction with a therapy dog dramatically reduced undergraduate students' self-reported perceived stress. A strength of this study is that it represents the first randomized controlled trial examining the causal effects of a large-scale, campus-based, universal, animal-assisted stress prevention program on college students' emotional well-being in naturalistic settings. The study demonstrated large effect sizes providing robust support for the utilization of such programs in, at least temporarily, promoting healthier emotionality in college students during an academically stressful time in the semester. These findings are further enhanced by the large sample size, which allowed for ample power to detect the presence of main effects, as well as increased confidence in generalizing results to the broader population of college students, beyond those previously studied.

Another strength of this study is its support of programmatic effects influencing momentary emotional experiences. Extended, highly intense, or contextually inappropriate experiences of negative momentary emotions are associated with higher instances of psychological disorders related to depression (Doane *et al.*, 2013), anxiety and other phobias (Kashdan & Collins, 2010) and eating disorders (Macht & Simmons, 2011). Additionally, a review of the literature by Lyumbomirsky, King, & Diener (2005) found greater experiences of positive emotions in an individual's day-to-day life was associated with better life outcomes (i.e., financial success, relationships, mental and physical health) in addition to supporting resilience (Tugade, Fredrickson, & Feldman Barrett, 2004). This study has demonstrated that it is possible to influence moment-to-moment emotional states after only 10 minutes of human–animal interaction.

Limitations

Although we believe that there are associated benefits with changes in moment-to-moment emotion in response to AAAs, this study is limited in that it only examines one outcome. Without additional measures of the physiological correlates of momentary emotion, we are unable to determine whether the 10-minute interaction produces a change in emotional state that is substantive enough to also affect trait-level characteristics of students' emotional functioning and/or stress physiology thought to play a role in the development of psychopathology. This question remains unanswered at this time, as prior work by Barker and colleagues (2016) found that neither the 15-minute interaction or a 15-minute attention control condition exhibited any effect on students' salivary alpha-amylase levels at post-condition despite effects on perceived stress. This is important as stress reduction has important links to achievement-related outcomes, such as executive functioning and attitudes towards learning (Cerqueira, Mailliet, Almeida, Jay, & Sousa, 2007). In addition to studying the physiological correlates of momentary emotion and stress it will be important to address the impact of the AAA activity at the behavioral level (i.e., how the activity might have impacted the student's ability to concentrate when studying for their final exams). Additionally, a limitation of the current study is that the measures used for depression and anxiety only measure the associated symptoms from the state level, not the trait level. Although it is imperative that we examine the effects of AAAs on additional outcomes, this limitation extends beyond the present study and represents a limitation more indicative of the status of the field.

Additional limitations in this study can be viewed in terms of its participants and design. The sample was predominantly female, which appeared to be due to a lack of male candidates in the classrooms researchers sampled, rather than lack of male interest in participation. Additionally, although this study examines human–animal interaction, it is limited in its focus by only examining human outcomes. Future work should more comprehensively examine the effects of such implementation practices on the well-being of the animal participants, in addition to identifying the mechanisms that underlie these interventions (e.g., the quality of interaction between human and animal). Finally, the design of this study was not conducive to establishing mechanisms by which animal-assisted college-based programs are most effective. In order to support evidence-based implementation practices, future research is needed to examine the role of dosage, in order to determine at what point the benefits of these interactions occur (e.g., 5 min, 10 min, 15 min, etc.) and whether exposure has a cumulative effect are needed.

Conclusion

In conclusion, this study demonstrates the effectiveness of 10 minutes of human–animal interaction in increasing feelings of contentment and decreasing feelings of anxiety and irritability among college students, compared to viewing photos of cats and dogs or waiting quietly. Although promising, given our very limited understanding of the underlying mechanisms informing the effectiveness of such programs, and the inability of this study to adequately address such questions, the results of this study, and its design, should not be used as a "go-ahead" for implementation of animal-assisted campus-based programs. We must further examine the wellbeing of the animals, dosage, different populations, and most importantly gain a better understanding of which mechanisms of the program may be most relevant to its success, particularly unpacking the role of observing others enjoying the interaction. Additionally, future studies addressing the growing concerns for animal well-being may inform the design of programs, incorporating different types of interactions with animals beyond just physical and verbal contact.

Author note

This work was supported by a grant provided to the first author through the Research Initiative in Human Sciences grant number 21441312 sponsored by Academic Programs, Washington State University's Office of Research and Extension.

We would like to acknowledge the Washington State University Office of the Dean of Students personnel and their program volunteers for coordinating the Pet Your Stress Away program who made each program successful. Additionally, we would like to acknowledge the Whitman County Humane Society and their volunteers for providing the dogs and cats who participated in each student visitation program. We also thank all the Pet Your Stress Away Study volunteers, research assistants, and participants, without whom this study would not have been possible. This study is registered with ClinicalTrials.gov, registration number NCT02758886.

References

American College Health Association. (2014). *American College Health Association-National College Health Assessment II: Reference group executive summary fall 2013.* Hanover, MD: American College Health Association.

Adam, E. K. (2012). Emotion—cortisol transactions occur over multiple time scales in development: Implications for research on emotion and the development of emotional disorders. *Monographs of the Society for Research in Child Development, 77*, 17–27. doi:10.1111/j.1540-5834.2012.00657.x

Adamle, K. N., Riley, T. A., & Carlson, T. (2009). Evaluating college student interest in pet therapy. *Journal of American College Health, 57*(5), 545–548.

Baran, M. (2003, December 8). College kids go to the dogs. *USA Today.* P. 6D.

Barker, S. B., & Wolen, A. R. (2008). The benefits of human-companion animal interaction: a review. *Journal of Veterinary Medical Education, 35*, 487–95. doi:10.3138/jvme.35.4.487

Barker, S.B., Barker, R.T., McCain, N.L., & Schubert, C.M. (2016). A randomized cross-over exploratory study of the effect of visiting therapy dogs on college student stress before final exams. *Anthrozoös, 29*, 35–46. http://dx.doi.org/10.1080/08927936.2015.1069988

Beck, A. T., & Steer, R. A. (1993). *Beck Anxiety Inventory: Manual (2nd ed.)*. San Antonio, TX: The Psychiatric Corporation.

Beck, A. T., Steer, R. A., & Brown, G. K. (1996). *Manual for the Beck Depression Inventory* (2nd ed). San Antonio, TX: The Psychological Corporation.

Binfet, J., & Passmore, H. (2016). Hounds and homesickness: The effects of an animal-assisted therapeutic intervention for first-year university students. *Anthrozoös, 29*(3), 441–454. doi: 10.1080/08927936.2016.1181364

Breslau, J., Lane, M., Sampson, N., & Kessler, R. C. (2008). Mental disorders and subsequent educational attainment in a US national sample. *Journal of Psychiatry Research, 42*(9), 708–716. doi:10.1016/j.jpsychires.2008.01.016

Brown, T. A., Antony, M. M., & Barlow, D. H. (1992). Psychometric properties of the Penn State Worry Questionnaire in a clinical anxiety disorders sample. *Behaviour Research and Therapy, 30*, 33–37. doi:10.1016/0005-7967(92)90093-V

Cavazos, J. (2010, May 4). Pets offer relaxing study break for VCU students. *Victoria Advocate.* Retrieved from https://www.victoriaadvocate.com/news/2010/may/04/jc_furry_friends_050510_95177/

Cerqueira, J. J., Mailliet, F., Almeida, O. F., Jay, T. M., & Sousa, N. (2007). The prefrontal cortex as a key target of the maladaptive response to stress. *The Journal of Neuroscience, 27*(11), 2781–2787.

Cohen, S., Kamarck, T., & Mermelstein, R. (1983). A global measure of perceived stress. *Journal of Health and Social Behavior, 24*(4), 385–396. doi:10.2307/2136404

Cohen, S., & Williamson, G. (1988). Perceived stress in a probability sample of the United States. In S. Spacapan & S. Oskamp (Eds.), *The social psychology of health.* Newbury Park, CA: Sage.

Crossman, M. K., & Kazdin, A.E. (2015). Animal visitation programs in colleges and universities: An efficient model for reducing student stress. In A. Fine (Ed.), *Handbook on Animal-Assisted Therapy: Theoretical Foundations and Guidelines for Practice* (4th ed.) (pp. 333–340). San Diego, CA: Academic Press.

Crossman, M. K., Kazdin, A. E., & Knudson, K. (2015). Brief unstructured interaction with a dog reduces distress. *Anthrozoös, 28*, 649–659. http://dx.doi.org/10.1080/08927936.2015.10 70008

Csikszentmihalyi, M., & Larson, R. (1987). Validity and reliability of the experience-sampling method. *The Journal of Nervous and Mental Disease, 175*(9), 526–536. doi:10.1097/00005053-198709000-00004

Daniels, M. (2010, December 16). Stressed-out students' best friend – Bringing dogs to campus ahead of semester finals is one way to help ease the academic pressures of college. *St. Paul Pioneer Press*, p. B6 de Beurs, E., Wilson, K. A., Chambless, D. L., Goldstein, A. J., & Feske, U. (1997). Convergent and divergent validity of the Beck Anxiety Inventory for patients with panic disorder and agoraphobia. *Depression and Anxiety, 6*, 140–146.

Devlin, R. (2011, May 4). Not a ruff day for KU students on eve of final exams. Reading Eagle. Retrieved from http://www2.readingeagle.com/article.aspx?id=305587

Doane, L. D., Mineka, S., Zinbarg, R. E., Craske, M., Griffith, J. W., & Adam, E. K. (2013). Are flatter diurnal cortisol rhythms associated with major depression and anxiety disorders in late adolescence? The role of life stress and daily negative emotion. *Development and Psychopathology, 25*(03), 629–642.

Eisenberg, D., Golberstein, E., & Hunt, J. B. (2009). Mental health and academic success in college. *The B. E. Journal of Economic Analysis & Policy, 9*(1), 1–35. doi: 10.2202/1935-1682.2191

Fine, A. H. (Ed.). (2015). *Handbook on Animal Assisted Therapy: Theoretical Foundations and Guidelines for Practice* (3rd ed.). London, UK: Elsiever Academic Press.

Fox, E. (2010, September 15). Sonoma state welcomes therapy dogs to campus. *Sonoma St. Star.* Retrieved from http://www.sonomastatestar.com/features/sonoma-state-welcomes-therapy-dogs-to-campus-1.1598761

Friedmann, E., Katcher, A. H., Lynch, J. J., & Thomas, S. A. (1980). Animal companions and one-year survival of patients after discharge from a coronary care unit. *Public Health Reports, 95*(4), 307–312.

Gaterud, A. (2011, May 5). Gone to the dogs. *Star Tribune*. p. 01E.

Gilbert, D. G., Stunkard, M. E., Jensen, R. A., Detwiler, F. R. J., & Martinko, J. M. (1996). Effects of exam stress on mood, cortisol, and immune functioning: Influences of neuroticism and smoker-non-smoker status. *Personality and Individual Differences, 21*(2), 235–246.

Grant, K. E., McMahon, S. D., Carter, J. S., Carleton, R. A., Adam, E. K., & Chen, E. (2014). The influence of stressors on the development of psychopathology. In M. Lewis & K. D. Rudolph (Eds.), *Handbook of Developmental Psychopathology* (pp. 205–223). New York: Springer Press. doi:10.1007/978-1-4614-9608-3_11

Hediger, K., & Beetz, A. (2015). The role of human-animal interactions in education. In J. Zinsstag, E. Schelling, D. Waltner-Toews, M. Whittaker, & M. Tanner (Eds.) *One health: The theory and practice of integrated health approaches* (pp. 73–84). Wallingford, UK: CABI. doi:10.1079/9781780643410.0073

Henry, F. (2008, March 8). Whole lotta solace in a fur coat: Kent students' worries fade when dogs arrive. *Cleveland Plain Dealer,* p. E1.

Hunt, J., & Eisenberg, D. (2010). Mental health problems and help-seeking behavior among college students. *Journal of Adolescent Health, 46*(1), 3–10. doi:10.1016/j.jadohealth.2009.08.008

Kashdan, T. B., & Collins, R. L. (2010). Social anxiety and the experience of positive emotion and anger in everyday life: An ecological momentary assessment approach. *Anxiety, Stress, & Coping, 23*(3), 259–272.

Kessler, R. C. (2011). The costs of depression. *Psychiatric Clinics of North America, 35*(1), 1–14. doi:10.1016/j.psc.2011.11.005.

Kruger, K.A., McCune, S., & Merrill, R. (2011). In J. Serpell & S. McCune (Eds.), *WALTHAM® Pocket Book of Human-Animal Interactions.* London, U.K.: Beyond Design Solutions. www.waltham.com/dyn/_assets/_pdfs/waltham-booklets/Human-AnimalInteractionsBookletElectronicversion.pdf

Lee, E. (2011). Review of the psychometric evidence of the Perceived Stress Scale. *Asian Nursing Research, 6*(4), 121–127. doi:10.1016/j.anr.2012.08.004

Lyubomirsky, S., King, L., & Diener, E. (2005). The benefits of frequent positive affect: Does happiness lead to success?. *Psychological Bulletin, 131*(6), 803–855. doi:10.1037/0033–2909.131.6.803

Macht, M., & Simons, G. (2011). Emotional eating. In I. Nyklíček, A. Vingerhoets, & M. Zeelenberg (Eds.) *Emotion regulation and well-being* (pp. 281–295). New York: Springer.

Meyer, T. J., Miller, M. L., Metzger, R. L., & Borkovec, T. D. (1990). Development and validation of the Penn State Worry Questionnaire. *Behaviour Research and Therapy, 28*, 487–495. doi:10.1016/0005-7967(90)90135-6

Montori, V. M., & Guyatt, G. H. (2001). Intention-to-treat principle. *Canadian Medical Association Journal, 165*(10), 1339–1341. Retrieved from http://www.cmaj.ca/content/165/10/1339.short

Nezu, A. M., Ronan, G. F., Meadows, E. A., & McClure, K. S. (Eds.) (2000). *Practitioner's guide to empirically based measures of depression.* New York: Kluwer Academic Publishers.

Ng, V., Koh, D., & Chia, S. E. (2003). Examination stress, salivary cortisol, & academic performance. *Psychological Reports, 93*(3), 1133–4. doi: 10.2466/pr0.2003.93.3f.1133

Ng, Z. Y., Pierce, B. J., Otto, C. M., Buechner-Maxwell, V. A., Siracusa, C., & Were, S. R. (2014). The effect of dog–human interaction on cortisol and behavior in registered animal-assisted activity dogs. *Applied Animal Behaviour Science, 159*, 69–81. doi:10.1016/j.applanim.2014.07.009

Novak, B. (2010, May 5). Finals stressing you out? See the 'Counseling Canines.' *Capital Times.* Retrieved from http://host.madison.com/news/local/education/university/finals-stressing-you-out-see-the-counseling-canines/article_58f36eee-56c4-11df-a80f-001cc4c03286.html

Palmateer, J. (2010, May 12). Dogs give students reason to smile before finals. *Daily Star.* Retrieved from http://www.thedailystar.com/news/local_news/article_3fa7c4d9-2a44-57ab-a891-947b28cfe00f.html

Papp, L. M., Pendry, P., & Adam, E. K. (2009). Mother-adolescent Physiological Synchrony in Naturalistic Settings: Within-Family Cortisol Associations and Moderators. *Journal of Family Psychology, 23*(6), 882–894. doi:10.1037/a0017147

Papp, L. M., Pendry, P., Simon, C. D., & Adam, E. K. (2013). Spouses' cortisol associations and moderators: Testing physiological synchrony and connectedness in everyday life. *Family Process, 52*, 284–298. doi:10.1111/j.1545-5300.2012.01413.x

Pendry, P., Carr, A. M., Smith, A. N., & Roeter, S. M. (2014a). Improving adolescent social competence and behavior: A randomized trail of an 11-week equine facilitated learning prevention program. *Journal of Primary Prevention, 35*(4), 281–293. doi:10.1007/s10935-014-0350-7

Pendry, P., Smith, A. N., & Roeter, S. M. (2014b). Randomized trial examines effects of equine facilitated learning on adolescents' basal cortisol levels. *Human-Animal Interaction Bulletin, 2*, 80–95.

Peterson, C., Park, N., & Seligman, M. E. P. (2005). Orientations to happiness and life satisfaction: The full life versus the empty life. *Journal of Happiness Studies, 6*, 25–41. doi:10.1007/s10902-004-1278-z

Reynolds, J. & Rabschutz, L. (2011). Studying for exams just got more relaxing—animal-assisted activities at the University of Connecticut library. *College & Undergraduate Libraries, 18*, 359–367. doi:10.1080/10691316.2011.624934

Riggenbach, A. (2010, January 25). Dogs on campus program brings a part of home to school. *eInside.* Retrieved from http://einside.kent.edu/?type=art& id=92387

Souter, M. A. & Miller, M. D. (2007). Do Animal-Assisted Activities effectively treat depression? A meta-analysis. *Anthrozöös, 20*(2), 167–180. doi: 10.2752/175303707X207954

Thomson, S. C. (2003, September 24). Furry Maryville U. visitors get their licks in – Pet "therapy" aids students. *St. Louis Post-Dispatch.* p. C8.

Trunnell, D. P. (2010, December 2). Cal State holds pet therapy event. *Redlands Daily Facts.* Retrieved from http://www.redlandsdailyfacts.com/general-news/20101202/cal-state-holds-pet-therapy-event

Tugade, M. M., Fredrickson, B. L., & Feldman Barrett, L. (2004). Psychological resilience and positive emotional granularity: Examining the benefits of positive emotions on coping and health. *Journal of Personality, 72*(6), 1161–1190.

Wheeler, E. A., & Faulkner, M. E. (2015). The "pet effect". *Society & Animals,* 1–14. doi:10.1163/15685306-12341374

Wilkes, J. K (2009). *The role of companion animals in counseling and psychology: Discovering their use in the therapeutic process.* Springfield, IL: Charles C Thomas Pub Ltd.

Wilson, E. O. (1984). *Biophilia: the human bond with other species.* Cambridge, MA: Harvard University Press.

9 Effect of Pet Interaction on Stress Reduction and Positive Mood Enhancement among Pet-Owners and Non-Owners

Aliya Khalid* and Saadia Dildar
Government College University, Lahore, Pakistan

Abstract
The present study investigated the effect of pet interaction on stress reduction and positive mood enhancement among pet-owners and non-owners. Sample of pet-owners (n = 90) and non-owners (n = 90) was taken from University of Veterinary and Animal Sciences, Lahore. Both male and female participants were included in the sample. The instruments used were Short Stress State Questionnaire (Helton, 2004), Brief Mood Introspection Scale (Mayer & Gaschke, 1988) and Pet Interaction Observation Checklist. Data was statistically analyzed by one way Analysis of Variance and Independent Sample t-test. Reduction in stress and increase in positive mood were found for both pet-owners and non-owners for the pet interaction groups as compared to control groups. However, no significant differences were found between the dog interaction group and cat interaction group for both pet-owners and non-owners. Moreover, pet-owners had lower scores on stress and higher scores on positive mood after pet interaction as compared to non-owners. Lastly, it was shown that individuals who interacted with pets for more than five minutes had lower scores on stress and higher scores on positive mood as compared to those who interacted for five minutes or less. The findings have implications for Animal Assisted Therapy for psychological well-being.

Keywords: pet interaction, stress reduction, positive mood enhancement, pet-owners, non-owners

The physical and psychological health both are indispensable for the effective functioning of an individual (Berli, Loretini, Radtke, Hornung, & Scholz, 2014; Coyne & van Sonderen, 2012; Goyal, Singh, & Sibinga, 2014). Researchers have tried to find different ways of dealing effectively with various health-related problems. Moreover, they have focused on finding ways to promote healthy behaviors and improve overall life quality. While many techniques and habits were found to be quite effective, there has been an increasing interest in how companion animals affected human health. Many studies have supported the positive association between human–animal interaction (HAI) and improved well-being.

With respect to the recent research trends in human–animal interaction, researchers carried out experimental studies to show the health benefits of interacting with pets. Among the various benefits, one was shown with regard to stress. Irrespective of ownership, pet interaction was associated with reduced stress in individuals

*Corresponding author: email:aliyakhalidpsy@gmail.com

(Hoffmann et al., 2009; Polheber & Matchock, 2014; Wells & Perrine, 2001; Wright et al., 2015). Moreover, companion animals (or pets) were found associated with experiencing more positive emotions and hence, having an overall enhanced positive mood (Johnson, Meadows, Haubner, & Sevedge, 2008; Kaminski, Pellino, & Wish, 2002; Lutwack-Bloom, Wijewickrama, & Smith, 2005). This was one of the reasons for pet keeping being more common. It was observed to be wide-spread among various societies (Serpell & Paul, 2011; Shipman, 2010).

Pets as attachment figures

With regard to differentiating between an untamed animal and a pet, Serpell (2011) provided a definition. According to him, a pet offered no particular function but was still adopted for a number of reasons. These included personal preference, status indication and simply being more appreciative of their presence in world. Attachment with pet also had certain characteristics. Melson (1989) viewed it as a distinctive relationship that an owner had with their pet. It included spending time, carrying out different activities, showing love and interest, having extensive knowledge about how to take care of pet and feeling responsible for their every need (Melson, 1989).

An individual's relationship with their pet had qualities similar to relationships found with other individuals. A number of studies showed that pets acted as attachment figures when it came to humans. Moreover, the pets reciprocated this relationship (Beck & Madresh, 2008; Zilcha-Mano, Mikulincer, & Shaver, 2011). Crawford, Worsham, and Swinehart (2006) proposed that pet attachment shared significant attributes of Bowlby's attachment theory (Bowlby, 1984).

It was previously believed that attachments among people were formed only with their primary care-takers. However, recently it was shown that attachment relationships were also newly formed in adulthood. In such cases, the partners functioned as attachment figures for one another (Doherty & Feeney, 2004; Feeney, 2004). Moreover, other comfort sources or figures also played a significant role in the attachment development for an individual. These included therapists (Mallinckrodt, Gantt, & Coble, 1995) and even different leaders belonging to organizations (Davidovitz, Mikulincer, Shaver, Izsak, & Popper, 2007). This attachment wasn't only limited to people; individuals formed significant bonds even with symbolic figures, such as God (Granqvist, Mikulincer, & Shaver, 2010; Rom & Mikulincer, 2003).

Zilcha-Mano et al. (2011) took into account these findings and suggested that the relationship between a pet and its owner was similar to the attachment relationship between humans. They also found out that pets fulfilled the four pre-requisites that defined an attachment figure. Pets served as safe haven for owners, provided a secure base, encouraged maintaining proximity and resulted in distress when separated (Zilcha-Mano et al., 2011).

Cohen's (1988) social buffering hypothesis highlighted how social support protected individuals from stressful situations under some conditions. This buffering role prevented the individual from appraising the situation as stressful. Secondly, social support promoted healthy behaviors that further reduced stress. Thus, pets served to provide support to individuals by functioning as effective protective figures.

With regard to pet-owners, it was found that they reported feeling close to their pets as well as actively seeking more closure and enjoying it (Kurdek, 2009). With pets, owners felt safe and confident enough to explore their environment (Kurdek, 2008). Pet-owners also felt that they could depend on their pets to provide comfort and relief when they felt distressed (Allen, Balscovich, & Mendes, 2002; McConnell, Brown, Shoda, Stayton, & Colleen, 2011). Losing a pet was actually distressing for most owners and even triggered a grieving period (Hunt, Al-Awadi, & Johnson, 2008; Kwong & Bartholomew, 2011).

Recently, pets were found to increasingly become an important part of many people's lives. Approximately 85% individuals considered pets to be a family member. Other family members also treated them as importantly in the household (Cohen, 2002). So, it was only natural to assume that they had such profound beneficial effects for their owners.

Cross-cultural variations in attitude towards pets

By taking into account anthropology literature, changes in pet keeping with respect to forms and popularity were observed. The term, pet, in itself has changed with respect to meaning in various societies across world with time (Herzog, 2014).

Many different animals were considered as pets, depending upon the specific society and region (Serpell, 2003). For most cultures, dog was most popularly kept as pet. Even then, differences existed in the way that dogs were treated. In a study by Gray and Young (2011), out of sixty cultures and societies, fifty-three kept dogs. However, only twenty-two reported bonding with their dogs as pets.

Differences in pet attachment were reported for Asian countries. According to Xiaoqiong (2008), Asians, particularly Chinese, had comparatively lower levels of pet attachment bonds. They mostly chose to keep pets for the purpose of protection. However, many accepted pets for reasons other than just providing protection. In a study by Kanamori, Kawashima, Kuwabara, and Macer (2001), 36% individuals reported pets as important members of their families; 17% individuals considered them as friends.

Pet keeping was found to be a common practice among Muslim countries. However, some animals were less likely to be kept as pets as compared to others. Moreover, health benefits associated with pet keeping were found to be fairly less. Among pets, dog was a point of controversy due to the religious beliefs. Muslims preferred dogs as pets less as compared to other religious groups. Al-Fayez, Awadalla, Templer, and Arikawa (2003) found that as compared to Americans, Muslims in Kuwait had lesser positive attitude toward pet keeping. In Tanzania, Christian families more readily adopted dogs as pets as compared to the Muslim families (Knobel, Laurenson, Kazwala, Boden, & Cleaveland, 2008).

The reason for this difference in attitude for Muslims toward pets was due to Islamic teachings. An animal was kept based on the purpose it served. This purpose was judged by important benefits that they provided for humans. These benefits at the simplest included assisting in hunting and providing protection. That is why dogs were generally condemned and people avoided keeping them at home for reasons other than herding and providing safety (Akhtar, 2013). It was also discouraged to form any emotional bond with dogs as they were considered unclean. Therefore, while pets were considered as important family members by people of many European countries, the same wasn't true for Muslim countries (Al-Fayez et al., 2003). However, this attitude toward pets among Muslims varied from region to region. Turkish individuals viewed pets more positively (Prokop, Ozel, & Usak, 2009).

Pet and stress reduction

Stress is an interaction between a person and their environment, appraised as demanding or exceeding available resources and that endangered overall well-being (Lazarus & Folkman, 1984). While many factors contributed to reducing stress, interacting with pets lowered the levels significantly. Studies showed that petting a companion animal resulted in reduced anxiety. It held true for even those individuals who had different attitudes and opinions toward animals (Barker, Knisely, McCain, Schubert, & Pandurangi, 2005; Lang, Jansen, Wertenauer, Gallinat, & Rapp, 2010; Shiloh, Sorekt, & Terkel, 2010; Tsai, Friedmann, Sue, & Thomas, 2015).

One of the major reasons for this stress reducing impact of pet interaction was attributed to oxytocin level changes within individuals. Oxytocin was a hormone associated with many positive effects on human body that included feeling relaxed and calm, experiencing greater closeness to others and feeling reduced stress. Interacting with a pet increased oxytocin levels as well as decreased heart rate (Friedmann, Thomas, Son, Chapa, & McCune, 2013; Miller et al., 2015).

Contrary to popular belief, pet-owners didn't benefit from only interacting with their pets. Interacting with an unknown pet also led to significant stress reduction (Wilson, 1991). A study by Raina, Waltner-Toews, Bonnet, Woodward, and Abernathy (1999) showed that interacting with pets kept both pet-owners and non-owners, physically active and led to reduced health deterioration.

Furthermore, this reduction in elevated levels of stress as a result of pet interaction was observed in first few minutes (Barker et al., 2005). Handlin et al. (2011) found that the levels of oxytocin significantly increased between one and five minutes after interaction with pet.

Pets also functioned as better supportive figures when compared to friends and spouses in certain conditions. This led to lowest reactivity to physical symptoms of stress and quicker recovery (Allen et al., 2002).

Pet and positive mood enhancement

According to Pychyl (2010), beneficial companionship developed between human and pet. Interacting with pets led to increase in positive affect, irrespective of history with pets (Johnson et al., 2008; Kaminski et al., 2002; Lutwack-Bloom et al., 2005). Pets reduced negativity among their owners and served as important social support resources (McConnell et al., 2011). Increase in oxytocin levels and decrease in cortisol, epinephrine and norepinephrine levels attributed to this increase in positive emotions (Cole, Gawlinski, Steers, & Kotlerman, 2007; Odendaal & Meintjes, 2003). Individuals involved in direct interaction with a dog reported significant increases in experiencing positive mood. However, all participants reported a decline in negative affect, irrespective of the condition (Picard, 2015).

Several reasons were found for this mood enhancing effect of interacting with pets. Pets provided unconditional love and support. They offered a sense of stability and security. Many people felt that they trusted their pets to help them in times of distress (Sharkin & Bahrick, 1990). Moreover, they caused significant biological changes. Beetz, Kotrschal, Hediger, Turner, and Uvnas-Moberg (2011) found that a friendly dog's support resulted in reducing the cortisol levels. And this decrease was found to be even more than when support was given by a human.

Differences between pet-owners and non-owners

Certain studies indicated differences between pet-owners and non-owners on different dimensions of well-being, including stress and mood. Staats, Sears, and Pierfelice (2006) reported that pet-owners believed in and experienced more health benefits as compared to non-owners. Owning and having a bond with one's pet provided well-being benefits for the owner just like any other person. Indeed, research showed that people viewed their pets as social supportive figures when they felt lonely, since pets served as important attachment figures (Zilcha-Mano et al., 2011). This led to buffering the impact of stressful situation and enhancing mood. Furthermore, pet-owners fared better when it came to individual differences as well as well-being. These included being more optimistic and active as well as having reduced health problems such as high blood pressure (McConnell et al., 2011).

Another possible explanation for the observed health benefits was the lifestyle of pet-owners. They were more physically active than non-owners, especially when the pet was a dog (Duncan & Fraser, 1997). Moreover, the bond with one's pet provided a sense of fulfillment and a purpose.

Differences between dog and cat owners

Smolkovic, Fajfar, and Mlinaric (2012) reported a higher frequency for ownership of dogs and cats as pets, with a higher pet attachment existing for dogowners. Winefield, Black, and Chur-Hansen (2008) also reported a higher frequency for dog-owners. Cats were not perceived as strongly a supportive pet as dog. However, they were found to be more effective at providing support as compared to other types of pets (such as birds or fish).

With respect to health benefits, Siegel (1990) found that dog-owners dealt better with stressful events in life. In addition, dog-owners spent more time with their pets as they found them an important part of their lives. As a result, dogs provided their owners with greater companionship as compared to other pets and acted as stronger attachment figures. Bao (2016) further found that dog-owners scored higher on all well-being measures as compared to cat-owners.

Personality and pet-preference

Among many attributes of an individual, personality also played an important role in determining the type of pet they kept or preferred. Orford (1994) explained how people interacted with others in a manner similar to their own personality traits. A dominant person interacted with individuals having more submissive personalities since it allowed for their dominant nature to shine through without any threat. Similarly, physically active individuals interacted with other active people because they engaged in the same consistent expression, without threatening each other.

With pets, people also interacted in ways consistent with their nature. An active person preferred dogs as it encouraged the active lifestyle. Similarly, an individual who didn't need as much of an active lifestyle preferred a cat as it fit in with their requirements and needs. Many other factors still influenced the interaction such as characteristics of pet (Houpt, Honig, & Reisner, 1996; New et al., 2000), individual differences and owner's lifestyle (Arkow & Dow, 1984). In addition, the owner's need for dominance in the pet-owner relationship dictated the quality of interaction. Less dominant owners showed more affection to their pets. Hence, the relationship depended on the owner's personality as well as the pet characteristics in accordance to the owner's needs (Woodwarda & Bauerb, 2007).

Indigenous Researches

With respect to indigenous researches, no work has investigated health benefits of interacting with pets. So far, only one published study with respect to human–animal interaction showed that pet-owners with higher pet attachment reported higher empathy as compared to those with lower pet attachment (Khalid & Naqvi, 2016). It was important to address this lack of indigenous published studies regarding the impact of animals as pets in order to better understand their impact with respect to the present culture.

Rationale

Many studies conducted with regard to human–animal interaction highlighted the beneficial effect of interacting with pets, especially with regard to reducing stress and enhancing mood (Berget, Ekeberg, Pedersen, & Braastad 2011; Handlin et al., 2011; Lutwack-Bloom et al., 2005; McConnell et al., 2011; Miller et al., 2015; Shiloh et al., 2010). Any country where pet keeping was fairly common needed to be considered for further studies. It was important to find out the role that pets played in the people's lives, rather than just being a static addition to their routine. Thus, the importance of investigating relevant hypotheses in a culture like that of Pakistan's couldn't be highlighted enough. It reflected other ways that the animal resources could be put to better and more humane uses (such as therapy and educational reform). Thus, this study examined the impact of interacting with pets on stress reduction and positive mood enhancement in the present society and context. It also compared this interaction effect for pet-owners and non-owners and highlighted any differences (or similarities) that existed respectively.

Furthermore, cultural differences existed with regard to pet-keeping and its possible beneficial effects. Individualistic cultures had greater pet attachment and resulting health benefits as compared to collectivistic cultures. Muslim societies, in particular, exhibited lower attachment to their pets and didn't experience as many benefits. Dogs were especially viewed unfavorably as pets (Al-Fayez et al., 2013; Knobel et al. 2008). Religious restrictions imposed on keeping dogs played a crucial role (Akhtar, 2013). On the other hand, dogs were kept popularly as pets in many other countries (Smolkovic et al., 2012; Winefield et al., 2008). The present study was carried out in a Muslim country and hence, it brought to light the current standing regarding pet preferences and identified health benefits.

Significance of the study

This study holds tremendous significance in the psychological as well as physical health area. The findings will be significant in highlighting the importance of companion animals as effective tools in therapeutic settings. They will also serve in increasing health benefits of individuals who may not actually own any pets and those individuals who find it hard to afford therapy (Shiloh et al., 2010).

Furthermore, it will lay down the foundation for human–animal interaction within the present society and culture which may be used further to establish grounds for Animal-Assisted Therapy (Nimer & Lundahl, 2007). These beneficial effects of pet interaction will also prove to be helpful in the educational settings. It has been shown that pets promoted emotional development and increased empathy among individuals (Daly & Morton, 2006; Thompson & Gullone, 2003). This will further prove to be helpful in the rehabilitation of individuals in correctional facilities such as jails. In addition, it will help individuals with limited social skills or those unable to function well socially, such as children with autism (Carlisle, 2014).

Method

Objectives

The objectives of the present study are as follows:

To investigate the effect of pet interaction on stress reduction and positive mood enhancement among pet-owners and non-owners.

To investigate time differences for pet interaction and its relationship with stress reduction and positive mood enhancement.

Hypotheses

The hypotheses of the present study are as follows:

Pet interaction will lead to stress reduction and positive mood enhancement for both pet-owners and non-owners.

Stress reduction and positive mood enhancement will be greater after interaction with dog as compared to cat.

Pet-owners will have greater stress reduction and positive mood enhancement as a result of pet interaction as compared to non-owners.

Participants interacting with pets for more than five minutes will have greater stress reduction and positive mood enhancement as compared to those interacting for less than five minutes.

Research design

It was an experimental pretest-posttest study with between-subject design. A pre- and post- measure was taken for stress and mood to highlight any changes that may have occurred as a result of the interaction.

Sample

A sample of 180 students was collected from the pet clinic and the BS (Hons) programs at University of Veterinary and Animal Sciences (UVAS), Lahore. It consisted of young adults in the age range of 18 to 26 years. The data was collected from the sample by using purposive sampling technique. Consent was taken from the participants. The inclusion and exclusion criteria were highlighted as follows:

Inclusion criteria

Participants should currently own a pet, based on their own interest rather than that of someone else's (such as family member); they should be actively involved in taking care of it (including giving food, playing, petting, financially investing, taking for regular medical check-ups etc.) (for pet-owners).

Participants should have a general favorable attitude (including interest, lack of fear, being able to pet etc.) toward animals (for non-owners). It was assessed with the help of verbal questioning before determining to include the participant in the study.

Participants should be at least within the age range of 18 to 26 years.

Exclusion criteria

Individuals with serious health problems (both physical and psychological) will not be included (for pet-owners and non-owners).

Individuals with severe animal phobias will not be included (for non-owners).

Demographic characteristics of the sample

The following table shows the frequencies and percentages for the demographic variables obtained for the sample. Table 9.1 illustrates the various demographics obtained for the sample of pet-owners ($n = 90$) and non-owners ($n = 90$). Age range was found to be 18 to 26.

Instruments

In addition to a demographic sheet, two instruments were used in the present study. Short

Table 9.1. Demographic Profile of the Sample (*N* = 180).

Variables	Pet-Owners (*n* = 90) *f*(%)	Non-Owners (*n* = 90) *f*(%)	Total (*n* = 180) *f*(%)
Gender			
Men	45(50)	45(50)	90(50)
Women	45(50)	45(50)	90(50)
Family Monthly Income (PKR)			
10,000 – 50,000	57(63.3)	76(84.4)	133(78.8)
50,001 – 100,000	30(33.3)	14(15.5)	44(24.4)
Above 100,000	3(3.3)	–	3(1.6)
Marital Status			
Single	88(97.8)	88(97.8)	176(97.7)
Married/In relationship	2(2.2)	2(2.2)	4(2.2)
Residential Area			
Rural	49(45.6)	51(56.7)	100(55.5)
Urban	41(54.4)	39(43.3)	80(44.4)
Type of pet (owned/preferred)			
Dog	32(28.3)	42(40.4)	74(34.1)
Cat	45(39.8)	44(42.3)	89(41.0)
Parrot	19(16.8)	5(4.8)	24(11.1)
Others (i.e. rabbit, pigeon, cow, lion, hen, horse)	17(15.0)	13(12.5)	30(13.8)
Level of comfort with pets			
1 – 4 (low comfort level)	1(1.1)	12(7.0)	13(7.2)
5 – 7 (moderate comfort level)	14(15.5)	51(56.6)	65(36.1)
8 – 10 (high comfort level)	75(83.3)	27(30)	102(56.6)
No. of pets at home			
1	45(50)	–	–
2 – 3	23(25.5)	–	
4 or more	22(24.4)	–	
Time spent with pet daily			
Thirty minutes to three hours	28(32.2)	–	
Four to six hours	32(35.5)	–	
More than six hours	29(32.2)	–	–
Duration of pet presence at home			
Six months to one year	41(45.5)	–	–
Two years	19(21.1)	–	–
More than two years	30(33.3)	–	
Money spent on pets monthly			
500 – 2000	19(21.1)	–	
2001 – 5000	51(56.6)	–	
More than 5000	20(22.2)	–	
Pet Interaction Observation Checklist			
Pet interacted with			
Dog	30(33.3)	30(33.3)	60(33.3)
Cat	30(33.3)	30(33.3)	60(33.3)
Control	30(33.3)	30(33.3)	60(33.3)
Time duration of interaction			
1 – 4 minutes	9(15.0)	10(16.6)	19(15.8)
5 – 7 minutes	28(46.6)	42(70.0)	70(58.3)
8 minutes or more	23(38.3)	8(13.3)	31(25.8)

Continued

Table 9.1. Continued.

Variables	Pet-Owners (*n* = 90) *f*(%)	Non-Owners (*n* = 90) *f*(%)	Total (*n* = 180) *f*(%)
Type of interaction			
Stroking	48(37.2)	49(52.1)	97(43.5)
Talking	39(30.5)	30(31.9)	69(12.5)
Hugging	34(26.3)	13(13.8)	47(21.1)
Kissing	8(6.2)	2(2.1)	10(4.5)
Level of proximity			
Holding the pet	57(95.5)	50(83.3)	107(89.2)
Sitting near the pet	3(5.0)	9(15.0)	12(10.0)
Standing near the pet	–	–	
Standing at short distance (less than five feet)	–		
Interacting from a greater distance (more than five feet)	–	1(1.6)	1(0.83)
Level of perceived comfort			
1 – 4 (low comfort level)	1(1.6)	–	1(0.83)
5 – 7 (moderate comfort level)	5(8.3)	6(10.0)	11(9.2)
8 – 10 (high comfort level)	54(90)	54(90)	108(90.0)

Note. % = Percentage.

Stress State Questionnaire was used to get a pre and post measure of stress. Brief Mood Introspection Scale was used to get a measure of the prevailing mood. In addition, a Pet Interaction Observation Checklist was used to observe and record the different behaviors of participants during the interaction.

Demographic sheet. The demographics were included in the demographic sheet after reviewing the available literature, which showed a significant relationship of the demographics with pet interaction, stress reduction and positive mood enhancement. The demographics included were age, gender, education, family monthly income, marital status, residential area, type of pet owned, level of comfort with pets/animals in general, number of pets, time spent with pets, duration of pet presence at home and amount spent on pet.

Short Stress State Questionnaire (SSSQ). SSSQ, developed by Helton (2004), is a self-report scale which measures level of stress before, during and after performance of a task. It has twenty-four questions each for state pre-questionnaire and state post-questionnaire. They are rated on a five-point Likert scale from "Not at all" to "Extremely". The three categories of the scale are task engagement ($\alpha = 0.77$), distress ($\alpha = 0.75$), and worry ($\alpha = 0.72$), each having eight number of items. There is no total score calculated for the instrument. Rather, the mean for each subscale is taken individually. Lower score on engagement and higher scores on distress and worry indicate higher level of stress. Confirmatory factor analysis provided a measure for construct validity. Items in each factor loaded higher than the cut-off value of 0.35. The three-factor structure was supported.

Brief Mood Introspection Scale (BMIS). BMIS, developed by Mayer and Gaschke (1988), is a mood scale consisting of 16 mood-adjectives. They are rated on a four-point Likert scale, from "definitely do not feel" to "definitely feel". With regard to scoring, responses for active, calm, caring, content, happy, lively, loving, and peppy are added up. The responses for drowsy, fed up, gloomy, grouchy, jittery, nervous, sad, and tired are reverse-scored and then added up. Finally, a total score for pleasant mood is obtained by adding the initial total and the reverse-scored items total. Higher scores indicate more pleasant mood. Cronbach's alpha reliabilities ranged from 0.76 to 0.83. The scale also has good factor validity with a value of 37.4%.

Pet Interaction Observation Checklist (PIOC). A Pet Interaction Observation Checklist was designed to observe and measure the time and different behaviors engaged in by the participants during pet interaction. It was designed keeping in views the behaviors that were commonly found to occur in the interaction between a pet and their respective owner. Development of PIOC guidance was taken from the theoretical and empirical literature on pet interaction (Handlin et al., 2011; Raina et al., 1999; Shiloh et al., 2010). Moreover, the checklist was then sent to three overseas researchers who were working in the area of human–animal interaction. Inter-rater reliability was determined based on whether the researchers thought the items needed revision or not. As per the feedback, suggestions were taken into consideration after careful evaluation, the necessary changes were made and the checklist was finalized. It was further refined after pilot testing. It included the pet interacted with, the time for which the participant interacted with pet, type of interaction (stroking, hugging, talking, kissing), level of proximity and level of observed comfort with pet animal.

Table 9.2 shows the inter-rater reliability for PIOC. It was found that the raters agreed sufficiently with respect to the items, except for items 3 and 4. Suggestions were provided which were then taken into consideration.

Operational definitions

Pet animal interaction (PAI). This was measured by PIOC and it referred to features of interaction between the participant and pet such as the time duration of interaction, the type of interaction carried out (including stroking, hugging, talking, kissing etc.), the level of proximity maintained while interacting and the level of comfort observed during interaction.

Stress. Stress was defined as the individual-environment relationship that the person assessed as exceeding the available resources and that endangered their well-being (Lazarus & Folkman, 1984). Scores obtained on Short Stress State Questionnaire (SSSQ; Helton, 2004) were the index of stress.

Engagement. This was predominantly a motivational factor that referred to how ready an individual was to act or how willingly they performed effectively.

Distress. This was a measure of the negative affect of the individual.

Worry. This cognitive factor referred to the level of self-focused attention, in addition to self-esteem. It also measured cognitive interference during thinking process.

Positive mood. Positive mood was a collection of pleasant attributes of mood of an individual. Score obtained on Brief Mood Introspection Scale (BMIS; Mayer & Gaschke, 1988) was the index of positive mood.

Procedure

The whole experiment was covered in various steps which are given as below:

Level one: obtaining permission. First of all, the experimenter took permission from the respective authors for using their instruments in the present study. Based on the nature of the study, the experimenter selected the University of Veterinary and Animal Sciences (UVAS) for carrying out the experiment. She explained the purpose of the study to the responsible authorities in order to get the required permission. In addition, participants provided their consent before being included in the study.

Level two: area selection for conducting research. The aviary garden behind the pet clinic

Table 9.2. Inter-Rater Reliability for Pet Interaction Observation Checklist.

Item	Rater 1	Rater 2	Rater 3	Agreement
1	1	1	1	3/3
2	1	1	1	3/3
3	0	1	1	2/3
4	1	0	0	1/3
5	1	1	1	3/3

provided a suitable place for conducting the experiment. This place afforded no distractions and it made sure that the study animals (dog and cat) were also comfortable. Moreover, the participants felt more comfortable interacting there. The experimenter set up a place in a secluded corner with chairs and a table for questionnaires and other materials.

Level three: selecting dog and cat. The experiment included interaction with either dog or cat (based on the experimental group). For dog, the experimenter selected a Russian Samoyed mix breed puppy (named Hachi) that was quite friendly and interactive. For cat, a Persian kitten (named Griffin) was selected. Many reports showed these breeds to be receptive to humans and overall friendly, without posing any threat. Selection of a puppy and kitten ensured the safety and comfort of the participants.

Level four: conducting experiment. The first step included random allocation of participants in any of the following five conditions:

Experimental Group 1 (pet-owners): Interaction with dog

Experimental Group 2 (pet-owners): Interaction with cat

Experimental Group 3 (non-pet owners): Interaction with dog

Experimental Group 4 (non-pet owners): Interaction with cat

Control Group (pet-owners and non-owners): Reading magazines

Random number table assisted in random allocation. Division of the digits (0–9) among the five conditions resulted in each group having two digits: 0,1 (group 1), 2,3 (group 2), 4,5 (group 3), 6,7 (group 4) and 8,9 (control group). To ensure random selection on basis of gender, within each group of two digits, the first digit represented man and the second digit represented woman. However, each individual fulfilled the required criteria to be part of the group before assignment. The pet clinic and university students provided the sample of pet-owners and non-owners. The sample selected from pet clinic also consisted of students within the identified age range.

The experimenter carried out the experiment for a period of three weeks, within the timings of 10:30 AM till 1:30 PM. Conducting the experiment involved group administration. The groups were heterogeneous, consisting of around seven to nine participants at a given time. The upcoming vacation and shortage of time due to ongoing examinations were important factors that needed to be taken into consideration. Moreover, people felt more comfortable in group administration. However, in spite of the group format, participants interacted individually with the study animal. The experimenter escorted the respective participant to the designated area for interaction which was sufficiently far from the other participants and ensured privacy. This controlled for social desirability bias to some extent.

After obtaining informed consent and assigning into respective group, the participants filled the demographic sheet and the two questionnaires, state pre-questionnaire of Short Stress State Questionnaire (SSSQ; Helton, 2004) and Brief Mood Introspection Scale (BMIS; Mayer & Gaschke, 1988). The participants received proper instructions, both verbally and in written text above the instruments. In case of any ambiguity, the experimenter provided further guidance. They were reassured that their responses will be kept confidential and that there were no right or wrong options within the instrument.

After that, they either interacted with a dog, a cat or read magazines, depending on which group they were assigned to. During the interaction, the experimenter filled out the Pet Interaction Observation Checklist while observing the different behaviors of the participant. The participants carried out the activity for the time duration they felt comfortable. Upon termination of interaction, the experimenter administered the two questionnaires again in order to get post measure scores.

At the end of the study, the experimenter debriefed the participants about the purpose of the study. She also thanked them for their participation in the research. In addition, the experimenter ensured that they felt no lasting stress or disturbance from interacting with the animals. The participants in the control group who reported increase in stress interacted with the pet animals, after making sure that they didn't have any phobias or health problems. They were asked to contact on the given email address in case of any problem that occurred later as a result of the experiment.

Ethical considerations

The following ethics were taken into consideration during the study:

Authors of the instruments were accessed for obtaining permission.

Written permission was obtained from the responsible authorities of the University of Veterinary and Animal Sciences (UVAS).

Informed consent was taken from the participants at start of the study.

Privacy and confidentiality of the participants' responses was ensured.

The participants were informed about their right to withdraw from the study at any time they wanted.

At the end of the study, the participants were debriefed about the purpose of the study and any queries that they had were properly addressed.

With regard to the animals involved in the study, it was ensured that they were not harmed in any way. The experimenter constantly provided fresh water and enough food at regular intervals throughout the day. The study animals had a sufficiently open area which was shaded and hence, was cool. The puppy was taken for a walk after the interaction was done with a group while the cat was engaged in playing with the cat nip, either by the experimenter or facilitator. The facilitator was a colleague to whom the purpose of the study was explained beforehand and who interacted with the study animals a number of times before the experiment was conducted in order to make sure that both parties were comfortable with each other. Break was provided after interaction with a group or whenever the animals seemed distressed. This was constantly monitored. The cat showed its distress by trying to go back in its carrier box or calling out. The puppy's distress was noted when its ears and tail drooped and it began whining. The experimenter and facilitator made sure that no participant treated the study animals with cruelty. In case any participant did try to cause any distress (on purpose or by accident), they were instantly stopped by taking away the animal. It was then explained that the behavior was unacceptable and how it was distressful for the animal. The animal was then given sufficient time to recover before continuing the experiment. The experimenter kept the study animals with her and had a sufficiently strong bond before the beginning of the experiment. Toys (cat nip, ball, chew toy) were also provided to them to assure their happiness. Both the puppy and kitten were vaccinated and dewormed. They were also taken for regular check-ups at the pet clinic. It was also ensured that they did not pose a threat to the well-being of the participants.

Results

The present research investigated the effect of pet interaction on stress reduction and positive mood enhancement among pet-owners and non-owners. In addition, it also investigated certain demographics for the variables. Analysis carried out included reliability estimates, Pearson Product Moment Correlation, One way Analysis of Variance and Independent Sample t-test.

Reliability estimates

In order to assess the reliability of the subscales of Short Stress State Questionnaire (Helton, 2004) and Brief Mood Introspection Scale (Mayer & Gaschke, 1988), alpha reliability coefficients were computed for the sample of the study ($N = 180$). The computation was done for both, pre and post measures of the instruments. In addition, descriptive statistics of the scales were calculated by computing their mean, standard deviation, skewness and kurtosis. The reliability estimates and descriptive of the scales are shown in Table 9.3.

In Table 9.3, alpha reliabilities and descriptive statistics are shown for the pre and post measures of stress subscales and mood scale. All three subscales of Short Stress State Questionnaire – engagement, distress and worry – had very good reliabilities for pre-measures, that were $\alpha = 0.87$, $\alpha = 0.92$ and $\alpha = 0.83$. For the post-measures of the three subscales, the reliability values were also found to be satisfactory, that were $\alpha = 0.88$, $\alpha = 0.90$ and $\alpha = 0.83$. For both the pre and post measures of the Brief Mood Introspection Scale, the reliability values were found to be highly satisfactory, that were $\alpha = 0.93$ and $\alpha = 0.92$.

One-way analysis of variance (ANOVA)

In the present study, three groups were present among both pet-owners and non-owners: two experimental groups (interaction with dog and

Table 9.3. Alpha Reliability and Descriptive Statistics for Short Stress State Questionnaire and Brief Mood Introspection Scale (N = 180).

Variables	k	α	Potential Range	Actual Range	Skewness	Kurtosis
Pre-Measures						
Engagement	8	0.87	8 – 40	11 – 40	–0.52	–0.08
Distress	8	0.92	8 – 40	8 – 37	0.86	0.09
Worry	8	0.83	8 – 40	8 – 38	0.04	–0.39
P/UP Mood	16	0.93	16 – 64	17 – 64	–0.45	–0.35
Post-Measures						
Engagement	8	0.88	8 – 40	17 – 33	–0.59	0.17
Distress	8	0.90	8 – 40	8 – 34	0.96	4.93
Worry	8	0.83	8 – 40	8 – 38	0.48	0.05
P/UP Mood	16	0.92	16 – 64	16 – 64	–0.80	4.09

Note. α = Alpha reliability; k = No. of items; P/UP Mood = Pleasant/Unpleasant Mood

interaction with cat) and one control group. One-way ANOVA was computed in order to find out the mean differences for stress subscales and mood scale for the experimental and control groups for the sample of pet-owners and non-owners. Results are shown in Tables 9.4, 9.5, 9.6 and 9.7.

Table 9.4 shows the results of one-way ANOVA for pre and post measures of stress subscales (engagement, distress and worry) and mood scale with the three groups (dog interaction, cat interaction and control) for pet-owners. It was shown that significant differences existed across the three groups for pre and post measures of stress and mood.

After applying post-hoc analysis (Bonferroni) the differences between the means of the different groups were observed. In the pre-measures, lower means were shown for dog interaction group for engagement and pleasant mood as compared to cat interaction and control groups (Table 9.5). Moreover, higher means for distress and worry were found among dog interaction group as compared to the other two groups. Additionally, it was found that the cat interaction group had lower means as compared to control group for both, engagement and pleasant mood. For distress and worry, cat interaction group had higher means as compared to control group. However, for the post-measures a significant difference was found for the study variables. It was found that dog interaction group had higher means for engagement and pleasant mood as compared to control group. Moreover, dog interaction group had lower mean for distress as compared to control group. Cat group also had significantly higher mean for pleasant mood as compared to control group. Hence, stress reduction and positive mood enhancement were found to be significantly higher for dog interaction group.

Table 9.6 shows the results of one way ANOVA for pre and post measures of stress subscales (engagement, distress and worry) and mood scale with the three groups (dog interaction, cat interaction and control) for non-owners. It was found that significant differences existed across the three groups for pre and post measures of stress and mood.

After applying post-hoc analysis (Bonferroni) the differences between the means of the different groups were observed. In the pre-measures, significant lower means were shown for dog interaction group for pleasant mood as compared to cat interaction and control groups (Table 9.7). However, for the post-measures a significant difference was found for the study variables. It was found that cat interaction group had higher means for engagement as compared to control group. Dog and cat interaction groups had lower means for distress and worry and higher means for pleasant mood as compared to control group. No significant mean differences were found between dog and cat interaction groups for post measures.

Independent sample t-test

Independent sample t-test was applied in order to find out whether significant differences exist between pet-owners and non-owners for stress

Table 9.4. One-way Analysis of Variance for Pet Interaction Types on Pre and Post Measures for Engagement, Distress, Worry and Pleasant/Unpleasant Mood among Pet-Owners (N = 90).

		SS	*df*	*MS*	*F*	*p*
Pre-Measures						
Engagement	Between Groups	626.60	2	313.300	8.66	0.00
	Within Groups	3146.30	87	36.164		
	Total	3772.90	89			
Distress	Between Groups	2216.82	2	1108.411	27.09	0.00
	Within Groups	3559.13	87	40.910		
	Total	5775.96	89			
Worry	Between Groups	1554.82	2	777.411	24.76	0.00
	Within Groups	2731.67	87	31.398		
	Total	4286.49	89			
P/UP Mood	Between Groups	5626.96	2	2813.478	38.15	0.00
	Within Groups	6415.37	87	73.740		
	Total	12042.32	89			
Post-Measures						
Engagement	Between Groups	120.56	2	60.278	5.84	0.00
	Within Groups	898.73	87	10.330		
	Total	1019.29	89			
Distress	Between Groups	163.62	2	81.811	4.61	0.01
	Within Groups	1544.03	87	17.748		
	Total	1707.66	89			
Worry	Between Groups	90.07	2	45.033	1.29	0.28
	Within Groups	3042.03	87	34.966		
	Total	3132.10	89			
P/UP Mood	Between Groups	909.36	2	454.678	8.32	0.00
	Within Groups	4751.63	87	54.616		
	Total	5660.99	89			

Note. $^{**}p < 0.01$; $^{*}p < 0.05$; SS = Sum of Square; df = degree of freedom; MS = Mean Square; P/UP Mood = Pleasant/Unpleasant Mood.

Table 9.5. Post Hoc Test for Pet Interaction Types on Pre and Post Measures for Engagement, Distress, Worry and Pleasant/Unpleasant Mood among Pet-Owners (N = 90).

					95% *CI*	
Dependent Variable	*i*	*j*	*MD (i-j)*	*SE*	*LL*	*UL*
Pre-Measures						
Engagement	Dog	Cat	−1.90	1.55	−5.69	1.89
		Control	−6.300*	1.55	−10.09	−2.51
	Cat	Control	−4.400*	1.55	−8.19	−0.61
Distress	Dog	Cat	5.033*	1.65	1.00	9.06
		Control	12.100*	1.65	8.07	16.13
	Cat	Control	7.067*	1.65	3.04	11.10
Worry	Dog	Control	9.933*	1.45	6.40	13.47
	Cat	Control	6.900*	1.45	3.37	10.43
P/UP Mood	Dog	Cat	−9.467*	2.22	−14.88	−4.05
		Control	−19.367*	2.22	−24.78	−13.95
	Cat	Control	−9.900*	2.22	−15.31	−4.49
Post–Measures						
Engagement	Dog	Control	2.833*	0.83	0.81	4.86
Distress	Dog	Control	−3.300*	1.09	−5.96	−0.64
P/UP Mood	Dog	Control	7.367*	1.91	2.71	12.02
	Cat	Control	5.867*	1.91	1.21	10.52

Note. $^{**}p < 0.01$; $^{*}p < 0.05$; MD = Mean Difference; SE = Standard Error; P/UP Mood = Pleasant/Unpleasant Mood; CI = Confidence Interval; LL = Lower Limit; UP = Upper Limit.

Table 9.6. One way Analysis of Variance for Pet Interaction Types on Pre and Post Measures for Engagement, Distress, Worry and Pleasant/Unpleasant Mood among Non-Owners (N = 90).

		SS	*df*	*MS*	*F*	*P*
Pre-Measures						
Engagement	Between Groups	27.756	2	13.878	0.50	0.61
	Within Groups Total	2405.133 2432.889	87 89	27.645		
Distress	Between Groups	65.489	2	32.744	1.00	0.37
	Within Groups Total	2837.133 2902.622	87 89	32.611		
Worry	Between Groups	26.689	2	13.344	0.51	0.60
	Within Groups	2296.467	87	26.396		
	Total	2323.156	89			
P/UP Mood	Between Groups	676.067	2	338.033	4.65	0.01
	Within Groups	6326.033	87	72.713		
	Total	7002.100	89			
Post-Measures						
Engagement	Between Groups	89.267	2	44.633	3.10	0.05
	Within Groups Total	1254.333 1343.600	87 89	14.418		
Distress	Between Groups	462.489	2	231.244	9.42	0.00
	Within Groups Total	2136.667 2599.156	87 89	24.559		
Worry	Between Groups	437.267	2	218.633	9.35	0.00
	Within Groups Total	2034.733 2472.000	87 89	23.388		
Post P/UP Mood	Between Groups	1606.067	2	803.033	17.93	0.00
	Within Groups Total	3897.533 5503.600	87 89	44.799		

Note. $^{**}p < 0.01$; $^{*}p < 0.05$; SS = Sum of Square; df = degree of freedom; MS = Mean Square; P/UP Mood= Pleasant/ Unpleasant Mood

Table 9.7. Post Hoc Test for Pet Interaction Types on Pre and Post Measures for Engagement, Distress, Worry and Pleasant/Unpleasant Mood among Non-Owners (N = 90).

					95% *CI*	
Dependent Variable	*i*	*J*	*MD (i-j)*	*SE*	*LL*	*UL*
Pre-Measures						
P/UP Mood	Dog	Cat	–5.567*	2.202	–10.94	–0.19
		Control	–6.033*	2.202	–11.41	–0.66
Post-Measures						
Engagement	Cat	Control	2.433*	.980	0.04	4.83
Distress	Dog	Control	–4.400*	1.280	–7.52	–1.28
	Cat	Control	–5.133*	1.280	–8.26	–2.01
Worry	Dog	Control	–4.933*	1.249	–7.98	–1.89
	Cat	Control	–4.367*	1.249	–7.41	–1.32
Post P/UP Mood	Dog	Control	7.633*	1.728	3.41	11.85
	Cat	Control	9.867*	1.728	5.65	14.09

Note. $^{**}p < 0.01$; $^{*}p < 0.05$; MD = Mean Difference; SE = Standard Error; P/UP Mood = Pleasant/Unpleasant Mood; CI = Confidence Interval; LL = Lower Limit; UP = Upper Limit.

reduction and positive mood enhancement. Table 9.8 illustrates the results obtained.

Table 9.8 illustrates the results obtained for pet status differences for stress reduction and positive mood enhancement after interaction. The third hypothesis of the study, "pet-owners will have greater stress reduction and positive mood enhancement as a result of pet animal interaction as compared to non-owners" was investigated. It was found that significant differences

Table 9.8. Difference between Pet-Owners and Non-Owners for Pre and Post Measures of Engagement, Distress, Worry and Pleasant/Unpleasant Mood (*N* = 180).

	Pet-Owners (*n* = 90)		Non-Owners (*n* = 90)				95% *CI*		
Variables	*M*	*SD*	*M*	*SD*	*t* (178)	*p*	*LL*	*UL*	Cohen's *d*
Pre-Measures									
Engagement	26.6	6.51	27.1	5.23	−0.54	0.59	−2.22	1.26	−0.08
Distress	19.0	8.06	16.2	5.71	2.67	0.01	0.72	4.83	0.40
Worry	22.5	6.94	22.8	5.11	−0.34	0.73	−2.10	1.48	−0.05
P/UP Mood	43.5	11.6	46.8	8.87	−2.09	0.04	−6.27	−0.18	−0.32
Post-Measures									
Engagement	26.7	3.38	26.3	3.89	0.78	0.44	−0.65	1.49	0.11
Distress	11.1	4.38	11.8	5.40	−0.95	0.34	−2.15	0.75	−0.14
Worry	16.4	5.93	19.0	5.27	−3.07	0.00	−4.22	−0.92	−0.46
P/UP Mood	57.0	7.98	54.7	7.86	1.93	0.06	−0.05	4.61	0.29

Note. P/UP Mood = Pleasant/Unpleasant Mood; *CI:* Confidence Interval; *LL* = Lower Limit; *UL* = Upper Limit

existed between pet-owners and non-owners for pre-measures of distress and pleasant mood. Pet-owners scored higher on distress and lower on pleasant mood as compared to non-owners. Significant difference was also found for the post-measure of worry. Pet-owners had significantly lower scores on worry as compared to non-owners. This supported the hypothesis to an extent.

In addition, Independent sample t-test was applied in order to find out whether significant differences exist between participants interacting for five minutes or less and more than five minutes for stress reduction and positive mood enhancement among. Table 9.9 illustrates the results obtained.

Table 9.9 illustrates the results obtained for pet interaction time difference for stress reduction and positive mood enhancement. It was found that significant differences existed between interaction for five minutes or less group and more than five minutes group for the premeasures of distress and pleasant mood. Participants interacting for five minutes or less had lower scores on worry and higher scores on pleasant mood as compared to those who interacted for more than five minutes. For post-measures, significant difference was found between the two groups for worry and pleasant mood. Participants interacting for more than five minutes had lower scores on worry and higher scores on pleasant mood as compared to those who interacted for five minutes or less. Moreover, the effect size was found to be medium in strength for both the variables (Cohen, 1988).

Discussion

The present study explored the effect of pet interaction on stress reduction and positive mood enhancement among pet-owners and non-owners. In addition, it explored certain demographic variables such as gender, pet ownership status and pet interaction duration.

Mean differences of stress and mood

Differences for stress and mood were observed for the four experimental groups and control group among both pet-owners and non-owners. The hypothesis, pet animal interaction will result in stress reduction and positive mood enhancement for both pet-owners and non-owners, was supported (see tables 9.4, 9.5, 9.6 and 9.7). Previous researches supported this finding (Friedmann et al., 2013; Handlin et al., 2011; McConnell et al., 2011; Shiloh et al., 2010). Researchers found that individuals benefitted from interaction with pets, even if it was a short-term interaction (Shiloh et al., 2010). In addition, the effectiveness remained even when interacting with an unknown pet. Moreover, even when there was no past experience with pets or

Table 9.9. Difference between Five Minutes or Less and More than Five Minutes Interaction for Pre and Post Measures of Engagement, Distress, Worry and Pleasant/Unpleasant Mood (N = 120).

	Five Minutes or Less (n = 70)		*More than Five Minutes* (n = 50)				95% *CI*		
Variables	*M*	*SD*	*M*	*SD*	*t* (178)	*p*	*LL*	*UL*	Cohen's *d*
Pre-Measures									
Engagement	26.3	4.96	25.2	5.86	1.10	0.27	–0.90	3.14	0.20
Distress	18.4	6.04	21.0	7.61	–2.11	0.04	–5.10	–0.16	–0.38
Worry	24.3	5.45	24.2	5.32	0.06	0.95	–1.92	2.04	0.02
P/UP Mood	43.8	8.23	39.9	10.5	2.32	0.02	0.58	7.36	0.41
Post-Measures									
Engagement	27.1	3.68	27.2	2.69	–0.28	0.78	–1.38	1.04	–0.03
Distress	10.6	3.92	9.8	3.09	1.38	0.17	–0.38	2.15	0.23
Worry	17.7	5.07	15.0	4.61	3.08	0.00	0.98	4.51	0.56
P/UP Mood	57.3	5.45	60.0	5.23	–2.65	0.01	–4.57	–0.66	–0.51

Note. P/UP Mood = Pleasant/Unpleasant Mood; *CI:* Confidence Interval; *LL* = Lower Limit; *UL* = Upper Limit

differing attitude, the beneficial effects of pet interaction were still observed (Wilson, 1991). Not only did interacting with pets reduce stress, but it also led to increasing an individual's positive mood (Kaminski et al., 2002). One of the reasons for this beneficial effect of pets has been attributed to the biological changes caused in the levels of oxytocin in individuals. Petting and stroking a pet increased the levels of oxytocin within the body, making one feel better (Miller et al., 2015). Furthermore, it significantly reduced the amounts of epinephrine as well as norepinephrine that were responsible for causing stress. Not only that, but interacting with pets also increased empathy, improved the functioning of the immune system and reduced aggressive tendencies. All these positive attributes resulted from the oxytocin system (Beetzl, Uvnas-Moberg, Julius, & Kotrschal, 2012). Interaction with pets also kept individuals active physically. This led to better overall health, reduced negative mood and better coping with life stressors. It also resulted in reduced reactivity, decreased heart rate and blood pressure (Allen et al., 2002). Thus, these beneficial effects highlighted the importance of pets in reducing stress and enhancing mood among other benefits, as also highlighted in the present study.

The second hypothesis of the study, stress reduction and positive mood enhancement will be greater after interaction with dog as compared to cat, was not supported (see tables 9.4, 9.5, 9.6 and 9.7). This was not in line with previous researches which had shown that interaction with dog resulted in greater health benefits as compared to interaction with cat (Handlin et al., 2011; Hoffman, 2009). This lack of a difference found was associated with an individual's preference, based on their personal traits. People usually related to others in ways in which they themselves preferred to interact. Hence, individuals who were dominant preferably interacted with submissive individuals, thus allowing them to do what they like. Likewise, active and friendly people preferred to interact with other friendly and active people, thus allowing them to express their traits (Orford, 1994). When people interacted with pets, many factors influenced the kind of interaction they had. It included the pet animal characteristics (Houpt et al., 1996; New et al., 2000), the lifestyle (Arkow & Dow, 1984) and individual differences among people (Brown & Katcher, 2001). Furthermore, the quality of interaction with pets depended upon how much the individual needed dominance in the relationship with pet. Those requiring less were more affectionate. Thus, the characteristics of the pet as well as the individual's needs dictated the interaction (Woodwarda & Bauerb, 2007).

In the present study, individuals were randomly selected to interact with either dog or cat. Even if interaction with dog produced greater positive effects, the beneficial effects of cat interaction were same in magnitude due to individual differences and characteristics of the pet. Hence, certain participants benefited more from interaction with cat as they fit in their preferred interaction style and they found the characteristics of cat more in line with their needs.

Pet status differences for stress and mood

The hypothesis, pet-owners will have greater stress reduction and positive mood enhancement as a result of pet animal interaction as compared to non-owners, was supported (see Table 9.8). Pet-owners had lower scores on worry after pet interaction as compared to non-owners. This was somewhat in line with previous researches (McConnell et al., 2011; Staats et al., 2006). The reason for this difference was that pet-owners considered their pets as part of the family. They related to them as attachment figures, since pets fulfilled the four prerequisites of an attachment figure (Zilcha-Mano et al., 2011). In fact, many owners considered their pets on level equivalent to their spouses and reported greater stress reduction when with their pets (Allen et al., 2002). Due to this, they more actively interacted with pets and took care of their needs, allowing them to benefit more from their presence due to physical, financial and emotional investment (Smolkovic et al., 2012). Furthermore, pet-owners benefitted from their pets just as they would from their relationship with other people. This was especially true when the pet-owners had healthier personalities. Even pet-owners with social or personal shortcomings were more open toward pets in order to address those shortcomings due to the positive qualities of pet interaction (McConnell et al., 2011). As a result, pet owners were more aware of the importance of pets in their lives. And they experienced more beneficial effects that came along with them, which was also shown in the present study.

Time differences for pet interaction and impact on stress and mood

The hypothesis, participants interacting with pets for more than five minutes will have greater stress reduction and positive mood enhancement as compared to those interacting for less than five minutes, was supported (see Table 9.9). However, the results were found to be significant for worry subscale of stress and nonsignificant for engagement and distress. Previous researches showed that the beneficial effects of interacting with a pet occurred after as little time as five minutes. Increasing the time to a specific period resulted in increase in the beneficial effects of the interaction, including stress reduction (Barker et al., 2005; Handlin et al., 2011). The activation of the oxytocin system attributed for this short time for experiencing the beneficial effects of pet interaction. The system activated few minutes after interaction with a pet, especially when it involved more petting and stroking. It reduced stress by decreasing the secretion of stress-causing hormones. Moreover, it increased the functioning of parasympathetic system, hence maintaining calm and restoring balance. It also increased positive qualities, including enhanced positive mood. Thus, the activation of the system resulted in significant beneficial effects for both, the individual and the pet.

Limitations and suggestions

The current study had certain limitations that played a role in the outcome. The sample was collected from only one university and one city, hence the results may not be generalizable to other areas due to the sample not being representative. The study may have been affected by subject bias. Moreover, due to group administration, there may have been social desirability bias among participants.

There are some suggestions that may be helpful for further studies. Samples from other provinces should also be included in order to make the sample more representative and increase the generalizibility of the results. Studies including follow-ups should be conducted in order to determine how long the beneficial effects of pet interaction lasted and whether there was difference for pet-owners and non-owners. Studies that take into consideration the pet preference of the individual and their personalities may shed light on the possible benefits of interacting with a pet suitable to one's personality.

Implications of the study

The present study is the first one to empirically investigate the effect of pet interaction on stress and mood in Pakistan. It has important implications for further studies. The two major animals with which interaction was done were dog and cat. Although results were significant, it would be interesting to carry out research with other animals that are also kept as pets in the society. It would provide further insight to measure and take into account the personalities of individuals. It would enable the investigation of the beneficial effects of pet interaction as a function of individual's traits. This study provided significant insight with regard to studying the variables in the present context – a collectivistic culture. It would help in better understanding what differences were found as compared to individualistic culture. The results also highlighted the importance of pets as effective therapeutic tools. It will be useful to carry out research in clinical settings to see whether the beneficial effects associated with pets were also consistent with clinical populations. Moreover, using pets as a complimentary teaching tool to encourage positive traits in individuals will be another useful outcome to study.

Conclusion

The present study revealed that pet interaction resulted in significant stress reduction and enhanced positive mood for both pet-owners and non-owners. In addition, pet-owners benefited more from this interaction as compared to non-owners. Moreover, the beneficial effect of pet interaction occurred within first few minutes. These results attributed to the physical and psychological health benefits associated with pets due to their many attributes including unconditional support and functioning as effective attachment figures (Kurdek, 2008; McConnell et al., 2011; Zilcha-Mano et al., 2011).

Clearly, there is ample opportunity and need for more investigation in the area of beneficial effects of pet interaction, especially in Pakistan. The literature in this area of research is non-existent, even though pets are part of many people's lives. This present study has made a modest contribution to this domain. By carrying out more empirical research on beneficial effects of pets, further valuable information and implications can be brought to light for the present society.

References

Akhtar, M. (2013). Place of dog in America and Islam. Retrieved from: http://muslimcouncilofamerica.org/place-of-dogs-in-america-and-in-islam/comment-page-1/

Al-Fayez, G., Awadalla, A., Templer, D. I., & Arikawa, H. (2003). Companion animal attitude and its family pattern in Kuwait. *Society and Animals, 11*, 17–28.

Allen, K., Blascovich, J., & Mendes, W. (2002). Cardiovascular reactivity and the presence of pets, friends, and spouses: the truth about cats and dogs. *Psychosomatic Medicine, 64*(5), 727–739. Retrieved from: http://journals.lww.com/psychosomaticmedicine/Abstract/2002/09000/Cardiovascular_Reactivity_and_the_Presence_of.5.aspx

Arkow, P., & Dow, S. (1984). The ties that do not bind: A study of human-animal bonds that fail. In R. K. Anderson, B. L. Hart, & L. A. Hart (Eds.), *The Pet Connection: Its Influence on our Health and Quality of Life* (pp. 348–354). Minneapolis, MN: University of Minnesota Press.

Bao, K. J. (2016). Is happiness a warm puppy?: examining the association between pets and well-being. Retrieved from: https://osf.io/2r8h6/

Barker, S. B., Knisely, J. S., McCain, N. L., Schubert, C. M., & Pandurangi, A. K. (2005). Exploratory study of stress-buffering response patterns from interaction with a therapy dog. *Anthrozoos, 23*(1), 79–91. Retrieved from: http://www.tandfonline.com/doi/abs/10.2752/175303710X12627079939341

Beck, L., & Madresh, E. (2008). Romantic partners and four legged friends: An extension of attachment theory to relationships with pets. *Anthrozoos, 21*, 43–56.

Beetz, A., Kotrschal, K., Hediger, K., Turner, D., & Uvnas-Moberg, K. (2011). The effect of a real dog, toy dog and friendly person on insecurely attached children during a stressful task: an exploratory study. *Anthrozoos, 24*, 349–368.

Beetzl, A., Uvnas-Moberg, K., Julius, H., & Kotrschal, K. (2012). Psychosocial and psychophysiological effects of human-animal interactions: the possible role of oxytocin. *Frontiers in Psychology, 3*, 234. Doi: 10.3389/fpsyg.2012.00234

Berget, B., Ekeberg, O., Pedersen, I., & Braastad, B. O. (2011). Animal-Assisted therapy with farm animals for persons with psychiatric disorders: effects on anxiety and depression, a randomized controlled trial. *Occupational Therapy in Mental Health, 27*(1), 50–64. Retrieved from: http://www.tandfonline.com/doi/full/10.1080/0164212X.2011.543641? src=recsys

Berli, C., Loretini, P., Radtke, T., Hornung, R., & Scholz, U. (2014). Predicting physical activity in adolescents: The role of compensatory health beliefs with the Health Action Process Approach. *Psychology & Health, 29*(4), 458–474. Doi:10.1080/08870446.2013.865028

Bowlby, J. (1984). *Attachment and loss* (Vol. 1). Harmondsworth: Penguin Books.

Brown, S. E., & Katcher, A. H. (2001). Pet attachment and dissociation. *Society & Animals, 9*(1), 25–41.

Carlisle, G. K. (2014). Pet dog ownership decisions for parents of children with autism spectrum disorder. *Journal of Pediatric Nursing, 29*(2), 114–23. Doi: 10.1016/j.pedn.2013.09.005.

Cohen, J. (1988). *Statistical power analysis for the behavioural sciences* (2nd ed.). Hillsdale, NJ: Lawrence Earlbaum Associates.

Cohen, S. P. (2002). Can pets function as family members? *Western Journal of Nursing Research, 24*, 621–638.

Cole, K. M., Gawlinski, A., Steers, N., & Kotlerman, J. (2007). Animal-assisted therapy in patients hospitalized with heart failure. *American Journal of Critical Care, 16*, 575–585.

Coyne, J. C., & van Sonderen, E. (2012). No further research needed: Abandoning the Hospital and Anxiety Depression Scale (HADS). *Journal of Psychosomatic Research, 72*(3), 173–174. Doi:10.1016/j.jpsychores

Crawford, H. K., Worsham, N. L., & Swinehart, E. R. (2006). Benefits derived from companion animals, and the use of the term 'attachment'. *Anthrozoos, 19*, 98–112.

Daly, B., & Morton, L. L. (2006). An investigation of human–animal interactions and empathy as related to pet preference, ownership, attachment, and attitudes in children, *Anthrozoos*, 19, 113-127. Retrieved from: http://dx.doi.org/10.2752/089279306785593801

Davidovitz, R., Mikulincer, M., Shaver, P. R., Izsak, R., & Popper, M. (2007). Leaders as attachment figures: Leaders' attachment orientations predict leadership-related mental representations and followers' performance and mental health. *Journal of Personality and Social Psychology, 93*, 632–650.

Doherty, N. A., & Feeney, J. A. (2004). The composition of attachment networks throughout the adult years. *Personal Relationships, 11*, 469–488.

Duncan, I. J. H., & Fraser, D. (1997). Understanding animal welfare. In M. C. Appleby & B. O. Hughes (Eds.), *Animal Welfare. CAB International* (pp. 19–31). Wallingford, UK.

Duvall Antonacopoulos, N. M., & Pychyl, T. A. (2010). An examination of the potential role of pet ownership, human social support and pet attachment in the psychological health of individuals living alone. *Anthrozoos, 23*(1), 37–54. Retrieved from: http://www.psychologytoday.com/blog/don'tdelay/201002/living-alone-can-canine-companionship-help-beat-loneliness

Feeney, J. A. (2004). Transfer of attachment from parents to romantic partners: Effects of individual and relationship variables. *Journal of Family Studies, 10*, 220–238.

Friedmann, E., Thomas, S. A., Son, H., Chapa, D., & McCune, S. (2015). Pet's presence and owner's blood pressures during the daily lives of pet owners with pre- to mild hypertension. *Anthrozoös*, 26(4), 535-550. Retrieved from: http://www.tandfonline.com/doi/abs/10.2752/175303713X13795775536138

Goyal, M., Singh, S., & Sibinga, E. M. S. (2014). Meditation programs for psychological stress and well-being: a systematic review and meta-analysis. *JAMA Internal Medicine,* 174(3). Doi: 10.1001/jamainternmed.2013.13018)

Granqvist, P., Mikulincer, M., & Shaver, P. R. (2010). Religion as attachment: Normative processes and individual differences. *Personality and Social Psychology Review,* 14, 49-59.

Gray, P. B., & Young, S. M. (2011). Human pet dynamics in cross-cultural perspective. *Anthrozoos, 24*, 17–30.

Handlin, L., Hydbring-Sandberg, E., Nilsson, A., Ejdebäck, M., Jansson, A., & Uvnas-Moberg, K. (2011). Short-term interaction between dogs and their owners – effects on oxytocin, cortisol, insulin and heart rate – an exploratory study. *Anthrozoos,* 24(3), 301-316. Retrieved from: http://www.tandfonline.com/doi/abs/10.2752/175303711X13045914865385?src=recsys

Helton, W. S. (2004). Validation of a short stress state questionnaire. *Proceedings of the Human Factors and Ergonomics Society,* 48(11), 1238-1242.

Herzog, H. (2014). Biology, culture, and the origins of pet-keeping. *Animal Behavior and Cognition, 1*(3), 296–308. Doi: 10.12966/abc.08.06.2014

Hoffmann, A. O. M., Lee, A. H., Wertenauer, F., Ricken, R., Jansen, J. J., Juergen Gallinat, J., & Lang, U. E. (2009). Dog-assisted intervention significantly reduces anxiety in hospitalized patients with major depression. *European Journal of Integrative Medicine,* 1(3), 145–148. Retrieved from: http://www.sciencedirect.com/science/article/pii/S1876382009000419

Houpt, K. A., Honig, S. U., & Reisner, I. R. (1996). Breaking the human-companion animal bond. *Journal of the American Veterinary Medical Association, 208*, 1653–1659.

Hunt, M., Al-Awadi, H., & Johnson, M. (2008). Psychological sequelae of pet loss following Hurricane Katrina. *Anthrozoos, 21*, 109–121.

Johnson, R. A., Meadows, R. L., Haubner, J. S., & Sevedge, K. (2008). Animal-Assisted Activity among patients with cancer: effects on mood, fatigue, self-perceived health, and sense of coherence. *Oncology Nursing Forum, 35*(2), 225–232.

Kaminski, M., Pellino, T., & Wish, J. (2002). Play and Pets: The Physical and Emotional Impact of Child-Life and Pet Therapy on Hospitalized Children. *Children's Health Care,* 31(4), 321-335. Doi: http://dx.doi.org/10.1207/S15326888CHC3104_5

Kanamori, S., Kawashima, T., Kuwabara, M., & Macer, D. (2001). Attitudes towards animals & animal loving week among Japanese young adults. Eubios *Journal of Asian and International Bioethics, 11*, 82–84. Retrieved from: http://www.eubios.info/EJ113/EJ113H.htm

Khalid, A., & Naqvi, I. (2016). Relationship between pet attachment and empathy among young adults. *Journal of Behavioral Sciences, 26*(1), 66–81.

Knobel, D. L., Laurenson, M. K., Kazwala, R. R., Boden, L. A., & Cleaveland, S. (2008). A cross-sectional study of factors associated with dog ownership in Tanzania. *Bio Medical Central Veterinary Research, 4*, 1–10. Doi: 10.1186/1746-6148-4-5.

Kurdek, L. A. (2008). Pet dogs as attachment figures. *Journal of Social and Personal Relationships, 25*, 247–266.

Kurdek, L. A. (2009). Pet dogs as attachment figures for adult owners. *Journal of Family Psychology, 23*(4), 439–446. Doi: http://dx.doi.org/10.1037/a0014979

Kwong, M. J., & Bartholomew, K. (2011). Not just a dog: An attachment theory perspective on relationships with assistance dogs. *Attachment and Human Development, 13*, 421–436.

Lang, U. E., Jansen, J. B., Wertenauer, F., Gallinat, J., & Rapp, M. A. (2010). Reduced anxiety during dog assisted interviews in acute schizophrenic patients. *European Journal of Integrative Medicine, 2*(3), 123–127. Doi: 10.1016/j.eujim.2010.07.002

Lazarus, R. S., & Folkman, S. (1984). *Stress, appraisal, and coping.* New York: Springer.

Lutwack-Bloom, P., Wijewickrama, R., & Smith, B. (2004). Effects of pets versus people visits with nursing home residents. *Journal of Gerontological Social Work, 44*(3–4), 137–159. Doi: http://dx.doi.org/10.1300/J083v44n03_09

Mallinckrodt, B., Gantt, D. L., & Coble, H. M. (1995). Attachment patterns in the psychotherapy relationship: Development of the Client Attachment to Therapist scale. *Journal of Counseling Psychology, 42*, 307–317.

Mayer, J. D., & Gaschke, Y. N. (1988). The experience and meta-experience of mood. *Journal of Personality and Social Psychology, 55*, 102–111.

McConnell, A. R., Brown, C. M., Shoda, T. M., Stayton, L. E., & Martin, C. E. (2011). Friends with benefits: on the positive consequences of pet ownership. *Journal of Personality and Social Psychology, 101*(6), 1239–1252. Retrieved from: http://www.apa.org/pubs/journals/releases/psp-101-6-1239.pdf

Melson, G. F., & Fogel, A. (1989). Children's ideas about animal young and their care: A reassessment of gender differences in the development of nurturance. *Anthrozoos, 2*(4), 265–273.

Miller, S. C., Kennedy, C. C., DeVoe, D. C., Hickey, M., Nelson, T., & Kogan, L. (2015). An examination of changes in oxytocin levels in men and women before and after interaction with a bonded dog. *Anthrozoos, 22*(1), 31–42.

New, J. C., Salman, M. D., King, M., Scarlett, J. M., Kass, P. H., & Hutchison, J. M. (2000). Characteristics of shelter-relinquished animals and their owners compared with animals and their owners in U.S. pet-owning households. *Journal of Applied Animal Welfare Science, 3*, 179–201.

Nimer, J., & Lundahl, B. (2007). Animal-Assisted Therapy: A Meta-Analysis. *Anthrozoos, 20*(3), 225–238.

Odendaal, J. S., & Meintjes, R. A. (2003). Neurophysiological correlates of affiliative behavior between humans and dogs. *Veterinary Journal, 165*, 296–301.

Orford, J. (1994). The interpersonal circumplex: a theory and method for applied psychology. *Human Relations, 46*, 1347–1375.

Picard, M. J. (2015). A study of the effect of dogs on college students' mood and anxiety. (Honors thesis, University of Maine, Orono). Retrieved from: http://digitalcommons.library.umaine.edu/cgi/viewcontent.cgi?article=1227& context=honors

Polheber, J. P., & Matchock, R. L. (2014). The presence of a dog attenuates cortisol and heart rate in the Trier Social Stress Test compared to human friends. *Journal of Behavioral Medicine, 37*(5), 860–7. Doi: 10.1007/s10865-013-9546-1.

Prokop, P., Ozel, M., & Usak, M. (2009). Cross-cultural comparison of student attitudes toward snakes. *Society & Animals, 17*(3), 224–240. Doi: 10.1163/156853009X 445398

Raina, P., Waltner-Toews, D., Bonnet, B., Woodward, C., & Abernathy, T. (1999). Influence of companion animals on the physical and psychological health of older people: An analysis of a one-year longitudinal study. *Journal of the American Geriatrics Society, 47*, 323–329.

Rom, E., & Mikulincer, M. (2003). Attachment theory and group processes: The association between attachment style and group-related representations, goals, memories, and functioning. *Journal of Personality and Social Psychology, 84*, 1220–1235.

Serpell, J. A. (2003). Anthropomorphism and anthropomorphic selection: Beyond the cute response. *Society and Animals, 11*, 83–100.

Serpell, J. A., & Paul, E. S. (2011). Pets in the family: An evolutionary perspective. In C. A. Salmon & T. K. Shackelford (Eds.), *The Oxford Handbook of Evolutionary Family Psychology* (pp. 298–309). New York: Oxford University Press.

Sharkin, B., & Bahrick, A. (1990). Pet loss: implications for counselors. *Journal of Counselling and Development, 68*(3), 306–308.

Shiloh, S., Sorekt, G., & Terkel, J. (2010). Reduction of state-anxiety by petting animals in a controlled laboratory experiment. *Anxiety, Stress, & Coping, 16*(4), 387–395. Doi: http://dx.doi.org/10.1080/1061580031000091582

Shipman, P. (2010). The animal connection and human evolution. *Current Anthropology, 51*, 519–538.

Siegel, J. M. (1990). Stressful life events and use of physician services among the elderly: The moderating role of pet ownership. *Journal of Personality and Social Psychology, 58*(6), 1081–1086. Doi: http://dx.doi.org/10.1037/0022-3514.58.6.1081

Smolkovic, I., Fajfar, M. & Mlinaric, V. (2012). Attachment to pets and interpersonal relationships: Can a four-legged friend replace a two-legged one?. *Journal of European Psychology Students, 3*(1), 15–23.

Staats, S., Sears, K., & Pierfelice, L. (2006). Teachers' pets and why they have them: an investigation of the human animal bond. *Journal of Applied Social Psychology, 36*, 1881–1891. Doi: 10.1111/j.0021-9029.2006.00086.x

Thompson, K. L., & Gullone, E. (2003). Promotion of empathy and prosocial behaviour in children through humane education. *Australian Psychologist, 38*(3) 175–182. Doi: 10.1080/00050060310001707187

Tsai, C., Friedmann, E., Sue, A., & Thomas, S. A. (2013). The effect of animal-assisted therapy on stress responses in hospitalized children. *Anthrozoos, 23*(3), 245–258.

Wells, M., & Perrine, R. (2001). Critters in the cube farm: perceived psychological and organizational effects of pets in the workplace. *Journal of Occupational Health Psychology, 6*(1), 81–7.

Wilson, C. C. (1991). The pet as an anxiolytic intervention. *Journal of Nervous and Mental Disease, 179*(8), 482–9. Retrieved from: https://www.ncbi.nlm.nih.gov/pubmed/1856711

Winefield, H. R., Black, A., & Chur-Hansen, A. (2008). Health effects of ownership of and attachment to companion animals, in an older population. *International Journal of Behavioral Medicine, 15*(4), 303–310. Doi: 10.1080/10705500802365532

Woodwarda, L. E., & Bauerb, A. L. (2007). People and their pets: a relational perspective on interpersonal complementarity and attachment in companion animal owners. *Society and Animals, 15*, 169–189.

Wright, H. F., Hall, S., Hames, A., Hardiman, J., Mills, R., PAWS Team., & Mills, D. S. (2015). A pet dog significantly reduces stress of primary carers for children with autism spectrum disorder: a prospective case control study. *Journal of Autism and Developmental Disorders, 45*(8), 2531–2540. Doi: 10.1007/s10803-015-2418-5

Xiaoqiong, H. (2008). The culture shock that Asian students experience in immersion education. *Changing English: Studies in Culture and Education 151*, 101–105. Doi: 10.1080/13586840701825378

Zilcha-Mano, S., Mikulincer, M., & Shaver, P. R. (2011). An attachment perspective on human–pet relationships: Conceptualization and assessment of pet attachment orientations. *Journal of Research in Personality, 45*, 345–357.

10 Oxytocin Responses After Dog and Cat Interactions Depend on Pet Ownership and May Affect Interpersonal Trust

Benjamin A. Curry[1], Brianne Donaldson[2], Moana Vercoe[1], Matthew Filippo[3] and Paul J. Zak[1,4*]

[1]*Claremont Graduate University;* [2]*Monmouth College;* [3]*Western University of Health Sciences;* [4]*Loma Linda University Medical Center*

Abstract

Although many of us interact daily with animals, we have little understanding of how this affects our interactions with people. This study assessed the physiological effects of human–animal interactions and tested if this affected interpersonal trust. Participants (N=141) were assigned to play with a friendly but unfamiliar cat or dog for 10 minutes or to rest quietly in a private room. Blood was obtained from human participants before and after animal interactions or rest, and videos of animal interactions were coded for encounter styles. Participants then made interpersonal monetary decisions to quantify trust and trustworthiness toward strangers. Although oxytocin (OT) fell on average after interactions with both dogs and cats, there was a positive and significant correlation between the change in OT after interacting with a dog and lifetime pet exposure. Participants who had lived with four or more dogs in their lifetimes had a positive increase in OT after interacting with an unknown dog. We found a negative correlation between the change in OT after interacting with a cat and cat ownership. Participants who had a reduction in stress hormones after a dog interaction showed increased trust in strangers. Specifically, a one-percentage-point decrease in the stress hormone adrenocorticotropin hormone increased trust in a stranger by 24 percent. Our findings show that the human OT response to animals depends on previous pet exposure.

Keywords: hormones, stress, attachment, neuroeconomics, trust

People live with pets for a variety of reasons and interact with them in different ways, but there is no universal human response to animals. Some people are inseparable from their cats and dogs, while others don't like animals at all. Studies have shown that patients with companion animals have lower blood pressures, heart rates, and stress levels, as well as improved emotional well-being (Jorgenson, 1997; Odendaal, 2000; Barker & Wolen, 2008; Barker et al., 2012). Interacting with a dog for as little as five minutes can lead to a reduction in the stress hormone cortisol, suggesting that animal-assisted therapy may be an effective anti-stress treatment (Odendaal, 2000; Barker & Wolen, 2008).

Chronic stress has been associated with cardiovascular disease, cancer, and depression (Maddock & Pariante, 2001), and the costs of work-related stress are estimated to be as high as four percent of GDP (Hoel et al., 2001). Some organizations have begun permitting employees to bring pets to work as a stress-reduction technique. Indeed, employee perceptions of pets in the office are positive, with the most commonly

*Corresponding author email: paul.zak@cgu.edu

cited benefit being a perceived lowering of stress (Wells & Perrine, 2001). Barker et al. (2012) found a significant reduction in perceived stress in pet owners who brought their dogs to work compared to those who had pets but did not bring them to work, and compared to employees who had no pets at all (Barker et al., 2012).

Interactions with animals may affect more than stress. For example, people who have dogs are judged to be more trustworthy than those who do not (Gueguen & Cicotti, 2008). Of particular interest is the finding that human–dog interactions have been associated with increases in oxytocin (OT; Odendaal, 2000; Odendaal & Meintjes, 2003; Nagasawa et al., 2009), although this effect may be non-robust due to factors like limited sample sizes and poor experimental controls (Beetz et al., 2012; Miller et al., 2009).

Neurochemicals like OT fluctuate to guide human and nonhuman animals' responses to their internal and external environments. Many hormones in human beings, including OT, adrenocorticotropin hormone (ACTH), cortisol (CORT), and testosterone (T), respond to social interactions. As social creatures, humans seek to balance the costs of social interactions (such as fear and danger) with its benefits (such as mating and alliance-building). Changes in neurochemicals affect this calculus, working at different time frequencies that range from milliseconds to hours.

OT is known to be released in women during labor and breastfeeding, and by both sexes during sex. Beyond peri-reproductive behaviors, over a decade of research on the behavioral effects of OT have shown that it increases when one is trusted (Zak et al., 2004; 2005), touched (Morhenn et al., 2008; 2012), watches an emotional movie (Barraza & Zak, 2009), or engages in a variety of group rituals (Zak, 2012). These studies have been confirmed by intranasal OT infusion studies showing that OT generally increases prosocial or moral behaviors (Zak, 2004; 2005; 2007; 2011; 2012; Kosfeld et al., 2005; Barraza & Zak, 2009; Barraza et al., 2011). OT is a rapid and unconscious signal that those around us appear to be safe, familiar, or trustworthy.

The effects of OT occur both on the central nervous system (primarily affecting activity in the amygdala, hypothalamus, and anterior cingulate cortex; Bethlehem et al., 2013; Kirsch et al, 2005), and the peripheral nervous system reducing sympathetic tone via the vagus nerve and inhibition of stress hormones such as ACTH and CORT (Meyer-Lindenberg et al., 2011; Norman et al., 2011). OT is synthesized in the hypothalamus within 1-2 seconds after a stimulus (Zak et al., 2004; 2005) and has a 3-5 minute half-life (Chard et al., 1970). Unlike most neurochemicals, a stimulus causes OT to be released in both the brain and, via the pituitary gland, the blood (Landgraf & Neumann, 2004). This means that a change in OT measured in the blood reflects a change in OT in the brain. Nevertheless, basal (unstimulated) plasma OT and OT in cerebrospinal fluid are unrelated (Dogterom et al., 1977).

Humans are gregariously social, and our neuroanatomy reflects this. Humans appear to have a larger number of frontal cortex OT receptors than other animals (Loup et al., 1991) though definitive cross-species studies have not yet been done. Human behaviors and brain structure suggest that people might use the same attachment system that evolved to care for offspring to attach to animals. The present study seeks to test this hypothesis using a large sample and an accepted methodology to measure the change in OT.

Others have tested this hypothesis but in much narrower ways than we do here. Odendaal (2000) tested N=16 participants and found a significant positive relationship between interacting with one's own dog and changes in plasma OT in both species. A similar study using N=10 females also found an increase in plasma OT in human participants when petting one's own dog (Handlin et al., 2011). Nagasawa et al., (2009) reported that a long gaze (but not a short gaze) at one's dog increased human urinary OT for N=55. Because of the short half-life of OT and the lack of published kinetics from OT synthesis in the brain to excretion in urine, Nagasawa et al.'s results are in question. Acute changes in OT are best measured through serial blood draws. The cited works also study only pets and their human caretakers. As a result, these studies are conditioned on a potentially long period of attachment between animals and humans than can be difficult to quantify. Conversely, our approach had people interact with unfamiliar but friendly dogs as a stark test of the neurochemical effects of dogs on humans. Our study used different dogs so that the findings were not dependent on interactions with a single animal.

Nothing in the brain happens in isolation. In the present study we also tested whether animal interactions affect the stress hormones ACTH and CORT. Odendaal & Meintjes, 2003 report such a finding for human CORT levels. Service dogs appear to decrease CORT in autistic children (Viau et al., 2010) and health care professionals (Barker et al., 2005). Because our experimental design used a short-duration (10 minute) interaction, we measured CORT along with the faster acting stress hormone ACTH. To rule out spurious findings from noisy physiologic measures, we also included an active behavioral task to assess if neuroendocrine changes in humans affect prosocial behaviors. That is, we tested if the neurophysiologic effect of interacting with an animal would carryover to interpersonal human interactions.

We also included a larger sample size than other studies as well as an active control condition. A total of N=62 participants interacted with unfamiliar dogs and N=47 interacted with unfamiliar cats. Including cats was a natural control since nearly as many households have cats (30.4%) as have dogs (36.5%; American Veterinary Medical Association, 2012). We also included a second control condition (N=32) of no animal interaction at all. Animal-human interactions were videotaped to test if the quantity and quality of these encounters were associated with physiologic changes.

We hypothesized that interactions with dogs, but not cats or quiet rest, would increase OT, decrease ACTH and CORT, and increase interpersonal trust.

Methods

Timeline

This study adapts the protocol in Zak et al. (2005) to accommodate animals in the experimental design. Six participants were recruited per session and, after baseline blood draws, were randomly assigned to one of three conditions: Dog, Cat, or Rest. In the animal conditions, participants interacted alone with an animal in small, closed rooms for 10 minutes. The Rest condition put participants in the same rooms but had them sit quietly for 10 minutes.

Immediately after the animal interaction or rest, a second blood draw was obtained and participants answered survey questions regarding their moods, pet experience histories, and attitudes. After completion of the surveys, participants were given instruction in the economic decision task and then made monetary transfer choices. After all decisions were made, participants were paid their earnings in private and dismissed. There was no deception of any type in this experiment.

Participants

Participants were recruited from the Claremont Colleges using fliers posted on campus, through social networking sites, and through word of mouth. Recruitment fliers and emails told potential participants that the study would examine the biological bases of decision-making and might involve interactions with dogs or cats. The Institutional Review Boards of Scripps College and Claremont Graduate University approved the study. All participants gave written informed consent prior to inclusion and were assigned an identity-masking code used to ensure anonymity. Experimental sessions were conducted in the early evening at the Center for Neuroeconomics Studies at Claremont Graduate University, and each session lasted approximately 60 minutes. A total of 141 participants were recruited, with 50 percent of them female. The average age of participants was 21.65 (SD = 4.64).

Blood Draws and Assays

Participants were taken to a private room where 28 ml of blood was drawn from an antecubital vein by a qualified phlebotomist. Two 8-ml EDTA whole-blood tubes and one 12-ml serum-separator tube were drawn maintaining a sterile field using Vacutainer® blood collection kits. The initial blood draw established basal OT, CORT, and ACTH.

A second 28-ml blood draw was obtained from each participant immediately following his or her 10-minute interaction with the animal or at the conclusion of the 10-minute rest period. All second blood draws occurred within two minutes after the rest or animal interaction ended. This design takes into account OT's short half-life and seeks to capture participants' physiologic states during the animal interaction.

After phlebotomy, each blood tube was immediately placed on ice before being put into to a refrigerated centrifuge and spun at 1500 rpm at 4°C for 12 minutes. Plasma and serum were withdrawn and placed into 2-ml polypropylene microtubes with screw caps. The microtubes were immediately placed on dry ice and then transferred to an −80°C freezer until analysis.

Hormones were assayed using either radioimmunoassays (RIA) or enzyme- linked immunosorbent assays (ELISA). Assays were performed at Biomarkers Core at Emory University in Atlanta, Georgia. ACTH and CORT were assayed using an RIA kit from Diagnostic Systems Laboratories (Webster, Texas), while OT was assayed using an ELISA from R&D Systems (Minneapolis, Minnesota). The inter- and intra-assay coefficients of variations were less than 15 percent for all tests. While recent advances in assay design have shown that an RIA with an extraction step measures OT more precisely than an ELISA (McCullough et al., 2013), this study was done in 2010 before the differences between the ELISA and RIA had been established. Since we focus on the change in OT after a stimulus and not OT levels, side-products that the ELISA may measure are likely to disappear when changes in OT are analyzed. As a result, we only report changes in OT.

Economic Decision Task

Participants were instructed in and made a single decision using a variation of the trust game (TG) developed by Berg et al. (1995). Each participant was randomly assigned to a dyad with another participant and then randomly assigned the role of Decision-Maker 1 (DM1) or Decision-Maker 2 (DM2). Both DMs were endowed with $10 at the start of the task and were extensively instructed about how their decisions would affect their earnings and the earnings of the other dyad member. Interactions between the participants were conducted exclusively through a computer interface.

The instructions stated that the amount transferred by DM1 would be removed from his or her account and would be tripled and placed in DM2's account. DM2 was then informed by the software of the tripled transfer received from the DM1 in his or her dyad and the total in his or her account. Then, DM2 was prompted by the software to enter an amount, including $0, that he or she would like to transfer back to the DM1 in the dyad. The amount sent by DM2 to DM1 would be subtracted from DM2's account and would transfer one-for-one into DM1's account. The instructions included several examples of DM1 and DM2 transfers and subsequent earnings. Participants were also prompted to ask questions prior to making decisions.

The transfer from DM1 to DM2 in this task is considered a measure of trust, and the amount returned by DM2 to DM1 is considered a measure of trustworthiness or reciprocity (Smith & Walker, 1993). The classical prediction in economics is that DM2 will return nothing to DM1 regardless of the amount she or he receives. However, in most studies in developed countries, 90-95% of participants show at least some trust and reciprocity (Zak, 2011; Camerer, 2003).

Video

Animal–human interactions were recorded on Sony digital cameras using tripods. Cameras were set up in such a way that both the animal and the human participant were in frame for the majority of the recording. Videos were transferred onto DVDs and given to four independent raters who had an inter-rater reliability of $b = 0.634$, $p < 0.001$. The coding quantified touch, visual gaze, and the use of toys during animal interactions.

Animals

Animals were recruited from lab members based on their friendliness toward strangers. Two animals were used at a time. The most-used dogs were named Rowdy, a Brittany, and Herriot, a beagle, though other dogs of various sizes and breeds were used as well. Cat interactions were conducted using two common housecats. The interaction rooms included toys and treats so that participants had several ways to engage with the animals. Multiple animals were used so that the results did not depend on the behavior of a single dog or cat.

In every experimental session, animals were accompanied by their owners or an animal rights observer. Our focus was on human physiology and behavior after animal interactions, not animal responses. As a result, blood samples were only obtained from people, not animals. Breaks were provided after every experimental session for animals to eat, drink, and use the litter box (cats) or walk in a grassy area (dogs). One dog in the first session appeared to be mildly distressed and was not used in subsequent sessions. All other animals appeared relaxed before, during, and after experimental sessions. Claremont Graduate University's Internal Review Board approved the animal handling protocol; IACUC approval was not necessary as the animals were not being studied.

Surveys

Trusting behaviors can be influenced by a number of underlying psychological factors. In order to untangle these interactions, we administered a number of surveys. These included Satisfaction With Life (SWL; Pavot & Diener, 1993) that provides a global assessment of one's flourishing, and the Affect Intensity Measure (AIM; Larsen, 1984) that measures the strength and valence of emotions. We also included a number of questions taken from the General Social Survey regarding attitudes about others (Gleaser et al., 2000) was well as demographic information. Questions regarding one's feelings about animals and pet ownership history were created for this study and can be found in the Appendix.

Results

Hormones

The physiologic effect of animal encounters was highly variable. The change in OT for those who interacted with dogs varied from +81% to −40%, while cat interactions produced changes in OT from +72% to −57%. As shown in Fig. 10.1, the average percentage change in OT was negative when participants interacted with both dogs ($M=-5.3\%$, $p=0.05$) and cats ($M=-9.5\%$, $p=0.003$). Average percentage changes in stress hormones did not statistically differ from zero after playing with dogs (two-tailed paired t-tests: CORT $M=0.6\%$, $p=0.89$; ACTH $M=8.0\%$, $p=0.18$) or cats (CORT $M=-3.3\%$, $p=0.42$; ACTH $M=4.1\%$, $p=0.45$).

Pet History

We found a positive and significant correlation between the percentage change in OT after interacting with a dog and the number of dogs ($r=0.275$, $p=0.04$), cats ($r=0.410$, $p=0.002$), and total number of pets one has resided with in one's lifetime ($r=0.403$, $p=0.002$; Figs. 10.2a-c).

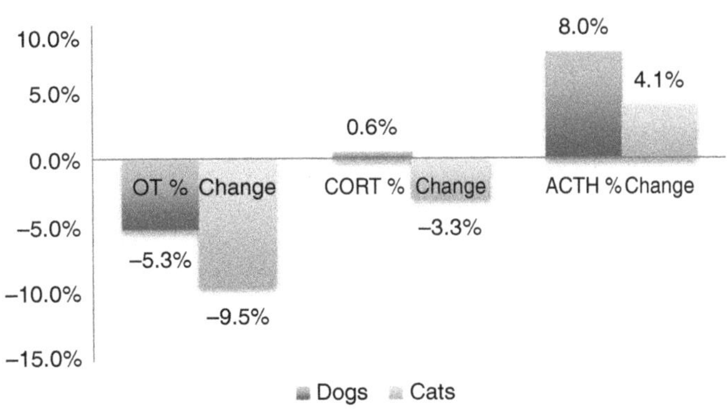

Fig. 10.1. Endocrine changes after animal interactions. Playing with an unfamiliar dog or cat caused a significant reduction in OT and insignificant changes in ACTH and CORT.

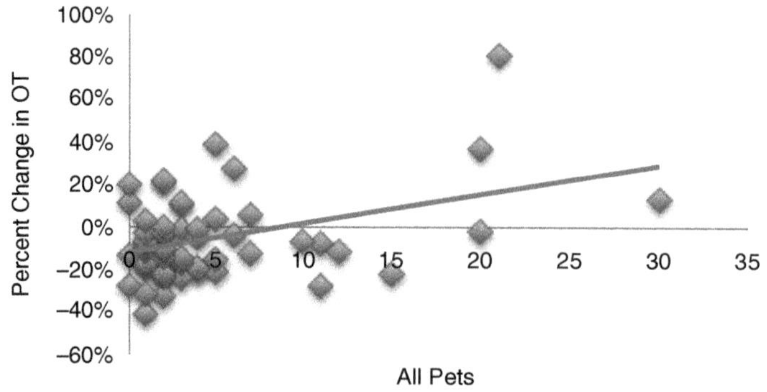

Fig. 10.2a. Percent change in OT and the total number of lifetime pets for people who interacted with a dog. Increases in oxytocin were associated with a higher number of pets owned in a participant's lifetime.

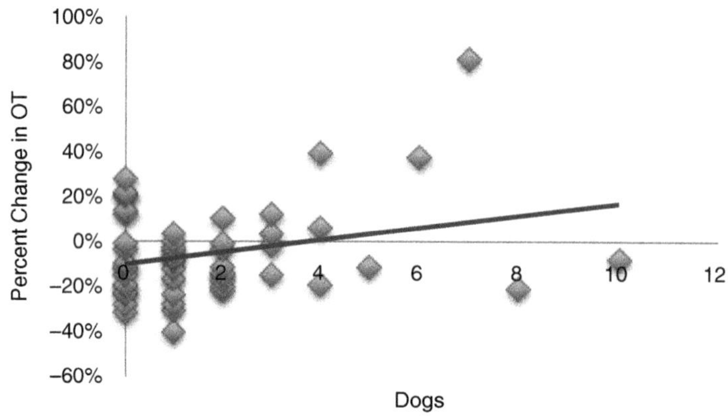

Fig. 10.2b. There was a positive association between the increase in OT and the total number of lifetime dog cohabitations for people who interacted with a dog.

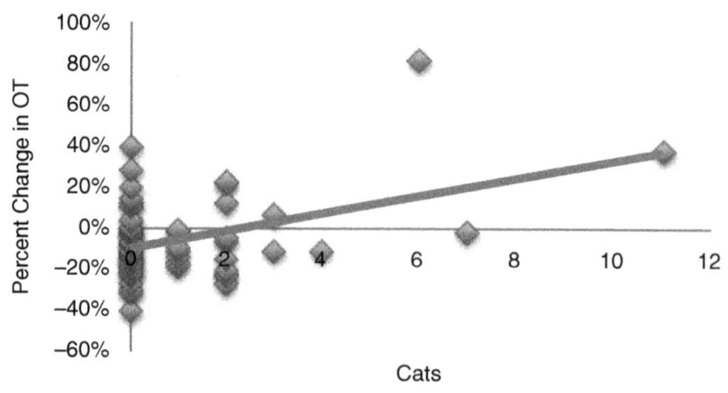

Fig. 10.2c. The number of cats a participant had lived with was positively associated with an increase in OT after interacting with a dog.

The significant relationship between the lifetime number of pets owned and the change in OT continues to hold after controlling for age and removing outliers (for instance, one individual reported 30 lifetime pets).

The opposite pattern was found for participants who interacted with cats: There was a negative relationship between the percentage change in OT and the number of cats a participant had lived with in his or her lifetime (r=–0.334, p=0.03; Fig. 10.3). The relationship between the lifetime number of cats owned and the percentage change in OT continued to be significant even after controlling for age (b = –3.9%, p = 0.02). The relationship between lifetime number of pets, lifetime number of dogs, and the change in OT after interacting with a cat did not reach statistical significance (Pets owned: r=–0.21 p=0.19; Dogs owned: r=0.21 p=0.18).

Interaction Types

While we coded for over two-dozen animal–human interaction variables, only a handful of them were significantly associated with changes in hormones. Table 10.1 shows the correlation and p-values for all coded variables. Significant correlations were found between petting a dog's belly and an increase in ACTH (r=0.34, p=0.01); the dog lying down away from the person and an increase in OT (r=0.26, p=0.05); and eye contact between the participant and the dog and an increase in OT (r=0.29, p=0.02). The correlation between the number of times a participant made eye contact with a dog and changes in OT replicates earlier work (Nagasawa et al., 2009). For participants who interacted with a cat, offering the cat a toy was associated with an increase in OT (r=0.30, p=0.05).

Trusting Behaviors

Overall, there were no significant differences among the three different treatment groups and the amount transferred by DM1s in the trust game (Dog: \$6.97; Cat: \$6.71; Control: \$6.28; F=0.14, p=0.86). Return transfers by DM2s also were statistically the same across groups (Dogs: 50.5%; Cats: 41.4%; Control: 57%; F=1.77, p=0.18).

When we looked at the relationship between stress hormones and trusting behaviors, we found that for DM1s who interacted with dogs, a reduction in ACTH marginally increased trust in a stranger (r=–0.349, p = 0.06; Fig. 10.4). For those in the dog group, the changes in OT and CORT were unrelated to trust (ps>0.05). The negative relationship between the change in ACTH and trust for those who interacted with dogs persists after controlling for changes in OT, age, and gender (b = –2.77, p=0.02, R^2=0.32).

For those who interacted with cats, a reduction in CORT increased trust (r=–0.495, p = 0.02; Fig. 10.5). Neither the change in OT nor the change in ACTH were associated with trusting behaviors for those who interacted with

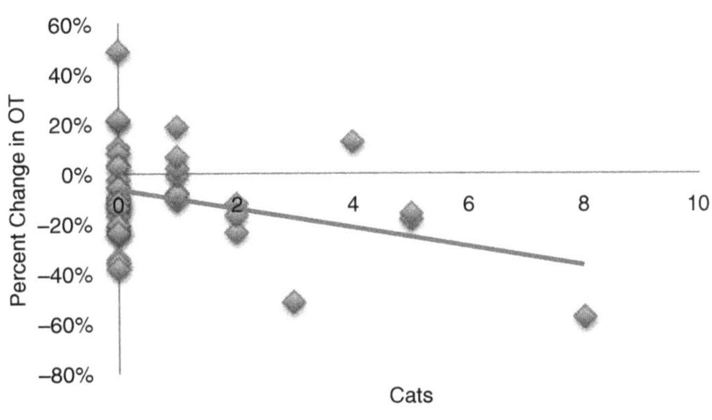

Fig. 10.3. Percent change in OT and the total number of cats one has had for participants who interacted with a cat. A larger number of cats was associated with a greater decrease in OT.

Table 10.1. Endocrine changes associates with human–animal interactions. All p values are two-tailed tests. For dogs, eye contact, petting, offering treats, and the number of times the dog lay down away from the participant were significantly correlated with hormone changes. For cat interactions, offering a toy during the session was positively correlated with changes in OT.

Dog Interaction Correlations				
% Change in		OT	CORT	ACTH
Petting - Total	*r*	0.09	0.04	0.22
# of times	*p*	0.49	0.75	0.10
Petting - Head	*r*	0.09	0.15	0.07
and face	*p*	0.49	0.27	0.60
Petting - Side	*r*	0.06	−0.03	0.17
and back	*p*	0.66	0.84	0.21
Petting - Belly	*r*	0.06	−0.08	0.34
	p	0.64	0.58	0.01
Toys (offers)	*r*	−0.12	0.12	0.12
	p	0.38	0.39	0.40
Treats (offers)	*r*	−0.10	−0.24	−0.13
	p	0.47	0.07	0.34
Lying down	*r*	0.00	0.15	0.16
(to engage person)	*p*	0.99	0.25	0.25
Lying down	*r*	0.26	0.06	0.05
away from person	*p*	0.05	0.68	0.71
Whining	*r*	−0.05	0.11	0.19
# of times	*p*	0.71	0.44	0.16
Facing door	*r*	0.18	0.15	−0.15
or window	*p*	0.18	0.27	0.28
Person says name	*r*	−0.07	−0.01	0.03
	p	0.60	0.96	0.85
Response to name	*r*	−0.12	−0.03	−0.20
	p	0.39	0.83	0.14
Response to non-	*r*	0.04	−0.16	−0.16
name verbal	*p*	0.77	0.24	0.24
Response to	*r*	0.02	−0.15	0.05
gesture	*p*	0.86	0.28	0.73
Person changes	*r*	0.06	0.01	−0.14
position	*p*	0.66	0.96	0.32
Animal initiates	*r*	0.03	0.08	0.05
contact	*p*	0.81	0.57	0.70
Eye contact	*r*	0.29	0.21	0.21
	p	0.02	0.12	0.12

Cat Interaction Correlations				
% Change in		OT	CORT	ACTH
Petting - Total	*r*	−0.05	−0.01	0.09
# of times	*p*	0.74	0.96	0.60
Petting - Head	*r*	0.02	−0.01	0.03
and face	*p*	0.90	0.94	0.87
Petting - Side	*r*	−0.03	−0.01	0.16
and back	*p*	0.84	0.96	0.32
Petting - Belly	*r*	−0.25	0.03	−0.01
	p	0.12	0.83	0.95
Toys (offers)	*r*	0.30	0.17	0.04
	p	0.05	0.28	0.80
Treats (offers)	*r*	−0.02	−0.25	0.02
	p	0.89	0.12	0.89
Lying down	*r*	−0.19	0.03	0.08
(to engage person)	*p*	0.24	0.87	0.62
Lying down	*r*	0.01	−0.03	0.14
away from person	*p*	0.94	0.83	0.38
Whining	*r*	0.26	0.06	−0.04
# of times	*p*	0.09	0.70	0.82
Facing door	*r*	0.14	−0.18	−0.26
or window	*p*	0.38	0.26	0.10
Person says name	*r*	0.00	−0.19	0.09
	p	1.00	0.25	0.58
Response to name	*r*	0.09	−0.01	0.00
	p	0.56	0.96	0.99
Response to non-	*r*	0.09	−0.23	0.05
name verbal	*p*	0.59	0.15	0.76
Response to	*r*	0.01	−0.15	0.08
gesture	*p*	0.95	0.35	0.61
Person changes	*r*	−0.22	0.05	0.08
position	*p*	0.17	0.78	0.64
Animal initiates	*r*	0.05	−0.18	0.21
contact	*p*	0.77	0.27	0.20
Eye contact	*r*	0.12	0.04	−0.15
	p	0.44	0.81	0.35

cats (ps>0.05). The negative relationship between changes in CORT and trust for participants who interacted with cats is also robust after controlling for the same variables as in the dog analysis (b=–7.10, p=0.06, R^2=0.30).

These findings caused us to further examine the relationship between stress hormones and trust. We found that 65% of DM1s had negative CORT changes after interacting with either animal, with an average percentage change of –17%. The increase in CORT for the other 35% only averaged 1.7%. Participants with a decrease in CORT did not exhibit a difference in trust from those whose CORT increased (Increase: $7.25; Decrease: $6.94; p=0.11). Similarly, 51% of DM1s had negative ACTH changes from animal interactions that averaged –28%, while the 49% of those with an increase in ACTH averaged just 2%. There was no difference in trust between groups (Increase: $7.15; Decrease: $6.48; p=0.40). These inconclusive results could be the result of measurement error from the assay. Indeed, we found a lack of the expected correlation between ACTH and CORT in participants who

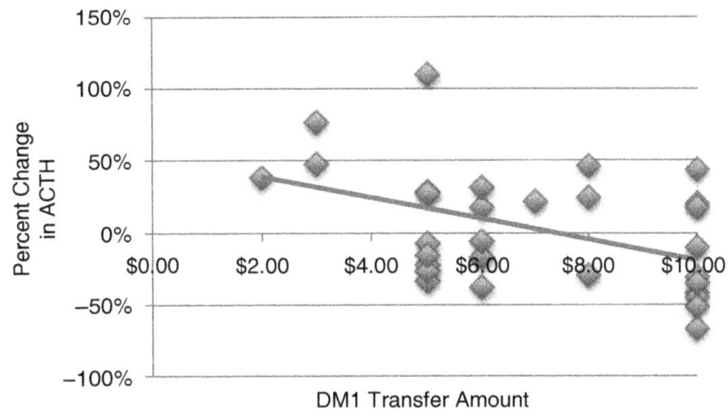

Fig. 10.4. Percent change in ACTH and DM1 transfer amount after dog interactions. For participants who interacted with a dog, larger reductions in ACTH were associated with higher DM1 transfer amounts.

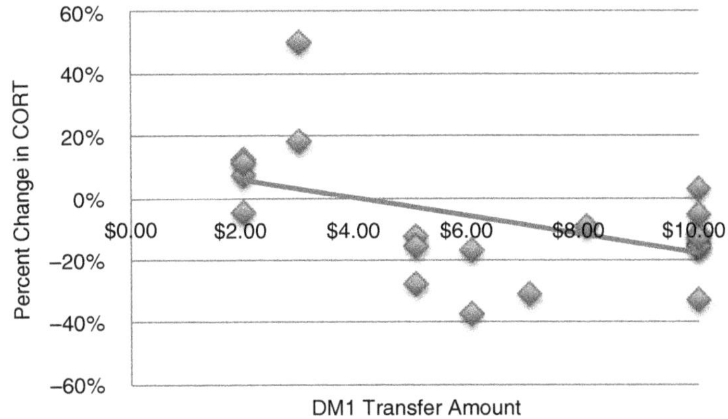

Fig. 10.5. Percent change in CORT and DM1 transfer amount after cat interactions. For those participants who interacted with a cat, larger reductions in CORT were associated with higher DM1 transfer amounts.

interacted with animals in our sample (r= −0.15, p=0.12). In order to derive robust results, we assessed trust in the 32% of participants who had reductions in both ACTH and CORT after animal interactions. We found that participants with reductions in both stress hormones demonstrated 25% higher trust compared to those who did not have an unambiguous reduction in stress ($8.11 vs. $6.48; p=0.02).

For DM2s who interacted with either type of animal, there were no significant correlations between hormone changes and trustworthiness. (Cats: CORT r=−0.13, p=0.57; OT r=−0.08, p=0.72; ACTH r=0.07, p=0.76; Dogs: CORT r=0.02, p=0.91; OT r=0.03, p=0.87; ACTH r=0.13, p=0.51). This was expected since the signal of trust DM2s receive from DM1s is likely to overwhelm the effects of dog or cat interactions (Zak et al., 2005; 2011). There was also no significant difference in DM2 trustworthiness for those with negative changes in CORT (Negative: 51%; Positive: 40%; p=0.11), ACTH (Negative: 46%; Positive: 46%, p=0.98), or both ACTH and CORT (Negative: 50%; Positive: 45%; p=0.59).

As in previous research (Zak et al., 2005), the trait and attitude surveys showed little association with trusting behaviors. Only those who thought money was very important showed less trust in strangers (r=–0.40, p=0.01). On the other hand, trustworthiness was positively correlated with emotional lability as measured by the AIM (r=0.51, p=0.001) and negatively associated with a desire to make money any way possible (r=–0.46, p=0.00) and a stated distrustof strangers (r=–0.29, p=0.06).

Discussion

This study sought to characterize the physiologic effects of human–animal interactions and to test if physiologic changes due to animals affected human–human interactions. As expected, our findings were more nuanced than were our hypotheses. Rather than interactions with dogs uniformly increasing OT, we found that only a subset of participants (27%) responded this way. If one owned a sufficient number of dogs, cats, or pets in one's lifetime, this increased the likelihood that interacting with an unfamiliar dog increased OT. For our data, if an average participant had resided with four or more dogs in his or her lifetime, then interacting with a dog in the lab produced an OT increase. This suggests that pet experience may prime the brain for physiologic attachment (an increase in OT) when one interacts with an unknown dog. There is evidence in rodents that rich social environments stimulate oxytocin receptor binding and result in increased social behaviors (Champagne & Meaney, 2007). It is possible that having pets in one's household has a similar effect on human beings.

We also tested the effect of human–animal interactions on interpersonal behaviors by asking participants to make a single monetary decision in which they could exhibit trust or trustworthiness through a computer-aided monetary transfer to a stranger. We found that a reduction in stress after playing with a dog linearly increased trust in a stranger. In our sample, a one percentage point decrease in ACTH increased trust by 24%, a substantial size effect. A further analysis revealed that a robust measure of stress reduction (a decline in both CORT and ACTH) from interacting with either a dog or cat was associated with 25% greater trust in a stranger. Playing with an animal reduced stress in approximately one-third of participants. Compared to those who did not get a stress reduction, this group of participants were more likely to self-identify as "dog people" (r=0.19, p=0.05) and report higher levels of religiosity in several questions (ps<0.05). Future studies should seek to understand the circumstances in which interacting with an unknown pet reliably reduces stress.

We did find several lines of evidence regarding the type of interactions with animals that affected OT. Eye contact with a dog was found to correlate with an increase in OT, confirming earlier work (Nagasawa et al., 2009). Given that both humans and dogs are social animals, intermittent eye contact can be interpreted as a display of trust and an engagement in a bonding activity. The dog lying down away from the participant also positively correlated with changes in OT. This behavior could indicate a degree of comfort the dog has toward the person in the room, enabling the human to feel more attached to the animal. In interactions between participants and cats, we found positive correlations between changes in OT and how many times a participant offered a toy to the animal. The lack of an increase in OT with other play styles may be due to the limited motivation by cats to socialize based on their generally solitary nature. By offering the cat a toy, a participant appears to be forming a connection with the animal, resulting in an increase in OT. The conditional nature of our findings is consistent with reports showing that OT infusion on human social interactions is conditional on set and setting (de Dreu et al., 2010).

For the scientific community, our discovery that an increase in OT after interacting with a dog was conditional on previous pet experience may help explain the inability of other labs to replicate Odendaal's (2000) findings of an increase in OT after interacting with one's own dog. The present study had a large number of participants interacting with unfamiliar dogs, setting the bar higher to find an OT effect from cross-species interactions. It is also interesting that previous cat ownership had a linearly decreasing effect on OT after interacting with a cat. This could be due the reduced quantity and quality of participant interactions in cats versus dogs. We hope that this research stimulates other studies on cross-species attachment, a phenomenon that may be more common than once thought (Zak, 2014).

Our findings may also prove useful to professionals using animal-assisted therapy. Encouraging patients to engage in eye contact, petting, and other bonding behaviors with service animals may be the most effective way to reduce stress and increase oxytocin. Our analysis also suggests that animal therapy may have a cumulative effect as we found for pet ownership on oxytocin release. Programs that provide live-in therapy dogs to warfighters who need emotional support, for example, due to post-traumatic stress disorder, may have a stronger therapeutic effect than short-duration visits with dogs (Altschuler, 1999). Patients who have a history of pet ownership may also achieve the benefits of animal-assisted therapy more rapidly than those who have not resided with pets. Our findings also support this use of animal therapy for other anxiety-related maladies such as autism spectrum disorder (ASD). Children with ASD have a diminished stress response when they hold guinea pigs (Kršková, Talarovičová, & Olexová, 2010; O'Haire, McKenzie, Beck, & Slaughter, 2015). Dog therapy for those with ASD may have even stronger effects (Solomon, 2010).

Dogs appear to have a special relationship with humans. This is reflected in the intense physiologic response to dogs for those who have a history of pet exposure. Our research elucidates the mechanism that is at least partially responsible for the positive effects of animal-assisted therapy and bring-your-dog-to-work programs. The benefits of dogs in our lives appear to grow the more we are exposed to them.

References

Altschuler, E. (1999). Pet-facilitated therapy for posttraumatic stress disorder. *Annals of Clinical Psychiatry, 11*(1), 29–30.

American Veterinary Medical Association. (2012). U.S. Pet Ownership & Demographics Sourcebook. Retrieved from https://www.avma.org/KB/Resources/Statistics/Pages/Market-research-statistics-US-pet-ownership.aspx.

Barraza, J., McCullough, M., Ahmadi, S., & Zak, P. (2011). Oxytocin infusion increases charitable donations regardless of monetary resources. *Hormones and Behavior*, *60*(2), 148–151.

Barraza, J., & Zak, P. (2009). Empathy toward strangers triggers oxytocin release and subsequent generosity. *Annals of the New York Academy of Sciences*, *1167*(1), 182–189.

Barker, R., Knisely, J., Barker, S., Cobb, R., & Schubert, C. (2012). Preliminary investigation of employee's dog presenceon stress and organizational perceptions. *International Journal of Workplace Health Management*, *5*(1), 15–30.

Barker, S., Knisely, J., McCain, N., & Best, A. (2005). Measuring stress and immune responses in health care professiona ls following interaction with a therapy dog: a pilot study. *Psychol. Rep.* 96, 713–72910.2466/pr0.96.3.713–729

Barker, S., & Wolen, A. (2008). The benefits of human–companion animal interaction: A review. *Journal of Veterinary Medical Education*, *35*(4), 487–495.

Beetz, A., Uvnäs-Moberg, K., Julius, H., & Kotrschal, K. (2012). Psychosocial and psychophysiological effects of human-animal interactions: the possible role of oxytocin. *Frontiers in Psychology*, *3*, 234.

Berg, J., Dickhaut, J., & McCabe, K. (1995). Trust, reciprocity, and social history. *Games and Economic Behavior*, *10*(1), 122–142.

Bethlehem, R., vanHonk, J., Auyeung, B., & Baron-Cohen, S. (2013). Oxytocin, brain physiology, and functional connectivity: a review of intranasal oxytocin fMRI studies. *Psychoneuroendocrinology*, *38*(7), 962–974.

Camerer, C. (2003). *Behavioral Game Theory: Experiments in Strategic Interaction.* Princeton University Press.

Champagne, F., & Meaney, M. (2007). Transgenerational effects of social environment on variations in maternal care and behavioral response to novelty. *Behavioral Neuroscience*, *121*(6), 1353–1363.

Chard, T., Boyd, N., Forsling, M., McNeilly, A., & Landon, J. (1970). The development of a radioimmunoassay for oxytocin: the extraction of oxytocin from plasma, and its measurement during parturition in human and goat blood. *Journal of Endocrinology*, *48*(2), 223–234.

De Dreu, C., Greer, L., Handgraaf, M., Shalvi, S., Van Kleef, G., Baas, M. and Feith, S. (2010). The neuropeptide oxytocin regulates parochial altruism in intergro up conflict among humans. *Science, 328*(5984), 1408–1411.

Dogterom, J., van Wimersma Greidanus, T., & Swaab, D. (1977). Evidence for the release of vasopressin and oxytocin into cerebrospinal fluid: measurements in plasma and CSF of intact and hypophysectomized rats. *Neuroendocrinology*, *24*(2), 108–118.

Hoel, H., Sparks, K., & Cooper, C. (2001). *The Cost of Violence/stress at Work and the Benefits of a Violence/stress-free Working Environment*. Geneva: International Labour Organization.

Guéguen, N., & Ciccotti, S. (2008). Domestic dogs as facilitators in social interaction: An evaluation of helping and courtship behaviors. *Anthrozoos: A Multidisciplinary Journal of The Interactions of People & Animals*, *21*(4), 339–349.

Glaeser, E., Laibson, D., Scheinkman, J., & Soutter, C. (2000). Measuring trust. *Quarterly Journal of Economics*, *115*(3): 811–846.

Handlin, L., Hydbring-Sandberg, E., Nilsson, A., Ejdebäck, M., Jansson, A., & Uvnäs-Moberg, K. (2011). Short-term interaction between dogs and their owners: effects on oxytocin, cortisol, insulin and heart rate—an exploratory study. *Anthrozoös, 24*(3), 301–315.

Jorgenson, J. (1997). Therapeutic use of companion animals in health care. *Image: the Journal of Nursing Scholarship*, *29*(3), 249–254.

Kirsch, P., Esslinger, C., Chen, Q., Mier, D., et al. (2005). Oxytocin modulates neural circuitry for social cognition and fear in humans. *Journal of Neuroscience*, *25*(49), 11489–11493.

Kosfeld, M., Heinrichs, M., Zak, P., Fischbacher, U., & Fehr, E. (2005). Oxytocin increases trust in humans. *Nature*, *435*(7042), 673–676.

Kršková, L., Talarovičová, A., & Olexová, L. (2010). Guinea pigs—The "Small Great" Therapist for Autistic Children, or: Do Guinea Pigs Have Positive Effects on Autistic Child Social Behavior? *Society & Animals*, *18*(2), 139–151.

Landgraf, R., & Neumann, I. (2004). Vasopressin and oxytocin release within the brain: a dynamic concept of multiple and variable modes of neuropeptide communication. *Frontiers in Neuroendocrinology*, *25*(3), 150–176.

Larsen, R., & Diener, E. (1987). Affect intensity as an individual difference characteristic: A review. *Journal of Research in Personality*, *21*(1), 1–39.

Loup, F., Tribollet, E., Dubois-Dauphin, M., & Dreifuss, J. (1991). Localization of high-affinity binding sites for oxytocin and vasopressin in the human brain. An autoradiographic study. *Brain Research*, *555*(2), 220–232.

Maddock, C., & Pariante, C. (2001). How does stress affect you? An overview of stress, immunity, depression and disease. *Epidemiologia e Psichiatria Sociale*, *10*(03), 153–162.

McCullough, M., Churchland, P., & Mendez, A. (2013). Problems with measuring peripheral oxytocin: can the data on oxytocin and human behavior be trusted?. *Neuroscience & Biobehavioral Reviews*, *37*(8), 1485–1492.

Meyer-Lindenberg, A., Domes, G., Kirsch, P., & Heinrichs, M. (2011). Oxytocin and vasopressin in the human brain: social neuropeptides for translational medicine. *Nature Reviews Neuroscience*, *12*(9), 524–538.

Miller, S., Kennedy, C., DeVoe, D., Hickey, M., Nelson, T., & Kogan, L. (2009). An examination of changes in oxytocin levels in men and women before and after interaction with a bonded dog. *Anthrozoos: A Multidisciplinary Journal of The Interactions of People & Animals*, *22*(1), 31–42.

Morhenn, V., Park, J., Piper, E., & Zak, P. J. (2008). Monetary sacrifice among strangers is mediated by endogenous oxytocin release after physical contact. *Evolution and Human Behavior*, *29*, 375–383.

Morhenn, V., Beavin, L., & Zak, P. (2012). Massage increases oxytocin and reduces adrenocorticotropin hormone in humans. *Alternative Therapies in Health and Medicine*, *18*(6), 11–18

Nagasawa, M., Kikusui, T., Onaka, T., & Ohta, M. (2009). Dog's gaze at its owner increases owner's urinary oxytocin during social interaction. *Hormones and Behavior*, *55*(3), 434–441.

Norman, G., Cacioppo, J., Morris, J., Malarkey, W., Berntson, G., & DeVries, A. (2011). Oxytocin increases autonomic cardiac control: moderation by loneliness. *Biological Psychology*, *86*(3), 174–180.

Odendaal, J., & Meintjes, R. (2003). Neurophysiological correlates of affiliative behaviour between humans and dogs. *The Veterinary Journal*, *165*(3), 296–301.

Odendaal, J. (2000). Animal-assisted therapy—magic or medicine?. *Journal of Psychosomatic Research*, *49*(4), 275–280.

Odendaal, J., & Meintjes, R. (2003). Neurophysiological correlates of affiliative behaviour between humans and dogs. *The Veterinary Journal*, *165*(3), 296–301.

O'Haire, M., McKenzie, S., Beck, A., & Slaughter, V. (2015). Animals may act as social buffers: Skin conductance arousal in children with autism spectrum disorder in a social context. *Developmental Psychobiology*, *57*(5), 584–595.

Pavot, W., & Diener, E. (1993). Review of the satisfaction with life scale. *Psychological Assessment*, *5*(2), 164.

Smith, V., & Walker, J. (1993). Rewards, experience and decision costs in first price auctions. *Economic Inquiry*, *31*(2), 237–244.

Solomon, O. (2010). What a dog can do: Children with autism and therapy dogs in social interaction. *Ethos*, *38*(1), 143–166.

Viau, R., Arsenault-Lapierre, G., Fecteau, S., Champagne, N., Walker, C., & Lupien, S. (2010). Effect of service dogs on salivar y cortisol secretion in autistic children. *Psychoneuroendocrinology*, *35*(8), 1187–1193.

Wells, M., & Perrine, R. (2001). Critters in the cube farm: perceived psychological and organizational effects of pets in the workplace. *Journal of Occupational Health Psychology*, *6*(1), 81.

Zak, P. (2011). The physiology of moral sentiments. *Journal of Economic Behavior & Organization, 77:* 53–65.

Zak, P. (2012). *The Moral Molecule: The Source of Love and Prosperity.* New York: Dutton.

Zak, P. (2014). Dogs (and Cats) Can Love. The Atlantic, April 22, Retrieved from http://www.theatlantic.com/health/archive/2014/04/does-your-dog-or-cat-actually-love-you/360784/

Zak, P., Kurzban, R., & Matzner, W. (2004). The neurobiology of trust. *Annals of the New York Academy of Sciences*, *1032*(1), 224–227.

Zak, P., Kurzban, R., & Matzner, W. (2005). Oxytocin is associated with human trustworthiness. *Hormones and Behavior*, *48*(5), 522–527.

Zak, P., Stanton, A., & Ahmadi, S. (2007). Oxytocin increases generosity in humans. *PLoS One*, *2*(11), e1128.

Appendix: Survey on Disposition Towards Animals

Have you even been threatened or physically assaulted by a dog? (y/n)

Have you ever been attacked by a cat? (y/n)

Have you ever interacted with a farmed animal (pig, chicken, goat, sheep, etc.)? (y/n)

If yes, on how many occasions?

Have you ever been to a zoo? (y/n)

If yes, on approximately how many occasions?

Have you ever observed animals in the wild? (y/n)

If yes, on approximately how many occasions?

Have you ever been to a circus? (y/n)

If yes, on approximately how many occasions?

Please indicate whether you agree with the following statements (1-5)

On the whole, I consider myself to be a "dog person."
On the whole, I consider myself to be a "cat person."
I would choose the company of animals over most people.
I have positive memories of dogs in my life.
I have positive memories of cats in my life.
I feel that dogs have unique personalities.
I feel like cats have unique personalities.
I feel that humans can treat animals anyway we want.
I think there is a connection between human violence towards animals and human violence towards other humans.
I think compassion towards animals can strengthen society.
I believe animals should receive moral consideration.
I feel that we should not inflict unnecessary suffering on animals.
I feel that animals should have legal protection.
In general, I feel that our society treats animals well.
I consider the treatment of animals when purchasing food.
I consider the treatment of animals when purchasing cleaning/beauty products.
I find it easier to interact with dogs than cats.
I find it easier to interact with cats than dogs.
I find it easier to interact with humans than animals.
I feel that dogs show emotional complexity.
I feel that cats display individual preferences.
I feel that cats can express their own likes and dislikes.

11 Effects of Canine-Assisted Intervention on the Mental Health of Higher Education Students: a Systematic Review

Karen Manville[1a*], Mark Coulson[2b], Michele A. Mulqueen[3c], Kirsty Neller[1d], Caroline Searing[4e], Sarah Welland[1f] and Gemma Reynolds[1g]

[1]*Middlesex University;* [2]*The University of East Anglia;* [3]*University of Derby;* [4]*University of the Arts, London*

Abstract

The aim of this systematic review was to evaluate existing literature exploring the effects of canine-assisted intervention (CAI) on the mental health of Higher Education (HE) students. A literature search was performed on 14th January 2021 for studies that investigated the effects of CAI on HE students. Thirty-three papers (6093 participants) encompassing 37 studies were included in this review. Study design varied in research objective, intervention type, timing, procedure, and measures. The Effective Public Health Practice Project Quality Assessment Tool found studies ranged in quality from moderate (n=7) to weak (n=30). The review identified CAI has a positive effect on levels of anxiety and stress in HE students. Key limitations of the studies include confounding influences during the intervention as well as a lack of control groups and standardized measures. Furthermore, intervention and procedures ranged substantially in design and application making direct comparisons difficult. The authors conclude two main outcomes from the review. Firstly, CAI improves mental health in HE students, in particular anxiety and stress. Secondly, CAI has a social benefit, encouraging communication and a shared experience. However, a number of methodological limitations of the studies are identified and reviewed. To conclude, this systematic review reveals strong support for the use of CAI in HE students as a form of therapy.

Keywords: Canine-assisted-intervention, Higher Education, Mental Health, Anxiety

Mental health is a growing public health concern. A recent longitudinal study (Kwong et al., 2021) found an increase in anxiety and a reduction in well-being as a result of the pandemic, particularly in young people and those with pre-existing health conditions. This is supported by Pierce et al. (2020), who found levels of mental distress increased in the UK population from 18.9% pre pandemic, to 27.3% just one month into the 2020 lockdown. Adolescents in particular, experienced an increase of symptoms related to depression (Wright et al.,

*Corresponding author: email: km1332@live.mdx.ac.uk
[a]Orcid ID 0000-0001-7489-616X
[b]Orcid ID 0000-0002-6760-8542
[c]Orcid ID 0000-0001-6206-178X
[d]Orcid ID 0000-0001-5461-8971
[e]Orcid ID 000-0003-3148-2690
[f]Orcid ID 0000-0001-1489-8240
[g]Orcid ID 0000-0003-2893-6380

2021), and Stewart et al., (2022) found clinical threshold levels of both anxiety and depression were exacerbated which negatively impacted mental health. Students in Higher Education (HE: education beyond secondary level, usually offered at a university or college) commonly suffer from mental health issues, in particular, stress, anxiety, and depression (e.g., Binfet & Passmore, 2016; Broglia et al., 2021; Daltry & Mehr, 2015; Dell at al., 2015; Pollard et al., 2021). Andrews and Wilding (2004) found that 9% of students without signs of depression prior to enrolment in HE developed clinical depression mid-way through the course, and 20% suffered clinically significant anxiety levels during their time in HE. Similarly, Richardson et al. (2015) revealed that 17% of UK university students suffered from depression and a further 12% experienced an anxiety disorder. More recently Savage et al. (2021) reported a decrease in HE students well-being levels alongside an increased in perceived stress, and Catling et al. (2022) found both anxiety and depressions levels increased as a result of COVID-19. One point of concern is that these studies only identify clinically significant depression and anxiety. These prevalence rates would be alarmingly higher if they also considered subclinical conditions.

HE students may experience periods of stress for a range of reasons (e.g., see Saleh et al., 2017). Specifically, Brown (2016) reports that increased tuition fees and student loans, alongside negative consequences of social media can increase risk of mental health issues in the current generation of university students. HE students may also experience greater levels of stress, anxiety, and depression than previous generations due to factors such as increased living costs or a lack of employment (Eisenberg, Gollust, Golberstein, & Hefner, 2007; Richardson et al., 2015). In addition, it has been suggested university students are at an age in which mental health issues are most likely to manifest (Richardson et al., 2015), a stage whereby young adults transitioning from childhood to adulthood poses an additional developmental challenge (Hunt & Eisenberg, 2009).

Currently the support for students struggling with mental health issues follows a traditional route (Kivlighan et al., 2021; Priestley et al., 2021; Rückert, 2015) which typically includes sessions with a trained professional schooled in the area of mental health issues (Adams et al., 2017; Brown, 2016; Goodman, 2017). However, these can often be restricted as they focus on issues within a particular moment in time (Goodman, 2017) or are time limited (Priestley et al., 2021) rather than providing on-going support. Given that 94% of HE institutions found the demand for counselling services had increased, and that less than 29% of universities had an explicit mental health or well-being strategy in place (Thorley, 2017), it is clear that much more is needed to support HE students with mental health issues. This is even before one considers the yet known effects of the Covid-19 pandemic on students' mental health (Son et al., 2020), and whether the current cohort of HE students who started their education during the pandemic will require even more additional support.

The use of animals in therapy or animal assisted therapy (AAT) is not uncommon, nor is it new. Beck (2000) cites Florence Nightingale as identifying that animals were a good companion for the sick, and Hart (2000), in a discussion on the psychosocial benefits of animal companions, argues that animals enhance quality of life and provide unconditional support. Within AAT, the use of canines is a growing area of interest (e.g. Binfet et al., 2018; Buttelmann & Römpke, 2014; Crossman et al., 2015; Elmaci & Cevizci, 2015; Smith, 2013), and much of the research to date focuses on the benefits of the interaction between humans and canines on mental health issues such as stress, anxiety, and depression (e.g., Buttelmann & Römpke 2014; Crossman et al., 2015; Dell et al., 2015). Other studies focus on benefits of this interaction on a range of medical conditions with more severe physical manifestations such as acute postoperative pain (Sobo et al, 2006), post-traumatic stress disorder (PTSD, Dietz et al., 2012), cancer (Johnson et al., 2008), and disability (Wrinkle et al., 2011). For the purpose of this review, the term 'canine assisted intervention' (CAI, Manville et al., 2022), see also Hartwig & Binfet, 2019a, 2019b; Silas et al., 2019) will be used to cover all dog or canine interaction used for therapeutic purposes.

The range of mental health issues HE students face during their time enrolled at university is wide (Brown, 2016; House of Commons, 2020; Kaparounaki et al., 2020; The Insight Network, 2020). In addition, the need for support is on the rise (The Insight Network, 2020; Thorley, 2017). Therefore, it is possible that CAI within the HE sector will benefit not only the mental health issues experienced by HE students, but also become an additional tool that universities can adopt to address the increased need for support. Despite the published studies and reviews discussing the benefits of human and canine interaction on student mental health (e.g., Adamle et al., 2009; Adams et al., 2017; Crump & Derting, 2015; Dell et al., 2015), to the author's knowledge existing literature has not been reviewed in a *systematic* manner in relation to the benefits of this interaction in HE students. As such, a review of the published work would be beneficial in order to amass existing findings in order to draw an overall conclusion on the effectiveness of CAI in this population. Furthermore, it would be useful to evaluate existing findings about specific elements of CAI, such as whether the duration or location of the intervention is important in its effectiveness. Therefore, using the PRISMA statement checklist as a guidance tool (Moher et al., 2009, PRISMA statement checklist, item number 4, objectives), this review will address three objectives:

> Objective 1: Identify, discuss, and evaluate existing evidence exploring the benefits of the interaction between human and canine on the mental health of students in HE, in particular anxiety, stress, and depression.
>
> Objective 2: Explore the individual's experience of positive psychological functioning, relationships with others, and an awareness of self.
>
> Objective 3: Examine whether current CAI studies are methodologically limited with specific focus on study design and specificity within this, participants, and sample size.

Methods

Literature search

Literature was searched for and identified in the form of journals from 1950 until 2021 (see Appendix 1 for search term). Seven databases were searched on 14th January 2021 to identify relevant papers: British Nursing Database, Cochrane Library, Education Research Complete, MEDLINE, PsycINFO, PubMed, and Web of Science. These databases were chosen based on the journals and types of papers published which includes medicine, mental health, and allied health care, education and psychology, zoology, veterinary science, interaction between animal and human, and all papers included physical interaction with a canine. No protocol was registered and therefore not included.

Study selection

Eligibility criteria was based on item 4 of PRISMA's statement PICO and included: (1) studies published in English (P), (2) use of real dogs (I), (3) HE students as participants (P), (4) addressed mental health (O), well-being (O), stress (O), anxiety or depression (O), (5) any sample size (P), and (6) any intervention involving a real canine (with or without a comparison group, (C)). Reviews, studies not published in English, all grey literature and repetitions were excluded. There were no relevant HE student meta-analyses or systematic reviews. As a final but vital exclusion, all studies, meta-analyses or systematic reviews using school children as participants were removed leaving only HE students. Studies were independently screened for relevance by KM and co-authors (KN, CS, MM, SW and GR), and disagreements resolved through discussion. Unresolved discrepancies were resolved between KM and GR. The search term resulted in a total of 4,011 papers. After applying the exclusion criteria this yielded 33 papers in total (see PRISMA flow diagram, Figure 11.1). Of these 33 papers, three are multi- study papers (Crump & Derting, 2015; McArthur & Syrnyk, 2018; Trammell, 2017), bringing the total number of studies to 37. It is important to note that this review included all papers where the intervention was a real canine regardless of study design (with or without control/comparator and pre-post measures). The authors felt the field of researching the impact of CAI in the mental health of HE students in empirically peer reviewed papers is in its infancy, therefore the results of any paper that had been peer reviewed held some value. As the field progresses, future research should focus on interventions with only control/comparator groups and pre/post measures, which provide more robust evidence that the intervention has changed mental health and wellbeing.

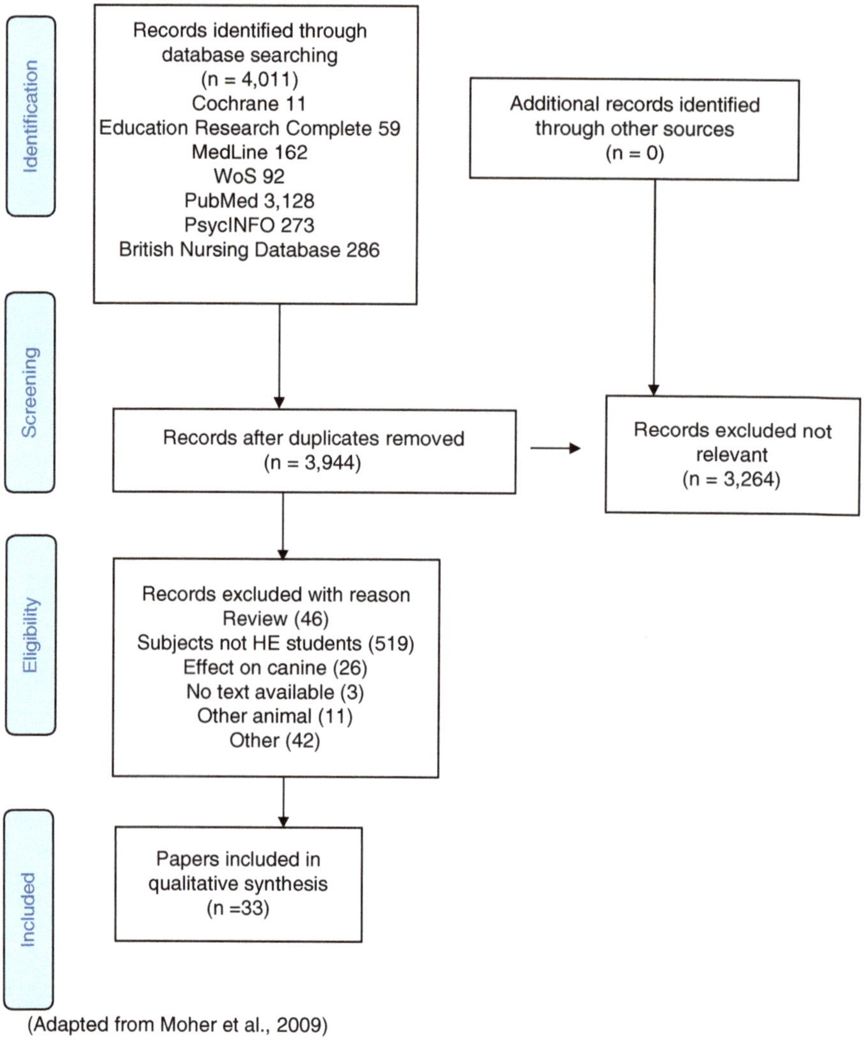

Fig. 11.1. PRISMA Flow Diagram.

Data extraction

Data was extracted from each of the 37 studies to identify key elements (Appendix 2). Using the *Data Collection Form for Intervention Reviews: RCT and non-RCT* (Cochrane, 2022) as a template, a data extraction tool was created to identify key characteristics/variables of each paper. These key elements fall into three main categories. Firstly, key characteristics of the study including country of origin, sample population size, age range, participant mental health, socioeconomic status, and whether they were rewarded for their participation. Secondly, study methodology including aims, study type, design and setting, interaction type and duration, use of control and/or comparison groups, inclusion/exclusion criteria, number of canines, canine- to-human ratio, perception of canine, effect size, power sample calculation, and statistical analysis used. Finally, study outcomes including results and limitations.

Assessment of study quality

The Quality Assessment Tool for Quantitative Studies from the Effective Public Health Practice Project was applied to assess the quality of studies to identify potential bias or confounding factors (Effective Public Health Practice Project, 2009). Study qualities were evaluated using six categories: selection bias, study design, confounders, blinding, data collection methods, and withdrawal and dropouts. For selection bias, 78% of studies were rated as fair (participants somewhat likely to represent the target population) and 22% as poor (participants not likely to represent the target population). 22% of the studies were rated as good in study design (randomized control trial (RCT) or controlled clinical trial), 65% as fair (cohort analytical or case control, cohort design or interrupted time series studies), and 13% as poor (any other, or method not stated). Confounders were rated as good in 78% of studies (controlled for 80% of relevant confounders), fair in 8% (controlled for 60-79% of relevant cofounders), and poor in 14% (controlled for 60% or less of relevant confounders, or confounders were not described). Blinding was rated as fair in 8% of studies (intervention status of participants are not made aware to the outcome assessor, or participants are not aware of the research question) and 92% were rated as poor (intervention status of participants is made aware to the outcome assessor, and participants are aware of the research question). The data collection method was rated as good in 46% of studies (data collection tools are valid and reliable), fair in 11% (data collection tools are valid but not reliable or reliability is not described), and poor in 43% (data collection tools are not valid, or neither validity nor reliability are described). Finally withdrawals/drop outs were rated as good in 16% of studies (follow up rate is 80% or above), fair in 22% of studies (follow up rates are 60-79%), and poor in 62% (follow up rates are 60% or less). Studies were rated by KM and co-authors KN, CS, MM, SW), and disagreements were resolved through discussion. Unresolved discrepancies were discussed between KM and GR.

Results

Appendix 2 presents a summary of the 37 studies.

Terminology

A range of terminologies were used to describe CAI. Seven of the 37 studies (18.92%) used AAT, and a further 12 (32.43%) used the term Therapy Dog. Three studies (8.11%) adopted the term Therapy Dog alongside an alternative term: Barker et al. (2016) used Therapy Dog Intervention, Daltry and Mehr (2015) Dog Therapy Outreach Program, and Dell et al. (2015) utilized Dog Therapy Program. Five studies (13.51%) used Animal Assisted Activities (AAA), two (5.41%) Canine Therapy, and Wilson (1987, 1991) applied the term 'effect of pet'. Two (5.41%) adopted a variation of 'dog-assisted': Grajfoner et al. (2017) used Dog-Assisted Intervention, and Wood et al. (2018) Dog-Assisted Therapy. The remaining six studies (16.22%) utilized a variation of animal, canine, dog, and pet. Adamle et al. (2009) used the term Pet Therapy, Crossman et al. (2015) Animal Visitation Program, Delgado et al. (2018) Canine Play Intervention, Silas et al. (2019) Canine Assisted Intervention (CAI), Stewart and Strickland (2013) Human–Animal Intervention, and Thelwell (2019) used dog interaction.

Sample

Sample size ranged from 44–1960 participants (M =183). Of the 37 studies, seven (18.92%) had fewer than 50 participants (M = 41), 24 studies (64.86%) between 51–150 (M = 85), and six (16.22%) used over 151 participants (M = 629). Ages ranged from 17–57 with a mean age of 21.17. Fifteen studies (40.54%) did not indicate ages and were therefore excluded from the calculations. Gender balance ranged from 100% to 55% females, 43% to 0% males, and 4.7% to 2% other. One study (2.70%) reported a transgender population and in five (13.51%) only female students were recruited. All participants were recruited within the university they were associated with.

Canine

Of the 37 studies, Wilson (1987, 1991) used a friendly dog, one study (2.70%) employed a companion dog (Stewart et al., 2014), and in Wood et al.'s (2018) study the canines were training to become Guide dogs. Buttelmann &

Römpke (2014) did not identify the canine's status, and Thelwell (2019) used a house-trained dog. In the remaining 31 studies (83.78%) all canines were classed as therapy dogs/canines. Handlers or canine owners were present during all data collection. Twenty-three studies (62.16%) gave specific canine breed and canine ages ranged from 10 months to 11 years, the remaining 14 (37.84%) did not include this information. Breeds included Collies, Golden Retrievers, Greyhounds, a Rhodesian Ridgeback, and Labradors alongside mixed breeds. Twelve studies (32.43%) utilized one canine in their research, one study (2.70%) 2 canines, and another (2.70%) three. One study (2.70%) had five canines, 18 studies (48.65%) used five or more canines, and in four studies (10.81%) the number of canines was unclear.

Study design

Within the 37 studies, there were five different study designs. Fifteen studies (40.54%) employed an intervention only design with no control or comparison group, and 13 studies (35.14%) had a control group alongside an intervention group. Two studies (5.41%) had a comparison group alongside an intervention group but no control group and six of the studies (16.22%) used a comparison design examining an intervention group against a comparison and control group. The last study, (2.70%) Shearer et al., 2016) was a two-phase study. Phase one had an intervention alongside a comparison group and phase two used a comparison, an intervention and a control group.

Using an intervention only design, Dell et al. (2015) had other well-being activities available at the same time including hand and body massages and snacks however these were not all available on all campuses that took part in the study. Two studies (5.41%) had a canine or a human in the room while participants watched a traumatic film and one (2.70%) asked participants in the experimental group to interact with a real canine while the comparison group viewed images of the same dog. In the two studies (2.70%) that had a comparison group but no control group, one asked the comparison group to read (Muckle & Lasikiewicz, 2017), and another had participants complete number and word tasks either with or without the canine present (Stewart & Strickland, 2013). Additionally, of the three papers (8.11%) that used a multi-study design, a combination of designs were adopted. Crump and Derting's (2015) first study consisted of both an experimental and control group and study two only used a canine group. Both of McArther and Syrnyk's studies (2018) used only a canine group, and in Trammell's (2017) three studies, study one had an experimental group and studies two and three had both experimental and control groups. Hall (2018) identified long term effects (16 weeks) as part of their discussion, while Binfet (2017) and Shearer et al. (2016) carried out follow up data collection sessions 2 weeks post-intervention, and Dell et al. (2015) and Ward-Griffin et al. (2018) 3 months and 10 hours respectively.

Study location

Of the 37 studies, 29 (78.38%) were carried out in a private room and five (13.51%) in a common area on campus where students could come and go. In two of the studies (5.41%) the location was unclear and one (2.70%) described the location as being in an *appropriate area*.

Measures and instruments

Thirty-one studies (83.78%) adopted quantitative measures, one (2.70%) qualitative measures and five (13.51%) adopted mixed methods. A total of 29 standardized measures were used (see Table 11.1 for full details). Of the 37 studies, 33 (89.19%) applied both pre and post measures. A further four (10.81% Adamle et al., 2009; Daltry & Mehr, 2015; Dell et al., 2015; McArther & Syrnyk, 2018) only used post measures.

Intervention duration

The duration of CAI ranged in all 37 studies from 2 minutes to 2.5 hours. Table 11.2 details intervention duration and the number of studies with this duration.

Twenty-seven of the studies (72.97%) had the intervention at only one time point, while ten (27.03%) had multiple interventions. Sessions

Table 11.1. Full list of standardized measures used including measure and the number of items per measure.

Anxiety	Audience Anxiousness Scale	12
Anxiety	Burns Anxiety Inventory	32
Anxiety	State Trait Anxiety Inventory	20
Stress	Perceived Stress Scale	10
Stress	Stress Arousal Checklist	2 (subscales)
Depression	Becks Depression Inventory	21
Anxiety and depression	Hospital Anxiety and Depression Scale	14
Life satisfaction of subjective well-being	Satisfaction with Life Scale	5
Well-being	Warwick-Edinburgh Mental Well-Being Scale	14
Mindfulness	Five Fact Mindfulness Questionnaire	39
Homesickness	Homesickness Questionnaire	33
Loneliness	University Of Philippines Loneliness Scale	25
Sense of belonging	Sense of Belonging in School	14
Connectedness to campus	Connectedness to Campus	1
	McAndrew's Measure of Rootedness	
Attitude towards animals	Animal Attitude Scale	20
Experiences with a canine	Experiences with Dog Inventory	13
Attitudes towards pets	Pet Attitude Inventory	18
Human animal bonding	Pet Attitude Scale	18
Happiness	Subjective Happiness Scale	4
Current mood, stress, and arousal	Affect Measure	3
Positive and negative affect	Positive and Negative Affect Schedule	10
Mood	UWIST Mood Adjective Check List	24
Mood	Mood Tracking Scale	10
Self esteem	Self-State Esteem Scale	20
Functional social support in chronically ill persons	Medical Outcomes Study Social Support Survey	8
Assesses attitudes	Semantic Differential	3 (dimensions)
Measures effective therapeutic relationships	Session Rating Scale	4
Credibility and expectancy	Credibility/Expectant Questionnaire	6

were spaced out over a two week to three month period with a minimum of two sessions (McArthur & Syrnyk, 2018; Trammell, 2019) and maximum of 16 sessions (Hall, 2018) available to participants.

Intervention activity

Of the 37 studies, 13 (35.14%) had participants take part individually. Buttelmann and Römpke (2014) assigned participants to a canine, fish, plant, or no interaction control group, Crossman et al. (2015) asked participants to play with a canine, view images of the canine, or be part of the control group by simply waiting, and Lass-Hennemann et al. (2014) assigned participants to one of four groups. All four groups watched a traumatic film however, the real dog group sat with a real dog, the toy dog group sat with a life sized toy Collie, and the friendly human group was accompanied by a previously unknown female graduate student. The alone group watched the film on their own. In their later study Lass-Hennemann et al. (2018) had all participants watch a traumatic film. Following this the dog group interacted with a canine for 15 minutes, the dog-film group watched a film clip of someone interacting with a dog for 15 minutes, and the alone group relaxed for 15 minutes. Stewart and Strickland (2013) allocated specific tasks to participants in the presence of a canine which included Monk and Conrad's clerical tasks (basic maths and proof reading), and Wilson (1987, 1991) had participants read quietly or out loud with a canine present. Grajfoner et al. (2017) had

Table 11.2. Summary of intervention duration and number of studies per duration.

Intervention duration	Number of studies
5 minutes	1 (2.7%)
10 minutes	3 (8.11%)
11 minutes	1 (2.7%)
13.5 minutes	1 (2.7%)
15 minutes	8 (21.62%)
20 minutes	4 (10.81%)
30 minutes +	14 (37.84%)
7–10 minutes	1 (2.7%)
2–30 minutes	1 (2.7%)
5–60 minutes	1 (2.7%)
5 minutes–2 hours	1 (2.7%)
No duration specified	1 (2.7%)

the intervention group interact with both the canine and handler, and the control group interact with the handler only. Thelwell (2019) had the intervention group interact with a canine and the control group watched a video of a dog, and Machová et al. (2020) had a canine intervention group, a relaxation comparison group who used anti-stress cubes, coloring books and a phone with music, and a no activity control group. Delgado et al. (2018), Fiocco & Hunse (2017) and Ward-Griffin et al. (2017) asked participants to simply interact and play with a canine.

Five of the studies (13.51%) chose to have participants interact with the canine in groups in a busy area on campus where students could choose the level of interaction. A further 19 (51.35%) had participants interact with the canine in groups in a private room. None of the studies reported following any pre-published report, manual or procedure. Of the 37 studies, only 5 (7.4%) employed pre and post measures alongside a canine intervention group, a control group, and a comparator group (studies described above). In exploring the effects of CAI on four different intervention groups, Buttelmann and Römpke's (2014) induced anxiety by having participants create a presentation on an unfamiliar subject. Following the intervention, all groups experienced a reduction in anxiety. This was greatest in the fish group (↓ 58.2%) when compared to the canine (↓ 56.2%) or plant (↓ 45.6%) groups, however the canine group showed more signs of enjoyment evidenced through laughter, and anxiety levels fell lower than the induced anxiety levels. Buttelmann and Römpke's (2014) were not alone in reporting CAI not as effective as a comparison group. In Lass-Hennemann et al.'s (2014) study, both the canine and friendly group were comparable in reducing anxiety, however in their later study (Lass-Hennemann et al., 2018), it was reported that the CAI group experienced a greater reduction in anxiety when compared against both the comparison and control group. Crossman et al.'s (2015) followed the results of Lass-Hennemann et al. (2018) reporting the greatest reduction in anxiety was experienced by the canine group when compared to the comparison and control groups. These results were also mirrored by Machová et al. (2020) who found participants that interacted with a canine experienced a greater reduction in stress when compared to the comparison and control groups.

Outcomes

Outcomes measured by the studies include anxiety, stress, depression, homesickness, and loneliness while social benefits included CAI taking on the role of a facilitator and encouraging social interaction.

Anxiety

Of the sixteen studies (43.24%) that measured anxiety, 13 identified that CAI effectively reduced anxiety (see Appendix 2 for a summary of details). Five of these studies applied a stressor to elicit higher levels of anxiety before then looking at whether that anxiety was reduced following the interaction. Eleven studies (29.73%) measured existing anxiety without applying a stressor.

Three of the studies (8.11%) did not report entirely supportive results. Stewart and Strickland (2013) demonstrated that not all participants experienced a decrease in state anxiety simply with the presence of a dog. Additionally, Buttelmann and Römpke (2014) reported a reduction in anxiety following CAI (↓ 56.2%) but also a decrease in anxiety in participants who interacted with a fish (↓ 58.2%) and plant (↓ 45.6%). While those in the fish group had a greater decrease in anxiety compared to the CAI group it was found that anxiety levels of participants who interacted with a dog dropped lower than induced anxiety levels and that the CAI group laughed more during interaction indicating a sign of enjoyment. Lass-Hennemann et al. (2014) also found CAI was not the most effective intervention as results from participants who were accompanied by a canine during the applied stressor were comparable to those who were accompanied by a friendly human.

Physiological measures as an indicator of anxiety were used in seven studies (18.92%), however only four (10.81%) recorded a decrease in BP as a result of CAI (Jarolmen & Patel, 2018; Muckle & Lasikiewicz, 2017; Wood et al., 2018; Wilson, 1987). Lass-Hennemann et al. (2014, 2018) found physiological and endocrine stress markers increased as a result of their applied stressor but were not moderated by the canine intervention. Buttelmann & Römpke (2014) removed all physiological measures (blood pressure (BP) and heart rate (HR)) as over 50% of participants did not indicate a positive effect in relation to anxiety, and it was felt BP and HR were influenced by other physical factors such as speech and movement.

Stress

Twenty-two (59.46%) of the studies explored the effect of CAI on stress, with 17 identifying a reduction in stress following CAI (see Appendix 2). Four of the studies (10.81%) did not find CAI to be effective in reducing self-reported stress levels (Barker et al., 2016; Crump & Derting, 2015 [study 1 and study 2]; Stewart & Strickland, 2013). An additional study, Griscti and Camilleri (2020), using physiological measures found that the presence of a canine had no effect on HR. Therefore, five studies failed to find CAI to be an effective intervention.

In addition to Griscti & Camilleri (2020), six other studies used a physiological measure (HR, BP, salvia nerve growth factor, (sNGF), heart rate variability (HRV)). Barker et al. (2016) found the majority of sNGF levels were undetectable and suggested that the stressor was not sufficient enough to cause an effect, therefore supporting their lack of an effect of CAI on self-reported stress. Similarly, Machová et al. (2020) found no significant reduction in systolic or diastolic BP in those who took part in a 10-minute canine interaction session compared to the control or comparison groups. Shearer et al. (2016) also found no significant change in HRV following CAI. Instead, the comparison (mindfulness) group showed higher HRV indicating the act of mindfulness may help students manage stress. As the only study to find any significant effect, Delgado et al. (2018) found all physiological markers of stress (systolic and diastolic BP, pulse, and salivary cortisol) decreased with the presence of a canine.

Depression

Depression was measured by two (5.41%) of the 37 studies. Shearer et al. (2016) found no significant difference between dog interaction and mindfulness groups as measured by the BDI. In addition, Hall (2018) excluded depression due to an abnormal distribute of the scores at the beginning and end of the semester.

Related to depression, two studies (5.41%, Dell et al., 2015; Stewart et al., 2014) identified a benefit of CAI on participants feelings of loneliness. The commonality between these studies was group rather than individual participation, therefore, not only did the participants benefit from the therapeutic value of CAI, but also the positive influence of social interaction with other humans.

Social benefits

Six studies (16.22%) found social factors had a positive influence on the benefit of CAI. Adamle et al. (2009) demonstrated CAI allowed students to build social relationships, and Binfet and Passmore (2016) identified CAI reduced feelings of homesickness. Participants found social interactions born from a non-judgemental environment allowed them to chat and make friendships that otherwise would not have been formed. Shearer et al. (2016) demonstrated the social environment supported short term anxiety and dysphoria reduction, and both Binfet (2017) and Stewart et al. (2014) found CAI provided social support. Additionally, Binfet (2017) found this social support element corresponded with improving stress buffers, Stewart et al. (2014) recognised a relaxed setting was created for the therapy session to take place, and participants in Dell et al.'s (2015) study felt CAI allowed them to meet new people however as this only represented 0.07% of participants (n=3) it is at best, a minor finding.

Discussion

The aim of this systematic review was to assess and evaluate existing research on the benefits of CAI on anxiety, stress, depression, and feelings of well-being in HE students. The search identified 33 papers from 20 peer reviewed journals totaling 37 studies. Both male and female participants took part with ages ranging from 17–57. The systematic review demonstrated that study design, intervention activities, intervention duration, and measurements of mental health used were diverse in approach and application. As a result of this, and the blend of comparisons of different treatments with different comparators, the many outcomes have been summarised under two main outcomes in relation to the benefits of CAI for HE students: (1) mental health benefits, and (2) social benefits. In addition, the systematic review identified a number of methodological limitations within the studies.

Outcome one: Mental health benefits

Thirty (81.08%) of the 37 studies reviewed found CAI effectively reduced a range of negative emotions. Sixteen studies explored the benefits of CAI on anxiety levels in HE students with thirteen identifying that in some capacity, interaction with a canine reduced participants' anxiety levels. The results are particularly compelling as studies varied substantially in how anxiety was measured (see Appendix 2). Another variation in study design were the number of canines used across studies which makes comparing studies difficult. While most studies recorded how many canines were used (Lass-Hennmann, 2014, 2018; Thelwell, 2019; Wood et al., 2018), others (e.g., Dell et al., 2015) did not record canine numbers, or for how long participant interaction lasted. Additionally, although Delagdo and Toukonen (2018) allocated one canine per participant, there were two dogs working in the data collection area. If one was not busy participants were allowed to interact with both dogs, however this frequency was not recorded adding another issue when comparing studies. As a result, it is difficult to infer whether the number of canines had an impact on the effect of CAI on anxiety levels.

In the thirteen studies that did indeed find a positive effect of CAI on anxiety levels, it is important to note some also demonstrated reductions in anxiety in non-canine comparison or control groups. For example, Shearer et al. (2016) found that while the canine group recorded a greater reduction in anxiety in comparison to a no-intervention control group, the comparison group receiving a mindfulness intervention, with activities including breathing and basic yoga, demonstrated significantly lower state anxiety than the canine group. Similarly, Spruin et al. (2020) on using a canine group, mindfulness therapy comparison group, and a control group found the mindfulness group to be as effective as the canine group in reducing student anxiety levels. Therefore, in comparison to other interventions, CAI may not always be the most effective intervention to address anxiety levels.

Stress was also consistently found to be significantly reduced following CAI with 16 studies that looked at stress indicating stress relief post CAI intervention. From the largest to the smallest, the studies varied in study design including the group size in which participants experienced CAI (see Appendix 2), whether participants took part individually (Delgado et al., 2018; Fiocco & Hunse, 2017), or in larger groups (Adamle et al., 2009; Binfet et al., 2018; Daltry & Mehr, 2015). Importantly, similar to the anxiety based studies, across a range of CAI designs, stress levels were reduced in 17 studies. One difficulty with drawing conclusions from these studies is the lack of control groups. While some (e.g., Barker et al., 2016; Griscti & Camilleri, 2020; Ward-Griffin et al., 2017) demonstrated reductions in stress in a canine group in comparison to a control group, many others (e.g., Binfet et al., 2018; Dell et al., 2015; McArthur & Syrnyk, 2018; Wilson, 1987, 1991; Wood et al., 2018) did not compare CAI to a control group.

Aside from the common theme that CAI has a beneficial effect on anxiety (e.g., Hall, 2018) and stress (e.g., Fiocco & Hunse, 2017) in studies who adopted a more rigorous approach with appropriate control groups, CAI sessions conducted with an informal and unstructured design also demonstrated a positive impact of CAI on stress (e.g., Daltry & Mehr, 2015) and anxiety (e.g., Stewart et al., 2014). This indicates that the best practice study design has yet to be identified and that components such as duration, human-to-canine ratio, or location need further research to identify optimum parameters for effective CAI.

While many of the studies in this review report on the positive impact of CAI on anxiety and stress, there is far less discussion in relation to the benefits on depression with only two of the 37 studies exploring this (Hall, 2018; Shearer et al., 2016). This may be because depression is often a long-term issue occurring throughout one's life, rather than a state issue, making it harder to address with a one off brief intervention. However, it is possible that long term CAI, used in a similar fashion to that of CAI in military personnel suffering with PTSD (Stern et al., 2013), may be beneficial to those suffering with depression. Future research is required to determine whether CAI can reduce depression in HE students.

Outcome two: Social benefits

The second main outcome of the systematic review was the evidence of social benefits as a result of CAI. Studies such as Shearer et al. (2016), identified the social element of CAI as being a strong contributing factor to reductions in anxiety levels, although ultimately the canine interaction was the key factor. It was also demonstrated that the social environment of CAI aided students in forming friendships that otherwise would not have been made by encouraging a less formal social environment (Binfet & Passmore, 2016). CAI may therefore be particularly suitable for first year students who are adjusting to a new life and community (Nauta et al., 2019), and for whom the transition to university can be particularly stressful.

A problem with many of the studies exploring CAI is that canine handlers were actively involved in the intervention, including answering questions about the canine (e.g., Barker et al., 2016; Binfet et al., 2018; Dell et al., 2015; Silas et al., 2019) or interacting with participants alongside the canines (e.g. Adamle et al., 2009). Some studies addressed the impact of having handlers actively involved in the canine sessions and the contribution towards CAI. For example, participants in Dell et al.'s (2015) study, described the handers as being *phenomenal* while another described 'the lady' as being *nice* suggesting handlers had a positive effect on the impact of CAI. Given the finding that social interaction may enhance the benefits of CAI, the fact that in some studies, handlers were actively involved has implications when drawing conclusions about the effectiveness of CAI. That is, it precludes the ability to ascertain how much of the benefit is a direct result of CAI itself as opposed to the social interaction between participants and handler. Furthermore, having handlers present and actively involved may have encouraged canines to better interact with participants (and vice versa) which could have had an effect on overall results.

An additional issue concerns studies conducted as an outreach program as students interacted with the dog in an informal setting, and both intervention and data collection were carried out in a busy common area of a popular residential hall with any number of external influences (Daltry & Mehr, 2015; Dell et al., 2015). In comparison, studies where data collection took place in a private room (e.g. Binfet, 2017) arguably provides more compelling evidence that any effect of CAI is a result of the intervention rather than social influences. In addition, participants in studies who did not complete pre-intervention measures (e.g. Daltry & Mehr, 2015; Dell et al., 2015) may have been more relaxed compared to those that did however without these pre-intervention results this is impossible to know. More importantly, the added benefit of a group and social element, as well as participants choosing to take part or being able to dictate the level and timing of the interaction, may have in turn resulted in a more positive outcome.

Methodological limitations

Despite the consistent finding that CAI is an effective intervention for HE students, many of the studies are limited by significant methodological limitations. Crucially, the lack of independent control groups limits the studies with only 20 of the 37 studies including some form of control group. While 14 of the 15 studies without a control group still concluded a benefit of CAI, these conclusions should be made with caution. The lack of a RCT design is also problematic. Only four studies (Binfet, 2017; Crossman et al., 2015; Griscti & Camilleri, 2020; Spruin et al., 2020), specifically state they followed a RCT design using pre and post standardized measures, with both an experimental and control group in a controlled laboratory setting. However it is of note that eleven others seem to adopt an RCT approach. As a final point, of the 37 studies reviewed, only seven (Buttelmann & Römpke, 2014; Crossman et al., 2015; Lass-Hennemann et al., 2014, 2018; Machová et al., 2020; Shearer et al., 2016; Spruin et al., 2020) applied both pre and post measures alongside a comparator and control group. While this does not deter from the results of the other 30 studies, it does mean these results are less robust in evidencing that CAI has had an impact on changes in mental health and well-being as there is no baseline to make comparisons to.

For four of the studies the impact of external influences in carrying out long term CAI over a number of weeks could be problematic. While longitudinal studies are essential for tracking long term benefits of CAI and are arguably ideal in allowing participants to become accustomed to the therapy method, it is impossible to control for what may take place between data collection sessions and subsequently impact the results. Additionally, there is the possibility of participants becoming too familiar with the study increasing the likelihood of demand characteristics and social desirability.

There are two further problematic elements within the 37 studies: age range and sample size. The age range in the 37 studies varied as the youngest participant was 17 and the oldest 57 (M = 21.17). This is problematic as different stages of life and development could affect the results with research supporting the claim that being older may allow one to deal with anxiety or depression by having better control of, or being better at regulating ones emotions (e.g., Lawrie & Phillips, 2016; Scheibe & Blanchard-Fields, 2009). Sample size is also a recurring issue as none of the studies include power calculations to demonstrate sufficient sample sizes. Further empirical research is therefore required on an HE population with adequate sample sizes focusing on appropriate age groups.

Internal factors with regards to participants' existing mental health are also often unaccounted for in the studies. In the 33 studies that carried out pre-intervention measures, some participants chose to take part if they self-identified with the study (for example, homesickness, Binfet & Passmore, 2016), and two studies excluded participants undergoing psychotherapeutic treatment (Lass-Hennemann et al., 2014, 2018). Only one study (Machová et al., 2020) reported whether participants had pre-existing mental health conditions or were undergoing other therapy which may affect how they approach and receive CAI and possibly impact results.

The lack of specificity in study design adds to the limitations of the studies reviewed. For example, some did not report how long each student spent with the canine (e.g., Daltry & Mehr, 2015; Stewart et al., 2014) and others (e.g., Dell et al., 2015) had large dropout rates introducing a possible issue of characteristic bias between those that stayed and those that dropped out. There may have been an issue with recruitment or the intervention itself may have, for the participant, been unsatisfactory, potentially skewing results if those finding CAI unhelpful subsequently dropped out. Additionally, the location in which data collection was carried out may limit the generalization of findings as five of the studies were conducted in a large busy area on campus introducing external influences which may have had an effect on canine behavior and participants experiences of CAI. Finally, data collection using informal evaluation forms or purpose created questionnaires (e.g., Daltry & Mehr, 2015; Machová et al., 2020; McArthur & Syrnky, 2018; Trammell, 2017) could also lead to results being left open to interpretation in comparison to studies using objective standardized measures that have a wealth of evidence supporting usage and validity.

To conclude, this systematic review identifies that despite the many differences in study design and intervention type, CAI generally has a positive effect on the mental health of HE students particularly in addressing anxiety and stress levels. It is clear that mental health issues are abundant in HE students during their time enrolled in university (Eisenberg et al., 2007; Richardson et al., 2015; The Insight Network, 2020; Thorley, 2017). Given the rise in the need for counselling support (Thorley, 2017) and the increase in stress, anxiety, and depressive thoughts, particularly due to the Covid-19 pandemic (e.g., Son et al., 2020), combatting mental health issues in this population requires significant attention. In light of this, the results from this systematic review are important as they identify strengths and areas of improvement within the field of CAI so that the use of canines as a therapy tool to support HE student's mental health can benefit from evidence that certain elements have been confirmed as being best practice. One significant limitation of this systematic review is the inability to carry out a meta-analysis. While this was one of the initial aims of the review, after reviewing the relevant studies it became apparent that study design, intervention activity and duration, location, and measurements used were far more diverse than expected. As a result of this diversity, and the mix of comparisons of different treatments with different comparators, it was decided that each combination needed to be considered separately. The second limitation relates to the number of studies that adopted both pre and post measures alongside a comparison and control group. Only seven studies applied comparison/control groups and pre/post measures, therefore it was decided to include all applicable study designs. As the field progresses, and more studies are published, a systematic review limited to only the most robust studies (i.e., with control/comparator groups and pre/post measures) would be useful. The outcomes themselves are also quite diverse, leading to further difficulties with a meta-analysis. Despite this weakness, the systematic review demonstrates that specific protocol, a manual or guidelines, has yet to be produced that can be followed when conducting CAI to ensure optimum results are achieved.

While determining these specific guidelines requires further research and experimentation, based on this review, the recommendation would be to focus on the use of a RCT study design, intervention activity and duration, the impact of a social environment in the form of individual versus grouped participants, and the location of the study. The involvement of the handler on the effectiveness CAI and would also benefit from further understanding. These could then be used to build a framework for effective and efficient CAI.

References

Adamle, K. N., Riley, T. A. & Carlson, T. (2009). Evaluating college student interest in pet therapy. *Journal of American College and Health*, *57*(5), 545–548.

Adams, T., Clark, C., Crowell, V., Duffy, K., Green, M., McEwen, S., Wrape, A. & Hammonds, F. (2017). The mental health benefits of having dogs on college campuses. *Modern Psychological Studies*, *22*(2), 50–59.

Andrews, B. & Wilding, J. M. (2004). The relation of depression and anxiety to life-stress and achievement in students. *British Journal of Psychology*, *95*(Pt 4), 509–21.

Barker, S. B., Barker, R. T., McCain, N. L., & Schubert, C. M. (2016). A randomized cross-over exploratory study of the effect of visiting therapy dogs on college student stress before final exams. *Anthrozoös*, *29*(1), 35–46.

Beck, A. M. (2000). The use of animals to benefit humans: animal-assisted therapy. In Fine., A.H. (Ed.), *Handbook on Animal Assisted Therapy, Foundations and Guidelines for Animal Assisted Intervention*, (21–40). Academic Press.

Binfet, J. T. (2017). The effects of group-administered canine therapy on university students' wellbeing: A randomized controlled trial. *Anthrozoös*, *30*(3), 397–414.

Binfet, J. T., & Passmore, H. A. (2016). Hounds and homesickness: the effects of an animal assisted therapeutic intervention for first year university students. *Anthrozoös*, *29*(3), 411–454.

Binfet, J. T., Passmore, H. A., Cebry, A., Struik, K., & McKay, C. (2018). Reducing university students' stress through a drop-in canine-therapy program. *Journal of Mental Health*, *27*(3), 197–204.

Brown, P. (2016). *The invisible problem? Improving students' mental health. - HEPI Report 88*. Oxford, Higher Education Policy Institute.

Broglia, E., Ryan, G., Williams, C., Fudge, M., Knowles, L., Turner, A., Dufour, G., Percy, A., Barkham, M., and on behalf of the SCORE Consortium. (2021). Profiling student mental health and counselling effectiveness: lessons from four UK services using complete data and different outcome measures. *British Journal of Guidance & Counselling*, https://doi.org/10.1080/03069885.2020.1860191

Buttelmann, D., & Römpke, A. K. (2014). Anxiety- reducing effect: dog, fish and plant in direct comparison. *Anthrozoös*, *27*(2), 267–277.

Catling, J. C., Bayley, A., Begum, Z., Wardzinski, C., & Wood, A. (2022). Effects of the COVID-19 lockdown on mental health in a UK student sample. *BMC Psychology*, *10*(118), https://doi.org/10.1186/s40359-022-00732-9

Cochrane. (2022). *Data extraction form. Cochrane. Developmental, Psychosocial, and Learning Problems*. https://dplp.cochrane.org/data-extraction-forms

Crossman, M. K., Kazdin, A. E., & Kundson, K. (2015). Brief unstructured interaction with a dog reduces distress. *Anthrozoös*, *28*(4), 649–660.

Crump, C., & Derting, T. L. (2015). Effects of pet therapy on the psychological and physiological stress levels of first year female undergraduates. *North American Journal of Psychology*, *17*(3), 575–590.

Daltry, R. M., & Mehr, K. E. (2015). Therapy dogs on campus: recommendations for counselling centre outreach. *Journal of College Student Psychotherapy*, *29*, 72–78.

Delgado, C., Toukonen, M., & Wheeler, C. (2018). Effect of canine play interventions as a stress reduction strategy in college students. *Nursing Educator*, *43*(3), 149–153.

Dell, C. A., Chalmers, D., Gillett, J., Rohr, B., Nickel C., Campbell, L., Hanoski, R., Haugerud, J., Husband, A., Stephenson, C., & Brydges., M. (2015). PAWSing student stress: A pilot evaluation study of the St. Johns ambulance therapy dog program of three university campuses in Canada. *Canadian Journal of Counselling and Psychotherapy*, *49*(4), 332–259.

Dietz, T. J., Davis, D., & Pennings, J. (2011). Evaluating animal-assisted therapy in group treatment for child sexual abuse. *Journal of Child Sexual Abuse*, *12*(6), 655–683.

Eisenberg, D., Gollust, S. E., Golberstein, E., & Hefner, J. (2007). Prevalence and correlates of depression, anxiety and suicidality among university students. *American Journal of Orthopsychiatry*, *77*, 534–542.

Effective Public Health Practice Project (EPHPP). (2009). Quality assessment tool for quantitative studies. Retrieved from http://www.ephpp.ca/tools.html

Elmaci, D. T., & Cevizci, S. (2015). Dog-assisted therapies and activities in rehabilitation of children with cerebral palsy and physical and mental disabilities. *International Journal of Environmental Research and Public Health*, *12*(5), 5046–5060.

Fiocco A. J., & Hunse, A. M. (2017). The buffer effect of therapy dogs exposure stress reactivity in undergraduate students. *International Journal of Environmental Research and Public Health*, *14*(7), 707.

Goodman, L. (2017). Mental health on university campuses and the needs of students they seek to serve. *Building Health Academic Communities Journal*, *1*(2):31.

Grajfoner, D., Harte, E., Potter, L. M., & McGuigan, N. (2017). The effect of dog -assisted interventional on student well-being, mood and anxiety. *International Journal of Environmental Research and Public Health*, *14*, 483.

Griscti, O., & Camilleri, L. (2020). The impact of dog therapy on nursing students' heart rate and ability to pay attention in class. *International Journal of Educational Research*, *99*, 101498.

Hall, D. (2018). Nursing Campus Therapy Dog: a pilot study. *Teaching and Learning Nursing*, *13*, 202–106.

Hart, L. A. (2000). Psychosocial benefit of animal companionship. In Fine. A.H. (Ed), *Handbook on Animal Assisted Therapy, Foundations and Guidelines for Animal Assisted Intervention* (59-78). Academic Press.

Hartwig, K. K., & Binfet, J. T. (2019a). What is important in canine-assisted intervention teams? An investigation in canine-assisted program online screening tools. *Journal of Veterinary Behavior*, *29*, 53–60.

Hartwig, K. K., Binfet, J. T. (2019b). *Canine-Assisted Interventions: A Comprehensive Guide to Credentialing Therapy Dog Teams*. New York, Routledge.

House of Commons (2020). *Support for students with mental health issues in Higher Education in England. Briefing Paper number 8592. 21 August, 2019*. Available at https://commonslibrary.parliament.uk/research-briefings/cbp-8593/

Hunt, J., & Eisenberg, D. (2009). Mental health problems and help seeking behavior among college students. *Journal of Adolescent Health*, *46*, 3–10.

Insight Network, The. (2020). *University Student Mental Health Survey 2020: A large scale study into the prevalence of student mental illness within UK universities*. The Insight Network, London.

Jarolmen, J., & Patel, G. (2018). The effects of animal-assisted activities on college students before and after a final exam. *Journal of Creative in Mental Health*, *13*(3), 264–274.

Johnson, R. A., Meadows, R. L., Haubner, J. S., Sevedge., K. (2008). Animal-assisted activity among patients with cancer: effects on mood, fatigue, self-perceived health, and sense of coherence. *Oncology Nursing Forum*, *35*(2), 225–232.

Kaparounaki, C. K., Patsali, M. E., Mousa, D. P. V., Papadopoulou, E. V. K., Papadopoulou, K. K. K., & Fountoulakis, K. N. (2020). *Psychiatry Research*, 290.

Kivlighan, D. M., Schreier, B. A., Gates, A., Hong, J. E., Corkey, J. M., Anderson, C. L., & Keeton, P. M. (2021). The role of mental health counselling in college students' academic success: An interrupted time series analysis. *Journal of Counselling Psychology*, *68*(5), 562–570.

Kwong, A., Pearson, R., Adams, M., Northstone, K., Tilling, K., Smith, D., Fawns-Ritchie, C., Bould, H., Warne, N., Zammit, A., Gunnell, D. J., Moran, P. A., Micali, N., Reichenberg, A., Hickman, M., Rai, D., Haworth, S., Campbell, A., Altschul, D., … Timpson, N. J. (2021). Mental health before and during the COVID-19 pandemic in two longitudinal UK population cohorts. *The British Journal of Psychiatry*, *218*(6), 334–343.

Lass-Hennemann, J., Peyk, P., Streb, M., Holz, E., & Michael, T. (2014). Presence of a dog reduces subjective but not physiological stress response to an analog trauma. *Frontiers in Psychology*, *5* (article 1010), 1–7.

Lass-Hennemann, J., Schafer, S. K., Romer, S., Holz, E., Streb. M., & Michael, T. (2018). Therapy dogs as a crisis interventional after traumatic events: an experimental study. *Frontiers in Psychology*, *9*(article 1627).

Lawrie, L., & Phillips, L. H. (2016). A maturing picture of emotions. *The Psychologist*, *29*(12), 908–911.

Machová, K., Procházková, R., Vadroňová, M., Součková, M., & Prouzová, E. (2020). Effect of dog presence on stress levels in students under psychological strain: a pilot study. *International Journal of Environmental Research and Public Health*, *17*, 2286.

Manville, K., Coulson, M., & Reynolds., G. (2022). A randomised controlled trial investigating canine assisted interaction effects on anxiety, stress and depression in higher education students. *Society and Animals*. doi: 10.1163/15685306-bja10101

McArthur, A. D, & Syrnyk, C. (2018). On-campus animal assisted therapy events, post-secondary students' reaction and mood. *Society &. Animals*, *26*(6), 616–632.

Moher, D., Liberati, A., Tetzlaff, J., & Altman, D. G. (2009). *Preferred reporting items for systematic reviews and meta-analyses: The PRISMA statement. PLoS Med*, *6*(7).

Muckle, J., & Lasikiewicz, N. (2017). An exploration of the benefits of animal-assisted activities in undergraduate students in Singapore. *Asian Journal of Social Psychology*, *29*(2), 75–84.

Nauta, M. H., aan het Rot, M., Schut, H., & Strobe, M. (2019). Homesickness in social context: an ecological momentary assessment study among 1st-year university students. *International Journal of Psychology*, *55*(3). 392–397.

Pierce, M., Hope, H., Ford, T., Hatch, S., Hotopf, M., John, A., Kontopantelis, E., Webb, R., Wessley, S., McManus, S., & Abel, K. (2020). Mental health before and during the COVID-19 pandemic: a longitudinal probability sample survey of the UK population. *The Lancet*, *7*(10), 883–892.

Pollard, E., Vanderlayden, J., Alexander, K., & O'Mahony, B. H. (2021). Student mental health and wellbeing: Insights from higher education providers and sector experts, June 2021. *Department for Education, Government Social Research*, https://www.employment-studies.co.uk/system/files/resources/files/Survey_of_HE_Providers_Student_Mental_Health.pdf

Priestly, M., Broglia, E., Hughes, G., & Spanner, L. (2021). Student perspectives on improving mental health support services at university. *Counselling & Psychotherapy Research*, https://doi.org/10.1002/capr.12391

Richardson, T. H., Elliott, P., & Roberts, R. (2015). The impact of tuition fees amount on mental health over time in British students. *Journal of Public Health*, *37*(3), 412–418.

Rückert, H. W. (2015). Students' mental health and psychological counselling in Europe, *Mental Health & Prevention* *3*(1-2), 34–40.

Saleh, D., Camart, N., & Romo, L. (2017). Predictors of stress in college students. *Frontiers in Psychology*, *8*(19), DOI: 10.3389/fpsyg.2017.00019.

Savage, M. J., Hennis, P. J., Magistro, D., Donaldson, J., Healy, L. C. & James, R. M. (2021). Nine months into the COVID-19 pandemic: a longitudinal study showing mental health and movement behaviours are impaired in UK students. *International Journal of Environmental Research and Public Health*, *18*(6), https://doi.org/10.3390/ijerph18062930

Scheibe, S., & Blanchard-Fields, F. (2009). Effects of regulating emotions on cognitive performance: What is costly for young adults is not so costly for older adults. *Psychology and Aging*, *24*(1), 217–223. doi:10.1037/a0013807.

Shearer, A., Hunt, M., Chowdhury, M., & Nicol, L. (2016). Effects of a brief mindfulness mediation intervention on students stress and heart rate variability. *International Journal of Stress*, *23*(2), 232–254. doi:10.1037/a0039814.

Silas, H. J., Binfet, J. T., & Ford, A. T. (2019). Therapeutic for all? Observations assessment of theory canine stress in an on-campus stress-reduction program. *Journal of Veterinary Behavior*, *32*, 6–13.

Smith, C. (2013). Comfort dogs aid healing in Newtown. *National Association of School Psychologists*, 41(8), 24.

Sobo, E., Eng, B., & Kasity-Krich, N. (2006). Canine visitation (pet) therapy: pilot data on decreases in child pain perception. *Journal of Holistic Nursing*, *24*(1), 51–57. DOI:10.1177/0898010105280112.

Son, C., Hegde, S., Smith, A., Wang, X., & Sasangohar, F. (2020). Effects of COVID-19 on college students' mental health in the United States: interview survey study. *Journal of Medical Internet Research*, *22*(9), e21279.

Spruin, E., Dempster, T., Islam, S., & Raybould, I. (2020). The effects of a therapy dog vs mindfulness vs a student advisor on student anxiety and well-being. *Journal of Further and Higher Education*, *45*(5), 588–600.

Stern, S. L., Donahue, D. A., Allison, S., Hatch, J. P., Lancaster, C. L., Benson, T. A., Johnson, A. L., Jeffreys, M. D., Pride, D., Moreno, C., & Peterson, A. L. (2013). Potential benefits of canine companionship for military veterans with posttraumatic stress disorder (PTSD). *Society & Animals*, *21*(6), 568–581.

Stewart, L. A., Dispenza, F., Parker, L., Chang, Y. C., & Cunnien, T. (2014). A pilot study assessing the effectiveness of an animal-assisted outreach program. *Journal of Creativity in Mental Health*, *9*(3), 332–345.

Stewart, T. M., Fry, D., McAra, L., Hamilton, S., King, A., Laurie, M., & McCluskey, G. (2022). Rates, perceptions and predictors of depression, anxiety and Post Traumatic Stress Disorder (PTSD)- like symptoms about Covid-19 in adolescents. *PLoS ONE*, *17*(4), e0266818.

Stewart, A., & Strickland, O. (2013). A companion animal in a work stimulation: the roles of task difficulty and prior companion-animal guardianship in state anxiety. *Society & Animal*, *21*(3), 249–265.

Thorley, C. (2017). *Not by Degrees: Improving Student Mental Health in the UK's Universities*. Institute for Public Policy Research, London.

Trammell, J. P. (2017). The effect of therapy dogs on exam stress and memory. *Anthrozoös*, *30*(4), 607–621.

Trammell, J. P. (2019). Therapy dogs improve student affect but not memory. *Anthrozoös*, *32*(5), 691–699.

Thelwell, E. L. R. (2019). Paws for thought: A controlled study investigating the benefits of interacting with a house-trained dog on university students mood and anxiety. *Animals*, *9*(10), 846.

Ward-Griffin, E., Klaiber, P., Collins, H. K., Owens, R. L., Coren, S., & Chen, F. S. (2018). Petting away pre-exam stress: the effects of therapy dogs sessions on student well-being. *Stress and Health*, *34*(3), 468–473.

Wilson, C. C. (1987). Physiological response of college students to a pet. *The Journal of Nervous and Mental Disease*, *175*(10), 606–612.

Wilson, C. (1991). The pet as an anxiolytic intervention. *The Journal of Nervous and Mental Disease*, *179*(8), 482–489.

Winkle, M., Crowe, T. K. & Hendrix, I. (2011). Service dogs and people with physical disabilities partnerships: a systematic review, *Occupational Therapy International*, *19*(1), 54–66.

Wright, N., Hill, J., Sharp, H., & Pickles, A. (2021). Interplay between long-term vulnerability and new risk: Young adolescent and maternal mental health immediately before and during the COVID-19 pandemic. *JCPP Advances*, *1*(1), https://doi.org/10.1111/jcv2.12008

Wood, E., Ohlsen, S., Thompson, J., Hulin, J., & Knowles, L. (2018). The feasibility of brief dog-assisted therapy on university students stress levels: the PAwS study. *Journal of Mental Health*, *27*(3), 263–268.

Appendices

Appendix 1

Search Terms used:

("animal therapy" OR "animal assisted activit*" OR "animal interaction" OR "animal visitation" OR "animal support" OR "animal assisted therapy" OR AAT OR "pet therapy" OR "pet assisted activit*" OR "pet interaction" OR "pet visitation" OR "pet support" OR "pet assisted therapy" OR "canine therapy" OR "canine assisted activit*" OR "canine interaction" OR "canine visitation" OR "canine support" OR "canine assisted therapy" OR "dog therapy" OR "dog assisted activit*" OR "dog interaction" OR "dog visitation" OR "dog support" OR "dog assisted therapy") AND (canine* OR dog) AND (anxiety OR stress OR depression OR mental health OR well-being) AND (school OR student OR college OR university OR campus OR educat*).

Appendix 2

Summary of participants, study design and outcome

First Author/Date	Terminology	Sample size	Participant age	Number of sessions	Timing (mins/ hours)	Group numbers	Canine per group	Study design	Measures used	Intervention activity	Outcome post intervention	Study quality (EPHPP)
Adamle, N. 2009	Pet Therapy	246	17–25	1	20 minutes + mingle session	50	5	Intervention only	Pet Therapy Program questionnaire	Canine interaction	Pet therapy program could be a temporary substitute to fill the void left by previous support systems for stressful periods and could be a catalyst to form new relationships	3
Barker, S. B. 2016	Therapy Dog Intervention	78	18+	1	15 minutes	Not specified	5	Intervention and control group	Perceived Stress Scale (PSS), stress VAS, sNGF	Intervention group: Canine interaction. Control group: drawing a diagram representing current life situation	A brief dog intervention therapy session statistically reduces students perceived stress	2
Binfet, J. T. 2016	AAT	44	18–22	8	45 minutes	3–4	1	Intervention and control group	McAndrew's Measure of Rootedness, Satisfaction with Life Scale, Connectedness to Campus, Focus group	Intervention group: Canine interaction. Control group: Informed they were on an 8 week 'wait list' and to continue with usual daily business	AAT reduced feelings of homesickness, increases feelings of satisfaction with life, feelings connected to campus and the well-being of 1st year students' experiences with homesickness	3
Binfet, J. T. 2017	Canine Therapy	163	17–49	1	20 minutes	3–4	1	Intervention and control group	PSS, Homesick ness Questionnaire, Sense of Belonging Scale	Intervention group: Canine interaction. Control group: Course based reading material	A 20 minute canine therapy session reduces stress and homesickness, and increases an affinity for campus community	3
Binfet, J. T. 2018	Canine Therapy	1960	–	6–7	20 minutes	3–4	1	Intervention only	VAS-Stress	Canine interaction	Canine therapy intervention reduces stress	3
Buttelmann, D. 2014	AAT	71	18.8–29.8	1	5 minutes	1	1	Intervention, comparison and control group	STAI, Audience Anxiousness Scale, Pet Attitude Scale, systolic/ diastolic BP and HR	Intervention group: Canine interaction. Comparison group: fish and plant interaction. Control group: No interaction, participants asked to 'wait'	All 3 conditions found anxiety reducing effects. The canine group was not more effective than the fish comparison group but was more effective than the plant group	2

Crossman, M. 2015	Animals Visitation Program	67	22–37	1	7 + 3 optional minutes	1	1	Intervention, comparison and control group	STAI, Positive and negative affect schedule (PANAS), Credibility/ Expectancy Questionnaire, Semantic Differential, Experiences with Dog Inventory	Intervention group: Canine interaction. Comparison group: Viewed images of the canine. Control group: No interaction, participants asked to 'wait'	AVP reduces anxiety and negative mood and increases positive moods. Supports existing AVP already in use	3
Crump, C. 2015	Study 1 - AAA	27	18–25	1	15 minutes	4	2	Intervention and control group	Stress Arousal Checklist, BP, HR	Intervention group: Canine interaction. Control group: took part in non-stressful activity including playing cards, listening to music, read and texting	AAA decreases psychological stress and increased psychological arousal. No significant effect on diastolic BP, HR or levels of salivary cortisol	3
	Study 2 - AAA	61	18–25	1	30 minutes	4	2	Intervention group only	Stress Arousal Checklist, BP, HR	Canine interaction	AAA decreases psychological stress and increased psychological arousal. No significant effect on diastolic BP, HR or levels of salivary cortisol	3
Daltry, R. M. 2015	Dog Therapy Outreach Program	54	18–32	15	2 hours	15-20 2	2 hours	Intervention only	Informal evaluation form	Canine interaction	Provides stress relief and comfort, and increases potential access to counselling services	3
Delgado, C. 2018	Canine Play Intervention	48	18–57	1	15 minutes	1	1	Intervention only	PSS, VAS-Mood, BP, Cortisol	Canine interaction	Dogs can moderate effects of stress. Improvement in mood and perceptions of stress and a positive change in psychological measures	3
Dell, C. A. 2015	Dog Therapy Program	403	–	2	5-60 minutes, no clear record	Not specified	–	Intervention only	PSS, VAS-Mood, BP, Cortisol	Canine interaction	Therapy dogs offer love and support and reduce stress	3
Fiocco, A. J. 2017	Therapy Dog	61	18–47	1	10 minutes	1	1	Intervention and control group	Therapy dogs offer love and support and reduce stress.	Intervention group: Canine interaction. Control group: No interaction, participants told to relax	Interacting with a dog for 10 minutes may significantly buffer stress response to a subsequent stressor	3

Continued

Continued.

First Author/Date	Terminology	Sample size	Participant age	Number of sessions	Timing (mins/ hours)	Group numbers	Canine per group	Study Design	Measures used	Intervention activity	Outcome post intervention	Study quality (EPHPP)
Griscti, O. 2020	Phase 1 –Dog Therapy	24	20–31	8	2.5 hours	24	1	Intervention and control group	Wrist HR monitor	Canine present during a lecture	The presence of a dog reduces stress	3
	Phase 2 –Dog Therapy	38	–	8	2.5 hours	38	1	Intervention and control group	Purpose written questionnaire	Canine present during a lecture	The presence of a dog has a calming effect on students	
Grajfoner, D. 2107	Dog-Assisted Intervention	132	17–34	1	20 minutes	1	1	Intervention and control group	Warwick-Edinburgh Mental Well-Being Scale (WEMWB S), STAI, UWIST Mood Adjective Check List (UMACL)	Intervention group: Canine + handler interaction. Control group: Handler interaction	20 minute session led to significantly greater improvement s in student well-being and anxiety	3
Hall, D. 2018	Therapy Dog	109	21–56	60	2-30 minutes, no clear record	Not specified	1	Intervention and control group	Hospital Anxiety and Depression Scale (HADS)	Intervention group: Canine interaction Control group: No canine interaction over the duration of the study	Therapy dogs on campus during a semester decrease anxiety symptoms	3
Jarolmen, J. 2018	AAT	86	18–39	1	15 minutes	Not specified	1	Intervention and control group	Systolic/diastolic BP	Intervention group: Canine interaction. Control group: No canine interaction, participants were asked to sit behind a privacy screen	Significant difference found in the reduction in BP levels between experimental and control group. BP viewed as an indication of anxiety levels	3
Lass-Hennemann, J. 2014	Therapy Dog	80	–	1	11 minutes	1	11	Intervention, comparison and control group	STAI-S, PANAS, systolic, diastolic BP, ECG, Cortisol, STAI-Trait, Pet Attitude Scale (PAS)	Activity: traumatic film clip Intervention group: Canine interaction. Comparison group: toy dog or friendly person companion. Control group: Alone	Presence of a dog reduces subjective experienced anxiety and negative affect after a traumatic film clip	2
Lass-Hennemann, J. 2018	Therapy Dog	60	–	1	15 minutes	1	1	Intervention, comparison and control group	STAI-State, PANAS, systolic, diastolic BP, ECG, Cortisol, STAI-T, PAS, Becks Depression Inventory (BDI)	Intervention group: Canine interaction. Comparison group: participants watched a video of canine interaction Control group: No interaction, participants told to relax alone	Presence of a dog reduces subjective experienced anxiety, less negative affect and more positive affect after a traumatic film clip	3

Machová, K. 2020	AAA	93	19-44	1	10 minutes	1	1	Intervention, compar ison and control group	Purpose written questionnaire. BP, HR.	Intervention group: Canine interaction. Comparison group: relaxing tasks Control group: No interaction, activity not given	AAA significantly improves mood and stress but not HR or BP was HAI	3
McArthur, A. D. 2018	Study 1 – AAT	80		1	90 minutes	Not specified	6	Intervention only	Purpose written questionnaire	Canine interaction	AAT improves self-reported perceived mood	3
	Study 2 – AAT	38		1	90 minutes	Not specified	6	Intervention only		Canine interaction	AAT improves mood (pre compared to post)	3
Muckle, J. 2017	AAA	62	–	3	60 minutes	Not specified	Unclear	Intervention and comparison group	Animal Attitudes Scale, PSS, STAI, State Self Esteem Scale, systolic and diastolic BP	Intervention group: Canine interaction. Comparison group: Quiet reading	AAA has a positive effect on psychological and physiological markers of stress. Reductions found in perceived anxiety, systolic BP and state self- esteem	3
Shearer, A. 2016	Phase 1-AAT	26	–	4	60 minutes	Not specified	1	Intervention and control group	STAI (mood inventory), PANAS, BDI, Five Facet Mindfulness Questionnaire, HRV,	Intervention group: Mindfulness meditation. Active control group: Canine interaction	AAT reduces anxiety	2
	Phase 2-ATT	48	–	4	60 minutes	Not specified	1	Intervention, comparison and control group	STAI (mood inventory), PANAS, BDI, Five Facet Mindfulness Questionnaire, HRV	Intervention group: Mindfulness meditation group. Comparison group: Canine interaction. Control group: no interaction, no activity given	AAT reduces anxiety	
Silas, H. J. 2019	CAI	754 students	–	1	90 minutes	126	15-17	Intervention only	VAS-Stress	Canine interaction	CAI reduces student and handler stress however canines stress increased (compared to measures of observed home stress) as a result of performing CAI	2
		40 handlers*	17-60	6								
		40 canines*	Bitches Mage = 4.75 Dog – not stated	6								

Continued

Continued.

First Author/Date	Terminology	Sample size	Participant age	Number of sessions	Timing (mins/ hours)	Group numbers	Canine per group	Study design	Measures used	Intervention activity	Outcome post intervention	Study quality (EPHPP)
Spruin, E. 2020	Therapy Dog	94	18-46	1	30 minutes	1	1	Intervention, comparison and control group	STAI, Mood Tracking Scale	Intervention group: Canine interaction. Comparison group: Mindfulness. Control group: Psychological support with a student advisor	Therapy dogs reduces anxiety as effectively as mindfulness therapy	3
Stewart, A. 2013	Human Animal Interaction	128	18-57	1	13.5 minutes	1	1	Intervention and comparison group	STAI	Activity: Clerical tasks Intervention group: Canine interaction Comparison group: No canine interaction during clerical task	Companion animals may provide stress relief for those in average stress jobs with positive feelings about companion animals but may have no effect for those in high stress jobs who do not already enjoy animal companionship	2
Stewart, A. 2014	AAT	55	–	20-24	2 hour drop in session	10-15	1	Intervention only	Burns Anxiety Inventory, University of Philippines Loneliness Scale, Session Rating Scale, Outreach program evaluation form	Canine interaction	AAT decreases self-reported anxiety and loneliness. AAT outreach intervention programs may be effective and efficient in supporting the demands of the expanding student body	2
Thelwell, E. L. R. 2019	Dog interaction	82	18-23	1	10 minutes	1	1	Intervention and control group	PAS, STAI, PANAS-Expanded form	Intervention group: Canine interaction Control group: Watch a video about dogs	Dog interactions reduced anxiety levels and improved mood scores.	3
Tramme II J. P. 2017	Study 1 – Therapy Dogs	127	–	1	2 hour drop in session	Not specified	7	Intervention only	Purpose written stress questionnaire	Canine interaction	Therapy dogs are associated with a small decrease in stress	3
	Study 2 – Therapy Dogs	44	–	1	15 minutes	Not specified	6	Intervention and control group	Purpose written stress questionnaire	Intervention group: Canine interaction. Control group: Watch a movie about dogs	Therapy dog group showed larger reductions in stress compared to the control group. There was no relation to exam performance	3

	Study 3 – Therapy Dogs	45	–	1	15 minutes	Not specified	5	Intervention and control group	Purpose written stress questionnaire	Intervention group: Canine interaction. Control group: Watched a movie about dogs	Therapy dog interaction immediately after a class had no effect on exam related stress reduction. However a (small) reduction in stress did predict better exam related performance	3
Trammell, J. P. 2019	Therapy Dog	44	–	2	Not specified	2	1	Intervention and control group	Affect measures, PSS	Activity: learning task Intervention group: Canine interaction. Control group: Alone	Interacting with a therapy dog decreases arousal and stress and increases happiness	3
Ward-Griffin, E. 2017	Therapy Dog	246	–	1	90 minutes	Not specified	7-12	Intervention and control group	Satisfaction with Life, Subjective Happiness Scale, PANAS, PSS, Medical Outcome Study Social Support Survey	Intervention group: Canine interaction. Control group: No canine interaction over the duration of the study	Therapy dogs on campus can have a positive effect on students well-being including reductions in stress and an increase in happiness and energy levels immediately post interaction. Negative affect and perceived stress decreased and perceived social support increased 10 hours post-intervention	3
Wilson, C. C. 1987	Effect of Pet	92	18-39	1	3 x 10 minutes	1	1	Intervention only	STAI, Pet Attitude Inventory, BP, HR	Reading aloud, reading quietly, and canine interaction	Interacting with a pet affects physiological and psychological response by lowering response levels and reduces anxiety levels	3
Wilson, C. 1991	Effect of Pet	92	18-39	1	3 x 10 minutes	1	1	Intervention only	STAI, Pet Attitude Inventory, BP, HR	Reading aloud, reading quietly, canine interaction (all participants)	Interacting with a pet affects physiological and psychological response by lowering response levels and decrease anxiety levels	3
Wood, E. 2018	Dog-Assisted Therapy	131	–	1	15 minutes	6	1-2	Intervention only	STAI, BP	Canine interaction	Decrease in state anxiety and systolic and diastolic BP	3

*excluded from data extraction figures

12 A Mixed-Methods Examination of an On-Campus Canine-Assisted Intervention by Gender: Women, Men, and Gender-Diverse Individuals' Self-Reports of Stress-Reduction and Well-Being

John-Tyler Binfet[1]*, Freya L.L. Green[1], Rebecca J.P. Godard[2], Madisyn M. Szypula[3], Camille X. Rousseau[1], and Jordy Decker[1]

[1]Okanagan School of Education, University of British Columbia, Okanagan; [2]Irving K Barber School of Arts, University of British Columbia, Okanagan; [3]Faculty of Engineering, University of British Columbia, Okanagan

Abstract

On-campus canine-assisted interventions (CAIs) provide opportunities for college students to interact with therapy dog-handler teams and are considered a low-cost and low-barrier way for students to reduce their stress and bolster their well-being. Across studies, we see participant samples comprised predominantly of women participants. The aim of this study was to assess the effects of a 20-min CAI on the well-being of women (n = 80), men (n = 54), and gender-diverse (n = 28; i.e., non-binary, genderfluid, and two-spirit) participants. Across all gender conditions, significant pre-to-post increases in well-being (i.e., campus connectedness, happiness, positive affect, or optimism) and decreases in ill-being (i.e., homesickness, loneliness, negative affect, anxiety, or stress) were found. Controlling for pre-test scores, there was no significant effect of gender on any of the well-being or ill-being. Findings corroborate previous research attesting to the efficacy of CAIs in enhancing the social and emotional well-being of students and suggest that CAIs are equally effective across participants of varied genders.

Keywords: canine-assisted interventions, gender, gender-diverse participants, therapy dogs, therapy dog-handler team, stress-reduction, well-being, college, university

Introduction

An increasingly common and popular way of reducing students' stress on-campus is seen in the proliferation of canine-assisted programming that provides opportunities for students to interact with therapy dogs and their handlers. Part of the appeal of such interventions may lie in their low cost, low barrier, and low stigmatization (Huber *et al.*, 2022) – students typically do not pay a fee, often a drop-in format is employed that requires no sign-up or appointment, and, as an adjunct or complementary mental health intervention (Fine *et al.*, 2019), there is little discomfiture around accessing this resource. From the perspective of students, it might be seen as "Well, it's not therapy. It's therapy-adjacent."

*Corresponding author email: johntyler.binfet@ubc.ca

Facilitating access to on-campus well-being resources is important in light of the prevalence of mental health challenges faced by post-secondary students, especially first-year students (Bruffaerts *et al.*, 2018; Cheung *et al.*, 2020). Supporting students' well-being and reducing factors contributing to ill-being is paramount to reducing the risk of students dropping out or underperforming academically (Pritchard and Wilson, 2003; Kotzé and Kleynhans, 2013; O'Keeffe, 2013; Miller *et al.*, 2017). For the purpose of our study, well-being was conceptualized as "a state of well-being in which every individual realizes his or her own potential, can cope with the normal stresses of life, can work productively and fruitfully and is able to make a contribution to his or her community." (World Health Organization, 2022, para. 1). As this definition incorporates both positive and negative dimensions of well-being, we designed our study to incorporate aspects of both well-being and ill-being.

Across studies, including randomized controlled trials, having students interact with therapy dogs has been shown to yield a number of favorable outcomes. This includes but is not limited to a reduction in stress (Barker *et al.*, 2016; Pendry and Vandagriff, 2019; Quintana *et al.*, 2019), homesickness (Binfet and Passmore, 2016), self-esteem (Muckle and Lasikiewicz, 2017), and anxiety (Kivlen *et al.*, 2022) and a corresponding boost to happiness (Ward-Griffin *et al.*, 2018; Sokal and Martin; 2021; Sokal *et al.*, 2021), positive affect (Peel *et al.*, 2023); and perception of connectedness to the campus community (Binfet *et al.*, 2022a). That is, we see evidence of a reduction in self-reports of ill-being and a corresponding boost in self-reports in varied indicators of social and emotional well-being. Certainly, there have been calls to increase the methodological rigor of studies assessing the effects of interacting with therapy dog-handler teams (see Rodriguez *et al.*, 2023); however, collective findings across studies, attest to several well-being benefits arising from such interactions (e.g., Crossman *et al.*, 2015; Barker *et al.*, 2016; Binfet *et al.*, 2018; Pendry *et al.*, 2020).

The question "Does it work?" has largely been addressed and researchers of late have explored the question "How does it work?" (e.g., Mueller *et al.*, 2021), identifying that touch between the visiting client and the therapy dog appears to be key to eliciting optimal well-being benefits (Beetz *et al.*, 2011; Pendry and Vandagriff, 2019; Binfet *et al.*, 2022a). Recent research has examined varied modes of delivery including virtual canine comfort modules (e.g., Dell *et al.*, 2021; Binfet *et al.*, 2022b) that assessed pre-to-post effects of spending virtual time with therapy dog-handler teams. Nascent findings from virtual interventions reveal that spending time virtually with therapy dogs is effective in reducing stress; however in-person sessions that afford students the opportunity to interact with dogs through touch, appears to be the more efficient modality for optimal stress reduction (Binfet *et al.*, 2022a). A question that merits further investigation is "For whom does it work?". This arises from an examination of participant samples that sees more women participate in on-campus canine-assisted interventions (CAIs) than other genders. Researchers have begun noticing these skewed participant samples too and as identified by researcher Dell *et al.* (2015, p. 353), "... there is a disproportionate presence of females in comparison to males in the study sample. There is also an underrepresentation of [transgender] individuals. It follows that the gender-specific findings require further investigation." It bears noting that, within the broader context of Canadian post-secondary enrolment and similarly in other countries, there tend to be more women students than other genders (i.e., 57% women, Statistics Canada, 2022). It could be that more women participate in CAIs as women are known to have more favorable views toward mental health care and openness to help-seeking compared to their male counterparts (Wendt and Shafer, 2016; Liddon *et al.*, 2018).

CAIs have been touted as an accessible way to provide opportunities for college students to spend time with therapy dogs as a means of reducing their stress, however, across studies, we see participant samples skew predominantly female (see Table 12.1) and there is a need to understand how CAIs differentially impact students by gender. As argued by Jensen *et al.* (2023, p. 7) in their recent examination of diversity, equity, and inclusion in HAI leadership, "... future research would benefit from increased nuance regarding varying facets of identity and diversity (e.g., diversity in gender, sexuality, disability, and religion.)" There is a skewed gender distribution evident in virtually all published

Table 12.1. Review of reported genders across recent canine-assisted intervention studies.

Citation	Sample size (*N*)	Female (%)	Male (%)	Non-binary (%)	Two-spirit (%)	Other genders (%)
Banks *et al.* (2018)	56	76.8	23.2	—	—	—
Barker *et al.* (2016)	78	76.9	23.1	—	—	—
Binfet (2017)	163	78	—	—	—	—
Binfet *et al.* (2022a)	284	77	21	2	—	—
Binfet *et al.* (2022b)	467	80.9	18.8	0.3	—	—
Binfet and Passmore (2016)	86	82.1	—	—	—	—
Dell *et al.* (2022)	140		Did not report sex/gender breakdown			
Dell *et al.* (2021)	94	92% women	—	—	—	—
	372	82% women	—	—	—	—
Fiocco and Hunse (2017)	61	77.1	22.9	—	—	—
Gebhart *et al.* (2020)	57	77.2	22.8	—	—	—
Grajfoner *et al.* (2017)	132	64.4	—	—	—	—
Haefelin et al. (2020)	165		Did not report sex/gender breakdown			
Hall and Duke (2021)	21	"Majority"	—	—	—	—
House *et al.* (2018)	343	71.7	26.7	—	—	0.6% did not disclose
Hunt *et al.* (2018)	57	74	26	—	—	—
Islam *et al.* (2017)	20	100	—	—	—	—
Kil (2021)	40	62.5	37.5	—	—	—
Kivlen *et al.* (2022)	26	92.3	7.7	—	—	—
Lalonde *et al.* (2020)	4	100	—	—	—	—
Lauriente and Kopp (2018)	206	—	—	—	—	—
Moores *et al.* (2022)	171	77	21	2	—	—
Peel *et al.* (2023)	265	63.0	35.8	—	—	1.1% did not disclose
Peña Gil *et al.* (2020)	64	89.1	—	—	—	—
Pendry *et al.* (2019)	307	61.9	—	—	—	—
Pendry *et al.* (2020)	309	78.6	—	—	—	—
Pendry and Vandagriff (2019)	249	83.5	—	—	—	—
Quintana *et al.* (2019)	530	63.6	—	—	—	—
Sarrafchi *et al.* (2022)	1155	70	30	—	—	—
Spruin *et al.* (2021)	94	60.6	39.4	—	—	—
Thelwell (2019)	80	47.5	52.5	—	—	0
Trammell (2019)	44	75	—	—	—	—
Ward-Griffin *et al.* (2018)	357	78	—	—	—	—
Williams *et al.* (2018)	39	69.2	30.7	—	—	—
Wood *et al.* (2018)	131	73.3	26.7	—	—	—

research examining the effects of CAIs on student well-being (e.g., 70% female in Sarrafchi *et al.*, 2022; 74% female in Trammell, 2019; 78% female in Ward-Griffin *et al.*, 2018; and 73% female in Wood *et al.*, 2018). Concomitantly, meta-analytic findings reveal low non-binary participant representation (Manville *et al.*, 2022). There remains, however, little research that has examined whether one's gender affects the well-being outcomes derived from participating in a CAI or whether participation in a CAI by gender-specific groupings would yield comparable outcomes across genders.

As our understanding of gender identity advances, it is important for researchers to design studies in ways that invite participants to accurately reflect their gender identity (Cameron and Stinson, 2019). Researchers must be mindful to collect demographic data in a way that does not imply a binary gender assumption (i.e., only providing options to identify as a "man" or a "woman"; see also Fraser, 2018). Further, language reflecting gender should be employed. For example, the use of "woman" versus "female" when asking participants for demographic information reflects inclusivity and more clearly refers to one's gender identity rather than biological sex. In order to capture participants' gender expression, researchers may consider adapting their demographic questionnaires to include an open-ended prompt, thus allowing participants to self-describe their gender identity (e.g., "Please describe your gender identity") rather than imposing uniquely binary gender options.

This research is focused on gender and CAIs within the post-secondary context; however, researchers within the broader context of human–animal interactions (HAIs) have recognized gender differences in research. This includes a review of effect sizes by gender across varied dimensions of HAIs including attitudes toward the protection of animals and attachment to pets (e.g., Herzog, 2007), the effects of companion animals on LGBTQ+ participants (see Diaz Videla *et al.*, 2023), and the protective role that animals play for transgender youth (see Wenocur *et al.*, 2022).

With respect to how CAI researchers incorporate and address participant gender within studies, a review of the extant research assessing on-campus CAIs reveals a dearth of findings elucidating the role gender plays in optimizing the well-being of students who spend time with therapy dogs. Ward-Griffin *et al.* (2018) conducted a study wherein undergraduate student participants ($N = 246$) completed pre- and post-test measures prior to, and after, attending a session that saw them interact with therapy dogs, handlers, and fellow attendees. Participants self-selected their dosage which was, on average, 30 min. The researchers found no gender differences in post-test stress, happiness, or energy after a drop-in style, mixed-gender, CAI.

Dell *et al.* (2015) conducted an exploratory pilot examination of interactions between undergraduate students ($N = 726$) and therapy dogs. Their analysis reviewed few differences across genders. Female students were more likely to strongly agree with statements such as "therapy dogs helped me to de-stress," "I feel comforted," and "I feel in control of my emotions" than their male counterparts. As only four participants identified as transgender, comparisons were not drawn. Participants' qualitative responses identified few differences by gender: "Overall, there were minimal differences between genders, but proportionately more females (29%) than males (14%) identified that they attended the event to destress; conversely, proportionately more males (52%) than females (30%) identified that it was just to be with the dogs" (Dell *et al.*, 2015, p. 344).

The present study is theoretically informed by Wilson's (1984) Biophilia hypotheses and Cobb's (1976) Social Support Theory. Biophilia hypotheses assert that humans are drawn to nature and life-like organisms that serve a calming and comforting effect. Animals in general, and therapy dogs in particular, are seen to provide a barometer of pending threat – if the animal is in a calm state it conveys to the human that no threat is imminent with the understanding animals are especially sensitive to environmental threats. Social support theory holds that humans' well-being is bolstered through interactions with others, that humans are social beings who thrive within a social dynamic. Collectively Biophilia hypotheses and social support theory informed both the design and delivery of the intervention employed in our study. Our inclusion of experienced therapy dogs who were accustomed to working within situations and contexts similar to those found in our study combined with the a priori behavior and temperament testing done in the B.A.R.K. (2023) program at the University of British Columbia (UBC), help ensure that dogs would behave in a calm and relaxed manner within sessions, thereby conveying a sense of safety and low-threat to participants. Social support theory was evident in our structuring of the intervention to occur within a social context comprised of the handler and 3–4 participants assigned to one dog-handler team. In doing so, we optimized the chances for participants to interact socially. The combination of providing access to calm and relaxed therapy dogs within a social context is thought to provide optimal stress-reduction conditions. The role of the handler was multifaceted and involved safeguarding their dog's welfare, introducing their dog to visiting students, and facilitating interactions between their dog and students.

The aim of this study was to assess whether there are gender differences in well-being outcomes as a result of participating in an on-campus CAI tailored to gender-specific groupings.

Methods

Procedure

Participants were recruited through posters placed around the campus, via social media, and via a student research portal offering modest course credit to participating students. Both university human (H14-00474) and animal ethics (A22-0185) certificates were issued and all participants provided written informed consent. All handlers attended training sessions to adequately prepare them for participation in this study. This included an overview of the procedure and protocols for the study; a training component wherein handlers were taught appropriate gender terminology and how to respectfully acknowledge participants' pronouns; a walk-through of the bank of questions that handlers could ask participants; and an opportunity to ask questions. Canine welfare was monitored throughout each session by a trained research assistant well-versed in identifying signs of canine distress/stress. Stress signals include, but are not limited to: excessive panting, turning away, whale eye, pawing, whimpering, trembling, yawning, pacing, or avoiding physical contact. No incidents of compromised welfare were reported in any of the sessions.

Intervention

Within their gender cohorts (i.e., women, men, and non-binary/ two-spirit/genderfluid individuals), participants were assigned on a first come first serve basis to sessions and once within a session, were randomly assigned to a dog-handler station along with other participants. The ratio of dog-handler team to participants was 1:3 or 1:4. Following protocols established to facilitate interactions at each dog-handler station, participants were asked to sit on floor markers to ensure that participants were at equal, pre-measured distance from the therapy dog and handler. Handlers were provided discussion guidelines to facilitate conversation at their station (see Fig. 12.1). A total of 11 sessions were offered, and the duration of visits was 20 min.

Participants

Student participants

A total of 163 participants were recruited from the undergraduate subjects' pool at a mid-size Western Canadian research-intensive university (student population > 11,000). Participants were comprised of 49% women (n = 80), 33% men (n = 54), and 17% non-binary and other genders (n = 28). Participants self-selected their gender group. Men and women could participate in either the group for their gender or the gender-diverse group, and gender-diverse individuals could participate in any of the three groups. The resulting group sizes were unequal with 74 in the women's group, 54 in the men's group, and 35 in the non-binary, two-spirit, and

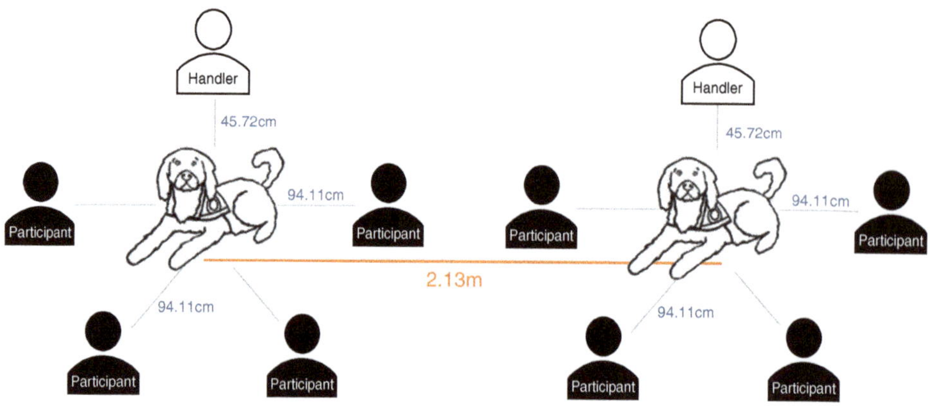

Fig. 12.1. Illustration of handler-dog-participant distancing protocol.

genderfluid individual's group. Participants' average age was 20.6 years (*SD* = 3.2, range = 17–46). Approximately half (54%, *n* =88) were White, followed by South Asian (15%, *n* = 25), two or more ethnic backgrounds (14%, *n* = 24), and other ethnicities (16%, *n* = 26).

Canine handlers

Chosen from a pool of 58 volunteer handlers from the B.A.R.K. program, 15 therapy dog handlers participated in this study. They were recruited through email sign-up, which is the standard process for volunteering for research within the program. Canine handler participants were comprised of 87% women (*n* = 13), 7% men (*n* = 1), and 7% (*n* = 1) who preferred to self-describe using open-ended prompts. All participants identified as White and the average age was 40.0 years (*SD* = 16.6, range = 23–69). On average, dog handlers had 4.5 years prior experience as therapy dog handlers (*SD* = 3.5, range = 6 months–12 years).

Therapy dogs

Chosen from a pool of 56 therapy dogs from the B.A.R.K. program, 15 therapy dogs were involved in this study working under the guidance of their handlers. Two-thirds of the therapy dogs were female (66.7%, *n* = 10; 33.3% male, *n* = 5) and the average age was 5.8 years (*SD* = 16.6, range = 1–10). Eight of the dogs were pure breeds (3 Golden Retrievers, 3 Labradors, 1 Border Collie, and 1 Bernese Mountain Dog) and seven were mixed (Boston Terrier X Pug, Labradoodle, Goldendoodle, Schnoodle, Lab/Husky Mix, Beagle mix, and one unknown mix). On average, therapy dogs had 3.5 years' prior experience working in canine-assisted programming (*SD* = 2.6, range = 6 months–9 years).

Self-report measures

Participants completed pre- and post-test survey packages. All measures were included in both survey packages, with the exception of the demographic questionnaire (pre-test only), the engagement questionnaire (post-test only), the session questionnaire (post-test only), and open-ended prompts (post-test only).

DEMOGRAPHIC QUESTIONNAIRE. Upon completion of the consent forms and prior to commencement of the intervention, participants were asked to provide their gender, age, ethnicity, hometown, year of undergraduate program, number of roommates, a description of any pets they had, and to rate themselves as low, medium, or high consumers of the on-campus CAI program.

Measures of well-being

CAMPUS CONNECTEDNESS SCALE. A single-item questionnaire was administered to assess participants' sense of connection to their campus community (*How connected do you feel currently to your 'campus community'?*) with participants indicating their self-rating of stress using a 5-point Likert-type scale ranging from "not at all connected" (1) to "very connected" (5).

HAPPINESS SCALE. A single-item questionnaire was administered to assess participants' happiness (*How happy do you feel right now?*) with participants indicating their self-rating of stress using a 5-point Likert-type scale ranging from "not at all happy" (1) to "very happy" (5).

POSITIVE AFFECT SCHEDULE. Administered as part of the 20-item Positive and Negative Affect Schedule (PANAS; Watson *et al.*, 1988), the positive affect subscale is comprised of 10 items (Interested, Excited, Strong, Enthusiastic, Proud, Alert, Inspired, Determined, Attentive, Active). Items are rated on a 5-point Likert-type scale ranging from "very slightly or not at all" (1) to "extremely" (5). In the present study, this scale was adapted to assess participants' positive affect in the moment (e.g., "Indicate to what extent you feel this way right now, that is, in this moment.") Cronbach's αs for pre- and post-session in this study were 0.83 and 0.91, respectively.

STATE-OPTIMISM MEASURE. The state-optimism measure (Millstein *et al.*, 2019) is comprised of seven items (e.g., "I am feeling optimistic about life's challenges"). Participants indicate to what extent they agree with each of the statements in that moment (i.e., "right now"). Items are rated on a 5-point Likert-type scale ranging from "disagree strongly" (1) to "strongly agree" (5). Higher total scores indicate higher levels of optimism. Cronbach's αs for each measurement occasion in this study were 0.89 and 0.93, respectively.

Measures of ill-being

HOMESICKNESS SCALE. A single-item questionnaire was administered to assess participants' perceptions of homesickness (*How homesick do you feel right now?*). Participants indicated their self-rating of homesickness using a 5-point Likert-type scale (1 = "Not at all homesick" to 5 = "Very homesick").

LONELINESS SCALE. Using a 5-point Likert-type scale (1 = "Not very" to 5 = "Very"), a single-item questionnaire (*How lonely do you feel right now?*) was administered to assess participants' perceptions of the extent to which they felt lonely.

NEGATIVE AFFECT SCHEDULE. Administered as part of the 20-item PANAS, the positive affect subscale of the PANAS is comprised of 10 items (Disinterested, Upset, Guilty, Scared, Hostile, Irritable, Ashamed, Nervous, Jittery, Afraid"). Items are rated on a 5-point Likert-type scale ranging from "very slightly or not at all" (1) to "extremely" (5). Higher total scores on this subset indicate higher levels of negative affect. In the present study, this scale was adapted to assess participants' negative affect in the moment (e.g., "Indicate to what extent you feel this way right now, that is, in this moment"). Cronbach's αs for pre- and post-session in this study were 0.80 and 0.71, respectively.

STATE–TRAIT ANXIETY INVENTORY STATE–5. The STAIS-5 (Zsido *et al.*, 2020), a shortened version of the state-trait anxiety inventory scale, comprised of five items (e.g., "I feel nervous"; Cronbach's α is 0.91 for the state subscale) was administered. Items are rated on a 4-point Likert-type scale ranging from "not at all" (1) to "very much so" (4) and participants indicate their responses based on how they feel in that moment, (e.g., *How do you feel right now?*). Higher total scores indicate higher levels of state anxiety. Cronbach's αs for each measurement occasion in this study were 0.71 and 0.48, respectively.

STRESS SCALE. To assess participants' current stress level, a single-item questionnaire was administered (*How stressed do you feel right now?*) with participants indicating their self-rating of stress using a 5-point Likert-type scale ranging from "not at all stressed" (1) to "very stressed" (5).

Experience questionnaires

ENGAGEMENT QUESTIONNAIRE. Upon completion of the intervention, participants were asked to rate their agreement with two single-items related to their engagement ("I made eye contact with the therapy dog" and "I physically touched/petted the therapy dog") which were rated on a 5-point Likert-type scale from "not often" (1) to "very often" (5). In addition, participants were asked to rate their physical proximity to the dog on a 5-point Likert-type scale from "not close" (1) to "very close" (5).

SESSION QUESTIONNAIRE. Upon completion of the intervention, participants were asked to indicate their agreement with three single-items related to the session itself ("this session was helpful," "the Covid-19 pandemic has reduced opportunities for me to interact with animals," and "I felt comfortable with the people in my group"). Participants indicated their agreement on a 5-point Likert-type scale ranging from "agree strongly" (1) to "disagree strongly" (5).

OPEN-ENDED PROMPTS. To capture participants' experiences in attending the on-campus CAI, a series of open-ended prompts were administered at the end of the post-test survey. These included the following questions: (1) *How did interacting with the therapy dogs make you feel?*; (2) *Did you make use any other well-being resources on campus? If so, please list the resources you use to take care of your mental health/well-being;* and (3) *Is there anything else you could share to help us understand your experience today?* Participants' responses to these open-ended prompts were coded using conventional qualitative content analysis (Hsieh and Shannon, 2005). Responses for each question were analyzed separately and read first for an overall general impression from which a series of general codes were identified. Next, these codes were clustered or winnowed (Wolcott, 1990) to reduce redundancy following which primary and secondary themes were assigned for each response.

Analytic strategy

Quantitative data were analyzed using ANCOVA. In each model, we used gender group as the predictor and post-intervention well-being/ill-being as the outcome, controlling for pre-intervention well-being/ill-being.

Qualitative data were analyzed using conventional content analysis (Hsieh and Shannon, 2005). This process involves numerous stages. First, all responses for each question were read in a single session by two trained qualitative coders to identify global themes that inform the development of the themes within the coding manual. Upon completion, a more exhaustive process was conducted wherein smaller segments of the responses were descriptively coded based on their key meaning. These codes are subsequently winnowed to form logical themes and sub-themes (Wolcott, 1990), which form a dynamic coding manual. This manual is then utilized to categorize the codes present in each of the participants' responses (see supplementary Appendices A and B). This process was repeated for each question or open-ended prompt. In order to ensure reliability in the content analysis, a second independent coder analyzed a 20% subset of all responses (Syed and Nelson, 2015). The inter-coder agreement rates for each question were 86.9, 97.4, and 90.9%, respectively. All disagreements that occurred were discussed between both coders and resolved.

Results

Quantitative findings

Well-being

Controlling for pre-intervention scores, there was not a significant effect of gender group on post-intervention connection, $F(2, 158) = 0.54$, $p = 0.58$, $\eta^2 < 0.001$, happiness, $F(2, 158) = 0.45$, $p = 0.64$, $\eta^2 < 0.001$, positive affect, $F(2, 158) = 0.52$, $p = 0.60$, $\eta^2 < 0.001$, or optimism $F(2, 159) = 0.42$, $p = 0.66$, $\eta^2 < 0.001$. Across all measures, participants experienced significant increases in well-being from pre-intervention to post-intervention (all $p < 0.001$; see Table 12.2); however, these effects were not dependent on gender group.

Ill-being

Controlling for pre-intervention scores, there was no significant effect of gender group on post-intervention stress, $F(2, 158) = 1.18$, $p = 0.31$, $\eta^2 = 0.01$, loneliness, $F(2, 158) = 0.23$, $p = 0.79$, $\eta^2 < 0.001$, homesickness, $F(2, 158) = 0.72$, $p = 0.49$, $\eta^2 < 0.001$, anxiety, $F(2, 158) = 0.02$, $p = 0.98$, $\eta^2 < 0.001$, or negative affect, $F(2, 158) = 0.48$, $p = 0.62$, $\eta^2 < 0.001$. Across all measures, participants experienced significant reductions in ill-being from pre- to post-intervention (all $p < 0.001$; see Table 12.2); however, these effects were not dependent on gender group.

Table 12.2. Pre- to post-intervention scores.

Variable	Pre-int. *M* (*SD*)	Post-int. *M* (*SD*)	Cohen's d_z
Connection	2.63 (1.01)	3.23 (0.97)	0.69
Happiness	3.16 (0.76)	4.11 (0.85)	1.00
Positive affect (PANAS)	2.98 (0.68)	3.25 (0.81)	0.55
Optimism	3.32 (0.79)	3.84 (0.74)	1.01
Stress	3.26 (0.98)	1.78 (0.80)	−1.46
Loneliness	2.59 (1.05)	1.74 (0.82)	−0.89
Homesickness	2.25 (1.26)	1.80 (1.01)	−0.59
Anxiety (STAIS)	1.67 (0.54)	1.20 (0.25)	−1.07
Negative affect (PANAS)	1.69 (0.54)	1.22 (0.29)	−1.16

Qualitative Findings

HOW DO THERAPY DOGS MAKE STUDENTS FEEL? Participants were asked: "How did interacting with the therapy dogs make you feel?" Of the 164 participants involved in this study, 163 responded to this question. Collectively, they wrote 4774 words, on average 29 words per participant. A total of 308 codes emerged from participants' responses during the analysis which were categorized into nine themes (see supplementary Appendix A).

The responses were initially coded based on their valence, (i.e., whether the feelings described in the participants' response were positive, negative, or neutral in nature). The majority of responses indicated that therapy dogs had made them feel something *positive* (91.6%). A small number (4.9%) reported something *neutral or could not be determined* or reported a *negative feeling* (3.6%). The most prevalent theme (55.8% of codes) indicated that the therapy dogs made participants feel *positive affect* in some way. Specifically, participants identified feeling *calm/relaxed* (38.4% of positive affect codes); *happy* (36.6%), *comfortable or at ease* (15.7%), *heard or valued* (4.7%), or *positive in general* (4.7%). These included examples such as "the therapy dogs really helped calm me down" (Participant 122; 19-year-old woman who self- clarified that their gender identity "can be determined on a day-to-day basis"; *calm/relaxed*); "As soon as I saw the dog I got a huge smile on my face and felt childlike giddy" (Participant 111; 32-year- old woman; *happy*); and "the therapy dog acted as a means to feel comfortable around others" (Participant 43; 22-year-old genderfluid individual; *comfortable/at ease*).

The second most prevalent theme that emerged from participants' responses was that spending time with the therapy dogs had *helped* in some way (15.9%). These responses indicated that the therapy dogs had provided help or an improvement in some way or another. As the descriptions of the help derived from the therapy dogs were rich and varied, these codes were categorized into the following sub-themes: *Helped – General, Improved mood, Reduced stress/anxiety,* and *Reduced homesickness/loneliness* (see supplementary Appendix A). Almost two-thirds of participants reported that the therapy dogs had helped to *reduce stress or anxiety* (61.2%) and included examples such as "I could feel my stress melt away" (Participant 111; 32-year-old woman), "helped reduce a lot of stress that I don't think I fully realized I had" (Participant 142; 21-year-old man), "It was like everything I was stressed about disappeared" (Participant 126; 18-year old genderfluid individual) and "I found that the therapy dog acted as a great form of stress relief" (Participant 43; 22-year old genderfluid individual). In addition, participants reported feeling that the dogs had helped to *improve their mood* (20.4%), such as: "Engaging with the therapy dogs really lifted my spirits" (Participant 36; 18-year-old woman) or *reduced their sense of homesickness or loneliness* (6.1%; e.g., "by interacting with the therapy dog, I felt less lonely and less homesickness"; Participant 104; woman, age not reported).

Other notable responses to this question indicated that the dogs had *engaged or grounded* participants (6.2%) such as: "It grounded me, I was focused on the present, not worrying about the future" (Participant 49; 19-year-old non-binary individual) or provided them with a *break or distraction* (5.8%).

In addition to the participants' responses being analyzed as a collective, we also looked at the prevalence of themes that emerged from each gender group (i.e., women vs. men vs. non-binary, two-spirit and genderfluid). As Table 12.3 illustrates, only very small discrepancies were noted between groups. Noteworthy findings emerged here indicating that participants in the non-binary/two-spirit/genderfluid group more often reported (10.9%) feeling *engaged, aware, or grounded* than those in the men's (6.9%) or the women's (3.5%). Equally, those in the men's group more often noted that spending time with the therapy dogs served as a *break or distraction* (9.9%) when compared to those in the women's (4.2%) or the non-binary/two-spirit/genderfluid group (3.1%).

Utilization of well-being resources

In order to gain insight into the resources that participants utilize in support of their mental well-being, they were asked: "Do you make use of any other well-being resources on campus?" A total of 160 participants responded to this forced binary "Yes/No" question. The majority

Table 12.3. Thematic analysis for the question "How did the therapy dogs make you feel?" by gender condition/group.

	women		men		Non-binary/two spirit/ genderfluid	
Themes	*n*	%	*n*	%	*n*	%
Break/Distraction	6	4.2	10	9.9	2	3.1
Dog characteristics	7	4.9	2	2.0	4	6.3
Engaged/Aware/Grounded	5	3.5	7	6.9	7	10.9
Helped – All	26	18.2	14	13.9	9	14.1
General	3	2.1	1	1.0	2	3.1
Improved mood	5	3.5	3	3.0	2	3.1
Homesickness/loneliness	2	1.4	1	1.0	0	0.0
Stress/anxiety	16	11.2	9	8.9	5	7.8
Negative	5	3.5	3	3.0	3	4.7
Neutral	1	0.7	1	1.0	0	0.0
Other	10	7.0	3	3.0	0	0.0
Positive affect – All	79	55.2	55	54.5	38	59.4
Calm/relaxed	33	23.1	21	20.8	12	18.8
Comfortable/safe	12	8.4	7	6.9	8	12.5
General	2	1.4	5	5.0	1	1.6
Happy	28	19.6	18	17.8	17	26.6
Heard/valued/loved	4	2.8	4	4.0	0	0.0
Socially connected	4	2.8	6	5.9	1	1.6
Total	143		101		64	

(65%) indicated that they did not use other resources on campus. Participants were also invited to list the resources or purposeful steps they take to take care of their mental health/well-being. Of the 164 participants in the study, 135 responded to this question and collectively identified 497 resources (*range* = 1–9 resources). On average, participants wrote 21 words, with a total of 2887 words being analyzed and coded into themes (see supplementary Appendix B). Figure 12.2 illustrates the themes that emerged from the participants' responses.

As depicted in Fig. 12.2, the primary resources identified were *social* in nature or involved *physical exercise*. *Social* resources included examples such as: "conversations with trusted individuals" (Participant 120; 21-year-old woman); "quality time with friends and family" (Participant 119; 17-year-old woman); "avoid draining my social battery and avoid negative people" (Participant 71; 24-year- old who identified as "woman leaning towards non-binary"); and "taking part in events and engaging in the community" (Participant 81; 18-year old woman). *Physical exercise* resources were varied and included attending a gym or working out, participating in group sports (volleyball, soccer, basketball, rugby), or individual activities (walking, hiking, yoga, stretching, running, cycling).

Open-ended responses

Finally, participants were asked: "Is there anything else you could share to help us understand your experience today?" to elicit open-ended, prompt-free descriptions of participants' experiences. Of the 164 participants in the study, 138 responded to this question although 8 responded with "No comments", thus 130 participants responded with a comment that could be analyzed. Collectively, participants wrote 2799 words in response, averaging 22 words per participant. A total of 203 codes emerged from the participants' responses, which were thematically categorized into 11 themes (see supplementary Appendix C). The majority of participants (65.0%) added additional comments that were *positive* in nature, 23.6% provided a *neutral* comment or a comment that *could not be determined*, and 6.4% reported something *negative*. Examples of these include: "It was really nice to interact with other non-binary/gender queer students! I feel like I have a bit more of a community now or

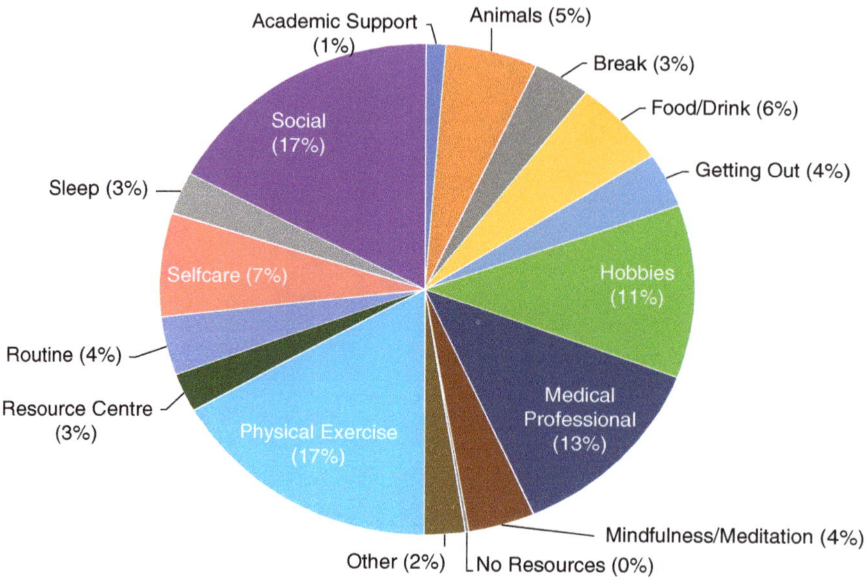

Fig. 12.2. Pie chart illustrating the utilized mental health resources identified by participants.

at least it was very nice to have a shared experience without having to express it in words" (Participant 151; 25-year-old non-binary individual; *positive*); and "I am quite hungry, so it distracted from the experience a little bit" (Participant 149; 18-year old man; *negative*).

The most prevalent theme that emerged indicated that participants found the session to be *beneficial* in some way (22.2%). Within this, several sub-themes emerged – participants cited benefits for their *emotional or mental health* (46.7% of the beneficial responses), *generalized benefits* (28.9%), or *social benefits* (24.4%). Examples of these include the following quotations from participants: "knowing that I was allowed to just be there and pet was very helpful for my anxiety" (Participant 40; 20-year old woman; *emotional or mental health*); "it helped me feel better about everything today" (Participant 140; 18-year old man; *general*); "I have autism and often feel more at ease with animals rather than people. In a way, this was more helpful than counselling" (Participant 132; 18-year old trans-masc, non-binary individual; *general*); "[The session] helped with the loneliness, and made me feel connected" (Participant 72; 20-year- old woman; *social*); and "Going to B.A.R.K. helped me gain a sense of community" (Participant 14; 19-year-old man *social*).

Almost a fifth of participants (19.2%) also provided *feedback*. Participants provided general feedback (38.5%), such as: "Please continue incorporating new and innovative methods involving dogs into education. It is a beautiful solution to so many complex problems" (Participant 61; man, age not reported) and "I will make an effort to utilize the B.A.R.K. program after today!" (Participant 119; 17-year old woman). In addition, 23.1% of those who gave feedback reported wanting more animals present at sessions or more time or additional sessions in future (15.4%). Additional participants (10.3% of feedback) also provided praise or positive feedback for the B.A.R.K. program on campus, such as "I'm very glad UBC has the B.A.R.K. program!" (Participant 123; 18-year old woman), and "You don't realize how much of an impact B.A.R.K. can have until you go" (Participant 63; 21-year-old man).

Other notable codes included that it was *good to have time with the dogs* (11.8%) and that it was a *great experience* (11.3%). In addition, it should be noted that 6.4% of participants reported a generalized *negative comment* about participating in the study, one such example of this was "my Tourette's causes me stress out in public, both suppressing it and worrying I'll tick" (Participant 68; 18-year-old non-binary individual) and "I was a bit distracted by wanting to meet the other dogs" (Participant 86; 19-year-old woman).

Discussion

This study assessed the effects of an on-campus CAI on self-reports of well-being in university students by gender and found a 20-min CAI did not differentially benefit students based on their identification as men, women, or non-binary, two-spirit, or genderfluid. The findings are discussed within the broader context of HAIs and the post-secondary setting.

First, these findings contribute to the growing body of literature attesting to the benefits of on-campus CAIs. The present study corroborated prior literature positing that CAIs are effective in reducing students' stress, loneliness, homesickness, negative affect, and anxiety as well as improve happiness, connection, and positive affect and our findings align with findings reported by other HAI researchers (e.g., Barker *et al.*, 2016; Binfet and Passmore, 2016; Crossman *et al.*, 2015; Ward-Griffin *et al.*, 2018; Pendry and Vandagriff, 2019).

Certainly, a key finding arising from our study is that there were no significant gender differences in well-being outcomes after participation in a CAI. As we illustrated at the outset of this article, there are gender differences in CAI studies with more women participants reported across studies than other genders (see Table 12.1). Although our study does not offer an explanation as to why there is such a strong skewed gender distribution, our findings do elucidate that CAIs within the post-secondary context appear to offer comparable benefits across genders. Future research might explore why, if CAIs work effectively across genders, are more women students inclined to participate in CAI on-campus research? As our study compared gender-specific groups to other gender-specific groups, a second future study might compare the outcomes for men, women, and gender-diverse students attending either a gender-specific group or a mixed-gender group to discern if comparable benefits arise across these groupings.

The findings from our study also hold implications within the post-secondary educational context for student well-being program developers as they seek to offer inclusive initiatives for a diverse range of students. Although quantitative findings indicated no significant differences by gender arising from the CAI, our qualitative analyses provide nuanced insights into participants' varied experiences across gender conditions. This was especially notable for the gender-diverse students who shared that they found the community and climate within this session to be a space that was comforting, safe, and trusted. This observation holds relevance for on-campus well-being programming seeking to introduce new support systems or resources for gender-diverse students. As our study drew a relatively robust subsample of gender-diverse students, it could be that offering gender-specific programming holds promise to increase engagement on campus.

A novel finding arising from our study identified students experiencing increased optimism after participating in a CAI. This finding in particular has implications for student well-being as increased optimism experienced by students' holds the potential to recalibrate how they think about their ability and potential as a student within the post-secondary context. This, in turn, may foster a more positive outlook on their university experience and their ability to cope with the academic demands being placed on them. Additional research examining the effects of CAIs on optimism and students' subsequent engagement in school work and the broader campus life is warranted.

Strengths and limitations

Our study was a first step in examining whether CAIs work equally well for varied genders and, in light of previous studies reporting participant samples comprised of predominantly women, our sampling of men, non-binary, genderfluid, and two-spirit participants, elucidates our understanding that the efficacy of CAIs does not appear to be gender dependent. The first strength of our study is found in our use of mixed methods with findings from our quantitative analyses supported by insights gleaned from our qualitative analyses. Second, we explored the effects of students interacting with therapy dogs on both varied dimensions of well-being and ill-being. In this regard, our collective findings provide a composite overview of outcomes impacting the mental health of students. A third strength of our study is found in the experienced therapy dog-handler teams who participated in the intervention. As reflected by our reporting of demographic characteristics of both therapy dogs and their handlers, the teams participating in the intervention had extensive experience in CAIs and were skilled in communicating and engaging with students and fostering canine–student interactions. A fourth strength is found in the handlers attending a training prior to the study (e.g., to familiarize handlers with gender terminology) and their following a bank of questions to help standardize the experience of participants across dog-handler teams. A final strength of our study is found in our successful recruiting of gender-diverse participants, especially given gender-diverse students typically have relatively low-representation across the larger student body.

Despite best intentions, there were limitations to this study. First, our cell sizes by gender were unequal with more women recruited than other genders. Although this reflects ecological validity in so much that it mirrors the gender distribution typically found on university campuses, we saw a disproportionate number of women in our study. A second limitation is found in the clustering of non-binary, genderfluid, and two-spirit participants. Given their relatively low numbers, these participants comprised a single group and future research could examine the effects of CAIs for a variety of genders grouped here under the gender-diverse umbrella. A final limitation is found in the potential variability in handlers – that is, pending the skills, experience, and demeanor of individual handlers, there may have been variability in the extent to which handlers were able to engage participants.

Conclusion

The findings from our study add to the body of literature extolling the benefits of providing opportunities for college students to bolster their well-being through interactions with therapy dogs. One aim of this study was to examine whether CAIs work equally well for all students. Our findings suggest that they do – regardless of gender, there appears to be no significant differences in well-being outcomes by gender. Extending our understanding of the benefits of CAIs, our qualitative findings provide insights into students' experiences within a session – that students largely make little use of other on-campus well-being resources and that the CAI is understood to be a time to relax and push aside the worries and pressures associated with being a university student.

Conflict of interest

The authors declare no conflict of interest.

Ethics statement

Both human and animal ethics approval for this study was granted by the University's (blinded for review) ethics committee (protocol numbers blinded for review). All relevant guidelines stated in the protocols were carefully followed. Participants reviewed the consent form and were provided with an opportunity to ask questions about participation prior to participating in this study. All participants provided written consent.

Funding statement

This research was funded from the Building Academic Retention through K9s (B.A.R.K.) program's research fund, University of British Columbia.

Author contributions

J.B, F.G., R.G., M.S., C.R., and J.D., conceptualized the study; J.B., F.G., M.S., and C.R., carried out the recruitment and methodological procedures; R.G., conducted the quantitative analysis and write-up of the quantitative results; F.G., M.S., and J.B. conducted the qualitative analysis and write-up of the qualitative results; J.B. and

F.G. carried out the original draft preparation; J.B., F.G. and R.G reviewed and edited the manuscript; J.B. supervised the study. All authors have read and agreed to the published version of the manuscript.

Data availability

All data undergirding the present study is available for researchers upon request by contacting the corresponding author.

References

Banks, J.B., McCoy, C. and Trzcinski, C. (2018) Examining the impact of a brief human-canine interaction on stress and attention. *Human-Animal Interaction Bulletin* 6(1), 1–13. DOI: 10.1079/hai.2018.0003.

B.A.R.K. (2023) Building Academic Retention through K9s. Available at: https://bark.ok.ubc.ca/ (accessed 11 October 2023).

Barker, S.B., Barker, R.T., McCain, N.L. and Schubert, C.M. (2016) A randomized cross-over exploratory study of the effect of visiting therapy dogs on college student stress before final exams. *Anthrozoös* 29(1), 35–46. DOI: 10.1080/08927936.2015.1069988.

Beetz, A., Kotrschal, K., Turner, D.C., Hediger, K., Uvnäs-Moberg, K. and Julius, H. (2011) The effect of a real dog, toy dog and friendly person on insecurely attached children during a stressful task: An exploratory study. *Anthrozoös* 24(4), 349–368. DOI: 10.2752/175303711X13159027359746.

Binfet, J.T. (2017) The effects of group-administered canine therapy on first-year university students' well-being: A randomized controlled trial. *Anthrozoos* 30(3), 397–414. DOI: 10.1080/08927936.2017.1335097.

Binfet, J.T. and Passmore, H.A. (2016) Hounds and homesickness: The effects of an animal-assisted therapeutic intervention for first-year university students. *Anthrozoos* 29(3), 441–454. DOI: 10.1080/08927936.2016.1181364.

Binfet, J.T., Passmore, H.A., Cebry, A., Struik, K. and McKay, C. (2018) Reducing university students' stress through a drop-in canine-therapy program. *Journal of Mental Health* 3, 197–204. DOI: 10.1080/09638237.2017.1417551.

Binfet, J.T., Green, F.L. and Draper, Z.A. (2022a) The importance of client– canine contact in canine-assisted interventions: A randomized controlled trial. *Anthrozoös* 35(1), 1–22. DOI: 10.1080/08927936.2021.1944558.

Binfet, J.T., Tardif-Williams, C., Draper, Z.A., Green, F.L., Singal, A., Rousseau, C.X. and Roma, R. (2022b) Virtual canine comfort: A randomized controlled trial of the effects of a canine-assisted intervention supporting undergraduate wellbeing. *Anthrozoös* 35(6), 809–832. DOI: 10.1080/08927936.2022.2062866.

Bruffaerts, R., Mortier, P., Kiekens, G., Auerbach, P., Cuijpers, K. et al. (2018) Mental health problems in college freshmen: Prevalence and academic functioning. *Journal of Affective Disorders* 225, 97–103. DOI: 10.1016/j.jad.2017.07.044.

Cameron, J.J. and Stinson, D.A. (2019) Gender (mis)measurement: Guidelines for respecting gender diversity in psychological research. *Social and Personality Psychology Compass* 13(11), e12506. DOI: 10.1111/spc3.12506.

Cheung, K., Tam, K.Y., Tsang, H., Zhang, L.W. and Lit, S.W. (2020) Depression, anxiety and stress in different subgroups of first-year university students from 4-year cohort data. *Journal of Affective Disorders* 274, 305–314. DOI: 10.1016/j.jad.2020.05.041.

Cobb, S. (1976) Social support as a moderator of life stress. *Psychosomatic Medicine* 38(5), 300–314. DOI: 10.1097/00006842-197609000-00003.

Crossman, M.K., Kazdin, A.E. and Knudson, K. (2015) Brief unstructured interaction with a therapy dog reduces distress. *Anthrozoös* 28(4), 649–659. DOI: 10.1080/08927936.2015.1070008.

Dell, C.A., Chalmers, D., Gillett, J., Rohr, B., Nickel, C. et al. (2015) PAWSing student stress: A pilot evaluation of the St. John ambulance therapy dog program on three university campuses in Canada. *Canadian Journal of Counselling and Psychotherapy* 49(4), 332–359. Available at: https://cjc-rcc.ucalgary.ca/article/views/61079.

Dell, C., Williamson, L., McKenzie, H., Carey, B., Cruz, M., Gibson, M. and Pavelich, A. (2021) A commentary about lessons learned: Transitioning a therapy dog program online during the COVID-19 pandemic. *Animals* 11, 914. DOI: 10.3390/ani11030914.

Dell, C.A., Mills, S., Goodfellow, H. and Cruz, M. (2022) A novel approach to supporting student mental health in the university classroom with therapy dogs. *Canadian Journal of Community Mental Health* 41(2), 97–101. DOI: 10.7870/cjcmh-2022-010.

Diaz Videla, M., Delgado Rodriguez, R., Martos-Montes, R., Ordonez Perez, D. and Calvo, P. (2023) The LGBTQ+ people-animal bond: A systematic review of the effects of companion animals on LGBTQ+ people. *Journal of Homosexuality*, 1–24. DOI: 10.1080/00918369.2022.2150920.

Fine, A.H., Beck, A.M. and Ng, Z. (2019) The state of animal-assisted interventions: Addressing the contemporary issues that will shape the future. *International Journal of Environmental Research and Public Health* 16(20), 3997. DOI: 10.3390/ijerph16203997.

Fiocco, A.J. and Hunse, A.M. (2017) The buffer effect of therapy dog exposure on stress reactivity in undergraduate students. *International Journal of Environmental Research and Public Health* 14(7), 707. Available at: https://hdl.handle.net/10393/38571.

Fraser, G. (2018) Evaluating inclusive gender identity measures for use in quantitative psychological research. *Psychology & Sexuality* 9(4), 343–357. DOI: 10.1080/19419899.2018.1497693.

Gebhart, V., Buchberger, W., Klotz, I., Neururer, S., Rungg, C. *et al.* (2020) Distraction-focused interventions on examination stress in nursing students: Effects on psychological stress and biomarker levels. A randomized controlled trial. *International Journal of Nursing Practice* 26(1), e12788. DOI: 10.1111/ijn.12788.

Grajfoner, D., Harte, E., Potter, L.M. and McGuigan, N. (2017) The effect of dog-assisted intervention on student well-being, mood, and anxiety. *International Journal of Environmental Research and Public Health* 14(5), 483. DOI: 10.3390/ijerph14050483.

Haefelin, N., Lange, N., Sweigert, B., Yonto, M. and Rivardo, M.G. (2020) Anxiety reduction in college students after brief interaction with a therapy dog or animatronic dog. *North American Journal of Psychology* 22(3), 411. Available at: https://link.gale.com/apps/doc/A637227331/HRCA?u=ubcolu mbia&sid=summon&xid=77158c99.

Hall, D. and Duke, G. (2021) Therapy dog effects on nursing student stress: A mixed methods study. *Nurse Educator* 46(4), E70–E74. DOI: 10.1097/NNE.0000000000000953.

Herzog, H.A. (2007) Gender differences in human–animal interactions: A review. *Anthrozoös* 20(1), 7–21. DOI: 10.2752/089279307780216687.

House, L.A., Neal, C. and Backels, K. (2018) A doggone way to reduce stress: An animal assisted intervention with college students. *College Student Journal* 52(2), 199–204. Available at: https://go.gale.com/ps/i.do?id=GALE%7CA544511706&sid=googleScholar&v=2.1&it=r&linkaccess=a bs&issn=01463934&p=AONE &sw=w&userGroupName=anon%7Ebb03f568&aty=open+web+entry#:~:text=Students%20were%20 encouraged%20 to%20interact,in%20perceived%20stress%20for%20students.

Hsieh, H.G. and Shannon, S.E. (2005) Three approaches to qualitative content analysis. *Qualitative Health Research* 15(9), 1277–1288. DOI: 10.1177/1049732305276687.

Huber, A., Klug, S.J., Abraham, A., Westenberg, E., Schmidt, V. and Winkler, A.S. (2022) Animal-assisted interventions improve mental, but not cognitive or physiological health outcomes of higher education students: A systematic review and meta-analysis. *International Journal of Mental Health and Addiction.* DOI: 10.1007/s11469-022-00945-4.

Hunt, M., Al-Braiki, F., Dailey, S., Russell, R. and Simon, K. (2018) Mindfulness training, yoga, or both? Dismantling the active components of a mindfulness-based stress reduction intervention. *Mindfulness* 9, 512–520. DOI: 10.1007/s12671-017-0793-z.

Islam, S., Spruin, E. and Fernandez, A. (2017) The benefits of therapy dogs on student well-being within a UK university. *Psychology and Behavioural Sciences International Journal* 7, 1–4.

Jensen, C.L., Ogeer, J., Beck, A.M. and O'Haire, M.E. (2023) Exploring diversity, equity, and inclusion perceptions among leadership in the field of human-animal interaction. *Human-Animal Interactions* 11(1), 1–9. DOI: 10.1079/hai.2023.0012.

Kil, T. (2021) Effects of the multimodal intervention program including animal-assisted therapy on depression and self-esteem among university students. *Journal of Animal Science and Technology* 63(6), 1443. DOI: 10.5187/jast.2021.e115.

Kivlen, C.A., Quevillon, A. and Pasquarelli, D. (2022) Should dogs have a seat in the classroom? The effects of canine assisted education on college student mental health. *The Open Journal of Occupational Therapy* 10(1), 1–14. DOI: 10.15453/2168-6408.1816.

Kotzé, M. and Kleynhans, R. (2013) Psychological well-being and resilience as predictors of first-year students' academic performance. *Journal of Psychology in Africa* 23(1), 51–59. DOI: 10.1080/14330237.2013.10820593.

Lalonde, R., Dell, C. and Claypool, T. (2020) PAWS your stress: The student experience of therapy dog programming. *Canadian Journal for New Scholars in Education/Revue canadienne des jeunes chercheures et chercheurs en éducation* 11(2), 78–90. Available at: https://journalhosting.ucalgary.ca/index.php/cjnse/article/view/69530.

Lauriente, T. and Kopp, D. (2018) Therapy dogs on campus: An exploration of how dog therapy services affect undergraduate students' stress levels. *Undergraduate Research Conference Proceedings* 12(1). Available at: https://publishing.bceln.ca/index.php/urcproceedings/article/view/346.

Liddon, L., Kingerlee, R. and Barry, J.A. (2018) Gender differences in preferences for psychological treatment, coping strategies, and triggers to help-seeking. *British Journal of Clinical Psychology* 57(1), 42–58. DOI: 10.1111/bjc.12147.

Manville, K., Coulson, M., Mulqueen, M.A., Neller, K., Searing, C., Welland, S. and Reynolds, G. (2022) Effects of canine-assisted intervention on the mental health of higher education students: A systematic review. *Human-Animal Interaction Bulletin* 13(1), 111–145. DOI: 10.1079/hai.2022.0012.

Miller, B., Fridline, M. and Bernert, D. (2017) Assessing the impact of undergraduate college student health on academic performance across academic year. *Psychology* 7(7), 408–417. DOI: 10.17265/2159-5542/2017.07.005.

Millstein, R.A., Chung, W.J., Hoeppner, B.B., Boehm, J.K., Legler, S.R., Mastromauro, C.A. and Huffman, J.C. (2019) Development of the state optimism measure. *General Hospital Psychiatry* 58, 83–93. DOI: 10.1016/j. genhosppsych.2019.04.002.

Moores, L., Button, P., Fawcett, E. and Whelan, B. (2022) Puppies, plants, painting, and popcorn: Evaluation of an integrated outreach program. *Journal of College Student Psychotherapy* 36(4), 410–425. DOI: 10.1080/87568225.2021.1881860.

Muckle, J. and Lasikiewicz, N. (2017) An exploration of the benefits of animal-assisted activities in undergraduate students in Singapore. *Asian Journal of Social Psychology* 20(2), 75–84. DOI: 10.1111/ajsp.12166.

Mueller, M.K., Anderson, E.C., King, E.K. and Urry, H.L. (2021) Null effects of therapy dog interaction on adolescent anxiety during a laboratory-based social evaluative stressor. *Anxiety, Stress, & Coping* 34(4), 365–380. DOI: 10.1080.10615806.2021.1892084.

O'Keeffe, P. (2013) A sense of belonging: Improving student retention. *College Student Journal* 47(4), 605–613.

Peña Gil, D., García García, M. and Camilli Trujillo, C. (2020) Dog- assisted intervention at a Spanish university: Pilot study. *Journal of Applied Research in Higher Education* 12(2), 344–356. DOI: 10.1108/JARHE-03-2019-0067.

Peel, N., Nguyen, K. and Tannous, C. (2023) The impact of campus-based therapy dogs on the mood and affect of university students. *International Journal of Environmental Research and Public Health* 20(6), 4759. DOI: 10.3390/ijerph20064759.

Pendry, P. and Vandagriff, J.L. (2019) Animal visitation program (AVP) reduces cortisol levels of university students: A randomized controlled trial. *Aera Open* 5(2), 1–12. DOI: 10.1177/2332858419852592.

Pendry, P., Kuzara, S. and Gee, N.R. (2019) Evaluation of undergraduate students' responsiveness to a 4-week university-based animal-assisted stress prevention program. *International Journal of Environmental Research and Public Health* 16(18), 3331. DOI: 10.3390/ijerph16183331.

Pendry, P., Carr, A.M., Gee, N.R. and Vandagriff, J.L. (2020) Randomized trial examining effects of animal assisted intervention and stress related symptoms on college students' learning and study skills. *International Journal of Environmental Research and Public Health* 17(6), 1909. DOI: 10.3390/ijerph17061909.

Pritchard, M.E. and Wilson, G.S. (2003) Using emotional and social factors to predict student success. *Journal of College Student Development* 44(1), 18–28. DOI: 10.1353/csd.2003.0008.

Quintana, S., Borckardt, M. and Aditya, T. (2019) Dog days of final exams: Using canine-assisted therapy to reduce stress and improve mood among community college students. *Quest* 3(1), 3. Available at: https://digitalcommons.collin.edu/quest/vol3/iss1/3.

Rodriguez, K.E., Green, F.L.L., Binfet, J.T., Townsend, L. and Gee, N. (2023) Complexities and considerations in conducting animal-assisted intervention research: A discussion of randomized controlled trials. *Human–Animal Interactions Journal*. DOI: 10.1079/hai.2023.0004.

Sarrafchi, A., David-Steel, M., Pearce, S.D., de Zwaan, N. and Merkies, K. (2022) Effect of human-dog interaction on therapy dog stress during an on-campus student stress buster event. *Applied Animal Behaviour Science* 253, 105659. DOI: 10.1016/j.applanim.2022.105659.

Sokal, L. and Martin, T. (2021) Post-secondary paw patrol: Effects of animal- assisted activities on students' stress, happiness, and well-being. *International Journal of Contemporary Education* 4(1). Available at: http://ijce.redfame.com.

Sokal, L., Bartel, B. and Martin, T. (2021) Effects of touch on students' stress, happiness, and well-being during animal-assisted activities. *Journal of Education and Development* 5(1), 111–122. DOI: 10.20849/jed.v5i1.887.

Spruin, E., Dempster, T., Islam, S. and Raybould, I. (2021) The effects of a therapy dog vs mindfulness vs a student advisor on student anxiety and well-being. *Journal of Further and Higher Education* 45(5), 588–600. DOI: 10.1080/0309877X.2020.1804535.

Statistics Canada (2022) Proportion of Male and Female Postsecondary Graduates, by Field of Study and International Standard Classification of Education. Available at: https://www150.statcan.gc.ca/t1/tbl1/en/tv.action?pid=3710013502.

Syed, M. and Nelson, S.C. (2015) Guidelines for establishing reliability when coding narrative data. *Emerging Adulthood* 3(6), 375–387. DOI: 10.1177/2167696815587648.

Thelwell, E.L. (2019) Paws for thought: A controlled study investigating the benefits of interacting with a house-trained dog on university students mood and anxiety. *Animals* 9(10), 846. DOI: 10.3390/ani9100846.

Trammell, J.P. (2019) Therapy dogs improve student affect but not memory. *Anthrozoös* 32(5), 691–699. DOI: 10.1080/08927936.2019.1645514.

Ward-Griffin, E., Klaiber, P., Collins, H.K., Owens, R.L., Coren, S. and Chen, F.S. (2018) Petting away pre-exam stress: The effect of therapy dog sessions on student well-being. *Stress and Health* 34(3), 468–473. DOI: 10.1002/smi.2804.

Watson, D., Clark, L.A. and Tellegen, A. (1988) Development and validation of brief measures of positive and negative affect: The PANAS scales. *Journal of Personality and Social Psychology* 54(6), 1063–1070. DOI: 10.1037/0022-3514.54.6.1063.

Wendt, D. and Shafer, K. (2016) Gender and attitudes about mental health help seeking: Results from National data. *Health & Social Work* 41(1), e20–228. DOI: 10.1093/hsw/hlv089.

Wenocur, K., Matthews, M. and Kotak, N. (2022) Personal and professional perspectives on the protective role of animals for transgender youth: A qualitative analysis. *Human Animal Interaction Bulletin* 13(1), 14–29.

Williams, C., Emond, K., Maynord, K., Simpkins, J., Stumbo, A. and Terhaar, T. (2018) An animal-assisted intervention's influence on graduate students' stress and anxiety prior to an examination. *Open Access Library Journal* 5(9), 1–16. DOI: 10.4236/oalib.1104831.

Wilson, E.O. (1984) *Biophilia*. Harvard University Press, Cambridge, MA.

Wolcott, H.F. (1990) *Transforming Qualitative Data: Description, Analysis, and Interpretation*. Sage, Thousand Oaks, CA.

Wood, E., Ohlsen, S., Thompson, J., Hulin, J. and Knowles, L. (2018) The feasibility of brief dog-assisted therapy on university students stress levels: The PAwS study. *Journal of Mental Health* 27(3), 263–268. DOI: 10.1080/09638237.2017.1385737.

World Health Organization (2022) Mental Health. Available at:https://www.who.int/news-room/fact-sheets/detail/mental-health-strengthening-our-response (accessed 18 September 2023).

Zsido, A.N., Teleki, S.A., Csokasi, K., Rozsa, S. and Bandi, S.A. (2020) Development of the short version of the spielberger state— trait anxiety inventory. *Psychiatry Research* 291. DOI: 10.1016/j. psychres.2020.113223.

13 Therapy Dogs, Stress-Reduction, and Well-Being Within the Detachment: Interviews with Law-Enforcement Personnel

Freya L. L. Green* and John-Tyler Binfet
Okanagan School of Education, University of British Columbia, Kelowna, BC

Abstract

Despite the increasing popularity of canine-assisted interventions (CAIs) across a variety of contexts, and the demonstrated efficacy they have on stress reduction, there is a paucity of research exploring the implementation of such programs within the context of law enforcement. Policing is known to be an environment in which personnel experience elevated occupational stress. As stress can compromise the overall well-being of law-enforcement personnel and their ability to serve the public, it is important to understand how CAIs involving therapy dog visitation are experienced by the very individuals for whom they are intended to help. This qualitative study explored Royal Canadian Mounted Police (RCMP) members' experiences of stress within a detachment and their perceptions of a CAI integrated within their workplace to support their well-being. Eight RCMP members (75% female, *Mage* = 49.21, *SD* = 6.12) from an urban RCMP detachment situated in the downtown core of a small city were interviewed. The interview focused on topics including members' experiences of stress within the workplace, their perceptions of the effects of stress, resources and sources of support, and their experiences participating in a weekly CAI within their detachment. Results indicated that organizational stressors were identified more often than operational stressors; that members most commonly reported that stress rendered them more irritable and impacted their sleep, and that the most commonly reported coping mechanism and resource are exercise and medical services, respectively. In discussing the CAI, participants were overwhelmingly positive in their experiences of the program, and demonstrated support for having CAIs within the detachment setting. Discussion of the impact of the sessions demonstrated that participants found that the program served as a break from work, relieved their stress, improved their mood, and helped them to change perspectives. Participants also identified the role of the dogs within the program, which included their role as a social being. The findings from the current study contribute to better understanding of the lived experiences of stress within RCMP members and of CAIs within an applied setting.

Keywords: law-enforcement, canine-assisted intervention, stress reduction, therapy dogs

As part of their routine duties, law-enforcement personnel regularly encounter dangerous situations and are often exposed to distressing events such as acts of mass causalities, deaths of colleagues, terrorism, homicides, and a constant, yet unpredictable, risk to life (Gershon et al., 2009; Gershon et al., 2002; Marmar et al., 2006; Westmarland, 2017). In addition to these potentially life-threatening

Corresponding author email: freya.green@ubc.ca
Conflict of Interest Statement: The authors report no conflicts of interest.

operational stressors, law- enforcement personnel may experience organizational stressors such as antisocial working hours and shift work, heavy workloads, intermittent work pace, and workplace discrimination (Gershon et al., 2009; Terpstra & Schaap, 2013; White & Robinson, 2014).

Given the stressors associated with the profession, law-enforcement is considered to be amongst the most stressful of all occupations (Anshel, 2000; Ménard & Arter, 2013; Ranta & Sud, 2008). For example, in a study by Queirós et al. (2020), 85% of Portuguese law-enforcement personnel (n = 2,057) exceeded the threshold for high operational stress levels and 28% presented as highly-distressed. Working in a high-stress profession places law-enforcement personnel at a heightened risk for compromised physical health including cardiovascular disease and obesity, social concerns such as distrust of others and isolation, familial issues including domestic violence and divorce, maladaptive coping mechanisms such as substance abuse and gambling, and overall compromised mental health (Bano & Talib, 2017; Carleton et al., 2018; Gershon et al., 2009; Terpstra & Schaap, 2013; Queirós et al., 2020; Zimmerman, 2012; 2014). In addition, it has been identified that increasing numbers of law-enforcement personnel are at risk of developing psychological disorders (Queirós et al., 2020). Mumford and colleagues (2015) found that post-traumatic stress disorder (PTSD) was disclosed by law-enforcement personnel (n = 184) at a rate of over double that of the general population (8.8% compared to 3.5%) and that anxiety and depression were reported almost twice as often in law-enforcement personnel compared to the general population. Specifically looking at Royal Canadian Mounted Police (RCMP), Carleton and colleagues (2018) conducted a survey of 5,813 public safety personnel (PSP; e.g., correctional workers, firefighters, paramedics, dispatchers, and police). In this study, the authors found that 50.2% of the RCMP members surveyed screened positive for an established mental health disorder (i.e., PTSD, major depressive disorder, generalized anxiety disorder, social anxiety disorder, panic disorder or alcohol abuse). Notably, a higher percentage of members screened positive for mental disorders than any other first responder including firefighters, paramedics, dispatchers, and municipal police. In addition, 24.4% of RCMP screened positive for three or more disorders – higher than any other PSP in the study (Carleton et al., 2018).

Literature Review

The literature review that follows will provide an overview of the literature on stress reduction in law-enforcement and on the efficacy of canine-assisted interventions for reducing stress.

Research on stress reduction in law-enforcement

As a result of this increasing concern for the personal well-being of employees, researchers are starting to examine the efficacy of well-being or stress-reduction programs for law-enforcement personnel. Generalized well-being programs have demonstrated efficacy in improving behavioral, emotional, social, and cognitive outcomes in law- enforcement personnel (Kuehl et al., 2014; 2016; McCraty & Atkinson, 2012) however the implementation of stress-reduction programs specifically is still lacking. Many law-enforcement detachments do not yet have wellness or stress-reduction programs in place to combat the stress or the resulting physical or mental health concerns that arise within the workplace (Crouch, 2014).

Furthermore, many of the programs that are targeted specifically at stress in law-enforcement are deemed to have limited efficacy. Patterson and colleagues (2014) conducted a meta-analysis of 12 stress-management interventions targeted at law-enforcement personnel published between 1984 and 2008. These interventions included stress-reduction or management programs, individual wellness counselling, stress- inoculation training, and writing interventions, amongst others. Patterson et al. (2014) concluded that, based on the effect sizes from these studies, the interventions were largely ineffective. More recently, Liakopoulou et al. (2020) conducted a randomized controlled trial to assess the effectiveness of the Pythagorean Self-Awareness Intervention (PSAI). The PSAI is a program in which a series of cognitive processes are practiced twice a day. These include a general recollection of the day's events followed by a focused recollection and evaluation of a specific event during the day. Finally, and upon completion of these recollections, individuals set specific goals for the following day based on their evaluation. Participants in the PSAI group (n = 27) demonstrated promising results for negative affect, cognitive speed, and verbal memory when compared with the control however, no significant results were found for a reduction in either organizational or operational stress.

The aforementioned study by Crouch (2014) established that 80% of law-enforcement officers were interested in participating in a program to improve their well-being if one were available. Given the negative ramifications of stress, the demands placed upon officers, and the lack of stress-reduction opportunities available to them, research is needed which explores the effective, feasible, and sustainable implementation of programs across agencies.

Research on canine-assisted interventions

One such opportunity to assist agencies in fostering employee well-being lies within the field of human–animal interactions (HAIs). Canine-assisted interventions (CAIs), a category of animal-assisted interventions that fall under the larger umbrella of HAIs (Binfet & Hartwig, 2019), remain under-utilized within law-enforcement despite their surge in popularity and efficacy in augmenting well-being across a variety of contexts and with a variety of clients (Binfet et al., 2018; Binfet & Passmore, 2016; Hoffman et al., 2009; Lang et al., 2010; Stevens et al., 2017). CAIs provide an opportunity for clients or visitors (often university students or seniors) to spend time and interact with certified therapy dog-handler teams (i.e. assessed and credentialed by a therapy dog organization) with the aim of reducing stress and improving well-being. Such interactions have been extensively studied within the post-secondary context and have been shown to be an effective means of increasing social interactions and reducing stress in a population known to experience elevated stress levels (e.g., Binfet, 2017; Binfet et al., 2017; Binfet & Passmore, 2016; Crossman & Kazdin, 2015; Dell et al., 2015; González-Ramírez et al., 2013; Pendry et al., 2018; Trammell, 2017; Ward Griffin et al., 2018).

Although the research is less prolific, there is evidence to suggest that CAIs are beneficial within other high-stress environments such as waiting rooms in emergency departments (Dell et al., 2019); for young children undergoing physical examinations (Nagengast et al., 1997) or residing in pediatric hospital wards (Braun et al., 2009; Tsai et al., 2010); and in forensic interviews with children (Krause-Parello & Friedmann, 2014).

One such example of this is the use of CAIs within the court system. Spruin et al. (2019) conducted an exploratory qualitative study wherein a therapy dog attended court to interact with individuals waiting in a magistrate's court waiting room. Court users (n =117) were interviewed during the visits and retrospective interviews were conducted with court professionals (n = 8). The thematic analysis from all participants confirmed that the experience of waiting to attend court was considered highly stressful due to the environment, the long waiting times, and the feeling of constant clock-watching (Spruin et al., 2019). Overall the CAI was perceived positively and court users identified the experience as having a positive and beneficial effect on them, including relaxation, reducing stress, eliciting happiness, and providing emotional support. Notably, only 4 participants reported no effect of the CAI and not a single court user felt that it had been a negative experience (Spruin et al., 2019).

Another notable example is that of CAIs for emergency medicine providers during their shifts (Kline et al., 2020). Kline and colleagues conducted a randomized control trial to examine the efficacy of a CAI during shift work. To do so, they compared the CAI versus colouring a mandala and versus a no-intervention control group. Emergency medicine providers' (n = 122) stress was assessed using a stress visual-analogue scale, a perceived stress scale, and salivary cortisol - each taken at the beginning, middle, and end of their shift. The 5-minute intervention (CAI or colouring a mandala) was administered 30-minutes before the second, mid-shift measurement. Results demonstrated that the post-shift self-reported stress levels increased for the control and the colouring conditions yet decreased significantly for the CAI group. In addition, the CAI group was associated with significantly lower salivary cortisol levels at the end of their shift when compared with the control group. This study demonstrates the potential for integrating a brief intervention during a regular shift of emergency medicine providers (Kline et al., 2020).

Despite the efficacy of CAIs to reduce stress in students or in high-stress contexts, there is a paucity of literature that has examined the efficacy of CAIs within a law-enforcement detachment. A careful review of the literature in psychology, sociology and anthrozoology revealed only one study examining the use of a CAI to support the well-being of law-enforcement personnel (Binfet et al., 2020). The aforementioned study, which was a preliminary study that preceded the present study, explored the effect of a CAI integrated within the workplace of law-enforcement personnel (Binfet et al., 2020). Seven therapy dog and handler teams were brought to an urban RCMP detachment, providing opportunities for RCMP members and civic staff to spend time dog-handler teams assessed and credentialed by the B.A.R.K. program. Participants spent, on average, 11 minutes visiting with B.A.R.K. therapy dogs and their handlers. Results demonstrated a significant effect of the intervention ($V = 52$, $p < 0.001$) with mean stress decreasing from 3.33 at T1 to 1.95 at T2. In addition, participants' descriptions of their work environment were significantly more positive after attending the CAI than before ($V = 2784.5$, $p < 0.001$). Notably pre-test self-reports of stress revealed that 47% of participating RCMP members reported feeling *somewhat-* to *very-stressed*, thus illustrating the importance of introducing an effective well-being initiative in this detachment (Binfet et al., 2020). This initial study helped illuminate our team's understanding around the uptake and the effects of a CAI within a busy detachment however we were left with an incomplete picture of how this CAI was experienced from the perspective of the participants who made use of this work-situated well-being initiative.

Further gaps in the literature have guided this study. It has been argued that organizational support for law-enforcement personnel is under-researched and that more research is needed to explore why police choose to, or not to, use stress-reduction services (Tucker, 2015). It has also been argued that qualitative research methods, which the present study utilizes, are considered valuable, yet underutilized within both occupational stress research (Mazzola et al., 2011; Moreto, 2015) and the field of HAIs (Fournier, 2019; Kazdin, 2017). HAI research could "gain tremendously by more qualitative evaluation of the experience of therapy involving an animal, that is, precisely how participants (children, parents, other adults, therapists, and handlers) experience the interaction" (Kazdin, 2017, p. 156). Finally, as there is an absence of knowledge surrounding law-enforcement personnel's experience of CAIs within a detachment setting, this study seeks to add valuable knowledge to the fields concerning HAIs and law-enforcement personnel stress/stress-reduction.

The present study was designed as a follow-up study to explore further the lived experiences of law-enforcement personnel stress and of a CAI within a detachment. The aim of this study was to explore Royal Canadian Mounted Police (RCMP) personnel's experiences of a CAI as an initiative to reduce stress within the detachment. The three research questions guide this study:

1. What are RCMP personnel's perceptions and experiences of stress within the workplace?
2. Do RCMP personnel gain anything from attending the CAI based in their detachment? If so, what are the benefits they experience?
3. What role do therapy dogs play within the context of the CAI based at the detachment?

Both Wilson's hypothesis of Biophilia (1984) and Cobb's social support theory (1976) serve as theoretical frameworks to guide this study and subsequent research questions. The Biophilia hypothesis posits that humans have evolved to pay particular attention to nature, living organisms and life-like processes and is suggested to have enhanced the chance of survival in humans (Wilson, 1984). In the early age of humans paying close attention to animals' behavior would have aided survival as animals would signal a pending threat or, if relaxed, would have implied that the surroundings were safe and secure, and thus, would have been relaxing for our human ancestors (Beetz, 2017). Today, although we no longer live amongst animals in the same way as our early ancestors, humans are still tightly connected to non-human animals. This connection is seen today in our affinity for spending more time at zoological parks than at major sports events (Wilson, 1992; 1993), and the popularity of having animals as companions (Serpell, 1996; 2017; Mornement, 2018). The theory of Biophilia has been supported in more recent research examining the efficacy of animal-assisted interventions (AAIs), in which animals have been found to relieve anxiety, pain, negative affect, and other unpleasant mental states (for a review see Waite et al., 2018).

Cobb's social support theory (1976) provides a second theoretical framework for this study. Social support is the information that "leads the subject to feel loved and cared for, [...] esteemed and valued, [... or] to believe that he belongs to a network of communication and mutual obligation" (Cobb, 1976, p.300). Cobb (1976) asserts that social support throughout one's life is protective against stress-related health concerns or crises. Social support is considered to be beneficial within the context of first responders wherein a relationship has been established between perceived social support and mental health (Prati & Pietrantoni, 2010). In addition, social support or social integration has been shown to mediate the impact and personal appraisal of stressful events (Joseph et al., 1995, Schwarzer et al., 2014). Further, social support theory is relevant to exploring the efficacy of therapy dog programs as research has proposed that canines provide social support equal to, or more beneficial than, humans (Kloep et al., 2017). Both the Biophilia and Social Support theories are relevant to the current study because the existing CAI within the RCMP detachment, which is explored in the present study, is designed to foster close, hands-on contact with therapy canines and to encourage social interactions within the workplace.

Methods

Phase I of this study was a preliminary pilot study that explored the effectiveness of a CAI within an RCMP detachment from a quantitative perspective (Binfet et al., 2020). It strove to answer the question – Do RCMP members and civic staff who attend a CAI hosted at the detachment report significant pre-to-post reductions in self-reports of stress? To do this, seven experienced B.A.R.K. handlers (85% female, *M*age =46.6 years, *SD* =13.3, *range* = 31–65) and their therapy dogs (60% male, *M*age = 4.64 years, *SD* = 1.65, range = 2–6 years) were brought into an urban law-enforcement detachment for 90-minute, weekly visits for 8 weeks. Participants (n = 120), who were RCMP members and civic employees, were able to visit during their working day for as long as they chose. Upon arrival and departure, they completed a visual analogue scale to assess pre- and post-test self-reports of stress. Throughout the session they were able to interact with the handlers, therapy dogs, B.A.R.K. program staff, and other attendees. The quantitative analysis, using a paired Wilcoxon signed-rank test demonstrated the efficacy of the CAI, with stress decreasing significantly from pre-to-post visit (Binfet et al., 2020). It is worth noting that this program was approved by both human and animal research ethics (H17-03306, A14-0134) as well as Divisional Research Project approval from the RCMP head office. In addition, a B.A.R.K. program staff member and RCMP liaison were present at all times to ensure canine, handler, and participant welfare.

The present study, Phase II, seeks to explore members' lived experiences of the CAI from a qualitative perspective and to provide context which was not obtained from Phase I. This phase strives to answer – What are the perceptions of RCMP members around workplace stress and the utility of participating in a within-detachment CAI? That is, we knew the intervention was effective in reducing members' self-reports of stress but we did not know why. In order to explore participants' insights and perspectives, we conducted individual, 60-minute interviews with eight RCMP members who had previously attended the CAI program situated within their detachment. These interviews were conducted and recorded by the first author who had prior experience and education in conducting qualitative research interviews. In addition, the first author had attended every CAI session held at the detachment and thus, had developed rapport with attendees. Interviews were transcribed verbatim by the first author and transcripts were analyzed using qualitative content analysis (Hsieh & Shannon, 2005).

Participants

Participants were recruited using posters placed throughout the detachment, seeking participants who had attended at least one CAI session held within the detachment. Participants were active members (of any rank) currently employed by the RCMP detachment situated in the downtown core of a mid-size Western Canadian city (population 152,000; Statistics Canada, 2017).

Eight participants were recruited for this study based on recommendations in prior interview-based studies (Guest et al., 2006; Morse, 1994, Creswell, 2007). Guest and colleagues (2006) sought to establish the optimal number of participants that should be recruited in interview studies. To do this, they interviewed 60 participants and analyzed the interviews in groups of six in order to determine at what point data saturation occurred – the point at which new information no longer adds value to themes or overall conclusions of the study. Their findings demonstrated that the majority of high-frequency codes (94%) that emerged from the full data set had already emerged from the first six interviews (Guest et al., 2006). As such, Guest and colleagues concluded that for a study seeking to focus on overarching themes emerging from the data, as is the case with the present study, six interviews would be sufficient to enable meaningful theme-development and useful interpretations (Guest et al., 2008, p.78). For the purpose of this study, the proposed sample size was eight to allow for potential participant attrition. The first eight participants to respond to the recruitment call were enrolled in the study.

Procedure

Human research ethics approval (H17-03306) and Divisional Research Project approval from the RCMP National Office in Ottawa and local detachment were obtained prior to the commencement of this study. Data for this study was collected through individual, in-person, semi-structured interviews with each participant. Semi-structured interviews were chosen because they can be utilized effectively when there is 'sufficient objective knowledge about an experience or phenomenon, but the subjective knowledge is lacking" (McIntosh & Morse, 2015, p.1). By interviewing a participant, as opposed to administering a series of surveys or questionnaires, the researchers were able to explore, in-depth, the lived experiences of members who choose to attend a CAI.

All interviews were conducted at the University of British Columbia, Okanagan campus at a time convenient to the participants between December 2018 and March 2019. The location of the university, as opposed to the local detachment, was chosen in order to help ensure confidentiality of the participants. Upon arrival at the interview session, participants read the informed consent form and reviewed the study information provided before providing written consent both to participate in the study and to have their interview audio-recorded. Participants were informed that they could withdraw from the study at any point until the data analysis phase after which time their data would be included in the analysis, although no participants did so. None of the participants declined to participate or refused to be audio-recorded. Next, participants completed a brief demographic questionnaire to collect descriptive information about the sample as a whole including age, gender, ethnicity, part-time/full-time status, and length of service with the RCMP. Once complete, participants had an opportunity to ask questions before the interview commenced. Upon completion of the interview, participants were given their remuneration gift certificate of $50 for a local coffee shop to thank them for their participation.

Measures

Demographic information. Of the eight participants (M_{age} = 49.21, SD = 6.12), 6 self-identified as female and 2 as male, all were full-time employees and active members of the RCMP detachment. Participants' average length of service was 20.25 years (*range*=10–28 years).

Interviews. Data for this study was collected through individual, in-person, semi-structured interviews with each participant. The interviews lasted, on average, 71 minutes (*range* = 63–77 minutes). All interviews were audio-recorded using a secure recording device (SONY voice recorder), were transcribed verbatim by the first author, and were imported into NVivo™. The audio recordings were imported, encrypted, and saved on a password-protected research computer of the first author. The recordings were deleted from the voice recorded immediately after import. A semi-structured interview guide, with 7 overarching themes and 15 open-ended questions, was used (see **Appendix**). Participants were asked to discuss the following themes: 1) levels of stress; 2) effects of stress; 3) coping mechanisms; 4) sources of support; 5) experiences of the B.A.R.K. program; 6) role of the therapy dogs; and 7) the potential of CAIs within law-enforcement detachments. All participants were assigned a pseudonym and the raw data was only accessible to the first author.

Data analysis

The data was analyzed using qualitative content analysis which has become widely used for participant-generated data and interview-based studies (Hsieh & Shannon, 2005; Robinson, 2014). This approach aims to examine the words within responses in depth so as to pay attention to the content and context of the text rather than simply counting words (Hsieh & Shannon, 2005). Conventional content analysis was chosen to interpret the data because it has been identified as an appropriate analysis method when there is limited pre-existing literature on the phenomenon at hand (Hsieh & Shannon, 2005). The conventional analysis approach allows the actual information from the data to inform and to help form categories rather than approaching the data with preconceived categories from prior literature (Hsieh & Shannon, 2005). As there is a paucity of literature examining the implementation of a CAI within a law-enforcement context, this approach is appropriate.

Firstly, the interviews were transcribed verbatim by the first author and transcribed interviews were imported into NVivo™, a computer software program that is designed for qualitative data analysis. NVivo™ was utilized as this software provides a visually-accessible format that indicates where codes are evident, thus aiding the researchers in the analysis. Secondly, the transcripts were read by the first author in a single session and global themes were identified. Upon completion, a more exhaustive analysis was conducted wherein smaller segments of each transcript were descriptively coded. These codes were subsequently reduced to form logical themes that accurately represented the key messaging from the data in a process called winnowing (Wolcott, 1990). The newly developed themes form dynamic coding manuals which are then used to conduct within- and cross-case analyses. Conducting both within-case and cross-case analysis allows researchers to examine each case in-depth but also to identify any shared themes across the participants (Ayres et al., 2003). As Ayres and colleagues argue, "neither across-case nor within-case approaches alone enable the researcher to interpret an experience both through its parts and as a whole, such that readers can recognize individual experience in a generalizable way" (Ayres et al., 2003, p.873). The final step in the data analysis was to establish inter-coder agreement by having a second graduate researcher independently code 20% of the interviews, which is a commonly used standard to ensure reliability in qualitative research (Syed & Nelson, 2015). The percentage agreement rate obtained in the present study was 88%. Any discrepancies in coding were reconciled through discussion. After the interview, member checking was conducted to confirm the researchers' interpretation of participants' responses and to verify understanding as well as reduce researcher bias. Detailed summaries of the interview were provided to the interviewee and they were asked to confirm, negate, or adjust the researcher's understanding. All participants actively engaged in the member checking process.

Results

As the findings from the cross-case analysis represent commonalities across participants and may be considered to carry additional weighting and be of shared importance, only cross-case findings are reported here. The salient themes in responses shared across participants have been organized into four main subject areas: 1) Police stress and coping mechanisms within the workplace; 2) Experiences of the canine-assisted intervention; 3) The role of the therapy dogs; and 4) The potential of CAIs within law- enforcement.

Subject area 1: police stress and coping

Participants' reports of stress were mixed. When asked to spend a few minutes reflecting on their stress level over the past 30 days, four of the participants identified that their stress was *high, or higher than usual*, however, three (37.5%) stated that their stress was *low-moderate*. In addition, three (37.5%) admitted that their stress levels, even over the past 30 days, had been *variable* or erratic, with one describing their stress as a "rollercoaster" (Participant 2).

Despite not being asked directly about stressors during the interview, all participants mentioned at least one source of stress when asked to describe their stress levels over the past 30 days. The most common stressor, and indeed the most common response to the question as a whole, was to identify a source of *organizational stress* (87.5%) including deadlines, heavy workloads and shortage of resources. One participant described organizational stressors as the "biggest source of stress" (Participant 2), another felt "overwhelmed by it all" (Participant 5) and one even described organizational stressors as a "life-sucker" (Participant 4). Across all participants, 39 stressors were identified which were categorized as *organizational* (48.7%), *operational* (e.g., negative interactions with the public, domestic violence cases; 28.2%), and *personal* (e.g., passing of a family member, home renovations; 23.1%).

The most prevalent themes that emerged when participants were asked how stress affects them were *irritability* (75%), reduced quality or quantity of *sleep* (62.5%), and that their mood was *affected* (37.5%). To cope with this stress, participants identified *exercise* such as using the gym or going for a walk (87.5%) and gaining or changing their *perspective* such as focusing on their goals or changing the approach to a task (75%). In addition, more than half of participants (67.5%) also identified having *breaks* as a way to cope including taking some time to be alone, taking time off from work, or getting up and having a break from a specific task.

Participants' views of where the responsibility laid for fostering well-being were variable, with 50% claiming it was *personal*, 50% claiming it was *collective*. In addition, 25% of participants felt that responsibility also fell onto the shoulders of the *RCMP* and that the organization should be putting energy and resources into ensuring that employees have the necessary tools and resources to improve their well-being. Interviewees (37.5%) also explicitly mentioned that their detachment was actively trying to improve wellness within the workplace.

The most prevalent responses for resources that participants utilized were *Psychologists/Medical Professionals* (87.5%), and *Other Resources* including Chaplains, the wellness committee, and online resources (87.5%). *Fitness/Gym, Employee Assistance Program, Peer-to-Peer Support Program, Events* such as detachment-led appreciation events, *and Social/Human contact* were also notable, with 62.5% of participants including each one of those categories when discussing the resources available to them as members. Over half of the participants (62.5%) also mentioned attending the *B.A.R.K. program* as a resource they utilize to relieve their stress.

The most common barriers to seeking well-being programs or initiatives included *other barriers*, such as being too senior, negative self-attitudes, and not recognizing the need (87.5%) and *stigma* either perceived or actual, and either self-imposed or imposed by others (62.5%). Other notable responses included *accessibility* (50%), *trust* (50%), and *lack of time* (37.5%).

Subject area 2: experiences of the CAI program

Participants were motivated to attend the program due to their *love of animals* (75%), *their prior knowledge or experience of CAIs* or canine-induced stress-relief (50%), or *other reasons* (50%) including curiosity and wanting to show support for the management team who brought the initiative into the detachment.

In order to delve deeper into the participants' experiences of the program, they were asked to describe what, if any, impact the program had on them. The most prevalent themes included that the program served as a *break* (87.5%) including that the CAI gave them a break from work or that the program helped them to recharge, refresh, or clear their mind. One participant even described the program as "a welcome relief" (Participant 5). Another common response from participants was that the program was *enjoyable* (75%). All participants stated that they had received *benefits* from attending the program, namely that it was *stress-relieving* (75%), that it helped them to *change perspectives* (75%), and that it *improved their mood* (50%). Specifically, participants stated that the program "lowers any existing stress or pressure you might have" (Participant 3; *stress-relieving*), "provides me with a better sense of reality" (Participant 4; *changed perspectives*), and that "you can feel that it has a positive impact on your mood" (Participant 7; *improved mood*). In addition, 25% of participants also felt that the program had helped to *improve the workplace climate*, citing more positive conversations with colleagues and improved faith in management's desire to improve well-being of colleagues, illustrated by the following participant's insight:

What I also really liked about it, and what I got from it, was that I felt like our senior management was doing something, you know actionable, that was a gesture of caring about their people [...] I believe it just shifts culture a little bit for us and, and I think it restores some people's faith in their management, that they care (Participant 2).

Three of the participants also explicitly drew attention to their view of the CAI being positive in contrast to the negative work environment in which it is situated (subsequently coded as *B.A.R.K. -work contrast*. One participant said "when you're coming from a negative, it's such a big positive to be in the presence of something that seems to want you there, and enjoys you [being] there" (Participant 4). Another added "B.A.R.K. is a positive experience to talk about and to dwell on as opposed to the regular norm of what we deal with on a regular basis which is 99.9% negative" (Participant 6).

Delving deeper into the aspects of the program that foster the beneficial outcomes, participants reported *physically touching the dogs* (75%), *dog characteristics* (such as the dogs being cute, loving or affectionate; 62.5%), or the dogs' ability to be *non-judgmental or unconditionally accepting* (37.5%). To this end, one participant stated that they felt that the therapy dogs had "innate sense of accepting you where you are, and for who you are, [and] you don't have to pretend" (Participant 5). In addition to unpacking the beneficial outcomes, participants were asked to reflect on how long the benefits lasted for them. Responses to this were variable in duration (i.e., *50 % reported less than a day; 37.5 % reported more than a day*) and often depending on what the participants would face in the remainder of their working day. Three participants also noted that thinking or talking about the session later on in the day or week brought some of the feelings back (*relived experiences impactful*). For instance, one participant said "you get another little boost from [thinking about B.A.R.K.] because you're remembering the feelings that it brought, and how you felt, [and] you were able to cope with the stress, just by thinking about it from when it happened before!" (Participant 5).

Subject area 3: the role of therapy dogs in CAIs

Three-quarters of the participants indicated that the therapy dogs' role was to be *social* including seeking attention, coming to greet participants, or "establishing the first contact" (Participant 3). Over half of the participants (67.5%) cited responses that were categorized as *other role* including "to be the centerpiece of the program" (Participant 3) and "to provide support" (Participant 8). The dogs' temperament was also a notable component to their role, with 50% of participants stating that the dogs' role was to be calm including Participant 6 who said that the role of the dog "is to remain nice and calm, and keep it a stress-free environment".

When discussing whether interventions similar to these would be as effective without the dogs, or with a replacement animal, participants overall were undecided. Half of participants felt that other animals would be possible (although often stated stipulations based on behavior or temperament), whereas the other half felt that other animals would not be as effective. When elaborating on their responses, 62.5% explicitly stated that *dogs were effective in the program due to their traits or characteristics* citing their reputation for being unconditionally loving, their disposition, or their unlikeliness to reject attention from a human. Participant 2 stated that "I think dogs have this reputation for being unconditionally loving [...] there's something about the way that they communicate with their eyes, their expressions on their faces and I think they're very affectionate".

Subject area 4: the potential of CAIs within law-enforcement

Participants demonstrated overwhelming support for having a CAI within their detachment. All participants felt that the program had a place within their workplace and stated that they would continue to attend sessions. Participants included a variety of reasons for why the program had a place within the detachment including: "because it's a work environment that can be stressful and I think it's a positive, proactive thing" (Participant 6) and because of the impact on both individual well-being and the detachment climate, as is evidenced in the following quote:

I think it helps to break down some of the stigma around mental health, it gives people an opportunity to do something themselves that assists their mental health, and it also generates conversation too amongst employees that, just due to geography of the building, they may not normally connect with (Participant 4).

The majority of participants (75%) explicitly endorsed the program and included testimonies such as "It's a positive part of a work day that not everybody gets to have" (Participant 2) and "I love them [B.A.R.K. sessions]. It's just a nice time away from my work and it's just a good-feeling time" (Participant 6). All but one of the participants (87.5%) stated that they intended to continue attending the program because they had gained a benefit, such as: "I can't change that I'm on a ten-hour shift, but I can at least make it as enjoyable as I can and taking 10 minutes to take a break and rub a dog's belly helps me" (Participant 1) and "I will continue to attend due to the fact of what they've given me back, they bring a calmness and just a different way of being" (Participant 8).

Discussion

The present study was a follow-up exploratory study to an initial investigation that examined the effects of a CAI on law-enforcement personnel's self-reports of stress. The aim of this study was to explore, in-depth, the perceptions and experiences of law-enforcement personnel who participated in a stress-reduction initiative that saw therapy dogs and their handlers visit an urban RCMP detachment as part of a well-being program. Our findings serve to elucidate the experiences and insights of eight participants as they shared their thoughts on stress and the role of therapy dogs in supporting well-being.

Situating our findings within the broader context of law-enforcement stress reduction, we see the insights of our participants corroborate previous descriptions of law-enforcement as a profession in which organizational stress arising from problematic scheduling (i.e., night shifts), variable shift schedules, burdensome workloads, and discrimination within the workplace, serve to collectively compromise employee well-being (Gershon et al., 2009; Terpstra & Schaap, 2013; White & Robinson, 2014). When asked to describe the toll of this stress, consistent with prior research, participants described heightened irritability, disrupted sleep, and diminished mood. As such, compromised well-being positions employees poorly to perform their work responsibilities, certainly with regard to serving the public and interacting with members of the public who, are themselves, often stressed.

We also see that exercise is a commonly reported coping mechanism and that members often report psychologists, medical doctors, and extended medical care as resources provided to them by the RCMP. These findings further corroborate existing literature (Cairney et al., 2014; Deb et al., 2008; Naz et al., 2014) and emphasize the importance of detachments providing opportunities for members to improve their well-being and cope with stress through exercise, medical coverage, and psychological services. It should be noted that these findings must be interpreted with caution, however, as although members are aware of many resources available to them, it remains unclear if they make use of these resources. There is a stark difference between being able to identify an available resource and utilizing these resources and finding them beneficial to their well-being.

The present study found that stigma and trust were the most notable barriers to making use of well-being resources. Stigma surrounding mental health is a well-documented barrier for seeking help, both within the general population and within law-enforcement (Lauber & Rossler, 2007; Lucia & Halloran, 2019) and this study further emphasizes the need for initiatives to reduce help-seeking stigma within a law-enforcement context. In addition, trust, specifically the fear of broken confidentiality, emerged as another notable barrier for seeking resources. This is in alignment with other studies within law-enforcement which have found that distrust for mental health professionals who do not work within law-enforcement and distrust in the confidentiality of the available resources are significant barriers to seeking help (Bryan & Morrow, 2011; Fox et al., 2012; Lucia & Halloran, 2019). The findings of the present study further strengthen the notion that law-enforcement personnel face trust concerns in their ability to seek well-being resources. The conclusions of the present study, and previous literature, should be taken into consideration by management personnel within law-enforcement settings. Building trust and reducing concerns over confidentiality should be a priority for law-enforcement agencies as this may help to improve the use of well-being resources and reduce the impact occupational stress has on the individual members and their ability to serve the public.

Accessibility concerns were also a notable barrier, as identified by half of the participants. There is a paucity of literature that addresses the issue of accessibility which, in the present study, encompassed a multitude of concerns working unusual hours outside of typical office hours, resources having a lack of capacity, being out on the road and away from resources, needing a referral from a medical professional, and not having rank-appropriate resources for more senior personnel. Future studies should explore further the accessibility barriers to ascertain resources that would address these concerns.

Examination of the salient themes that emerged when participants were asked for their views on the CAI introduced within their detachment, participants shared that the CAI program was stress relieving or had a calming effect. This is in alignment with prior research examining the impact of CAIs both within a detachment setting and in other contexts (Binfet & Passmore, 2016; Binfet et al., 2020; Barker et al., 2016; Crossman & Kazdin, 2015; Pendry & Vandagriff, 2019). Specifically, the findings from this study further corroborate the findings from emerging research on CAIs in law-enforcement conducted by Binfet and colleagues (2020). The aforementioned study found a significant reduction in pre-to-post-test self-reports of stress of members attending a within-detachment CAI. It follows that participants interviewed in this follow-up study would identify a stress-relieving benefit from attending the program having reported lower levels of stress upon leaving the session.

Three-quarters of the participants reported that the CAI has helped them to change their perspective, including feeling more positive, resilient, or having a different motivation having attended a session. McCullough and colleagues (2016) postulate that "because pets, including dogs generally give individuals feelings of positivity, it can help to improve individuals' moods and reduce stress" (p.4), however, to date, research has yet to examine participants' self-perceived positivity in terms of their outlook. Further, more research is warranted to examine the potential for CAIs to boost positivity as an outcome in visitors. In addition, there is a dearth of literature examining the effect of CAIs and therapy dogs on self-perceived resiliency. CAIs have been combined with resilience training workshops (Kjellstrand Hartwig, 2017), although the effect of the therapy dog alone on resilience has not been examined specifically. Finally, the notion that participants identified the CAI as helping them to change perspective is a notable finding as it links into participants' coping mechanisms. Three quarters of participants identified gaining perspective as one of the ways they cope with stress. It is possible that one of the reasons that participants viewed the program as beneficial and successful was because the program assisted them with one of their pre-existing coping mechanisms.

Participants also identified that the program was enjoyable to attend. One possible explanation is that attending a CAI provides a novel way to improve their well-being and have a break from work and work-related stressors. The concept of a CAI being enjoyable has been found in other studies with different clientele including children (Harris & Binfet, 2020) and in patients with aphasia (Macauley, 2006). CAIs provide a novel and enjoyable modality through which participants' well-being may be enhanced. This is noteworthy within the context of law-enforcement where members are known to report a number of barriers for seeking help. A well-being resource that is deemed to be enjoyable is likely to be utilized more than other, more formalized opportunities.

Further, participants shared that a CAI is a nonthreatening and accessible program that serves to reduce the stigma around help-seeking. This is especially important as law-enforcement personnel report numerous barriers to seeking well-being resources and tend to under-utilize available resources (Blum, 2000; Bryan & Morrow, 2011; Downs & Eisenberg, 2012; Tanielian & Jaycox, 2008; White et al., 2016). Relatedly, at the core, participants revealed that the therapy dogs played a key role within the CAI and their view was that dogs needed to be concomitantly social (i.e., outgoing) yet calm. This informs our understanding of temperament testing of therapy dogs and their training. It further informs the nature of interactions between visitors to sessions and handlers and suggests that at the outset of a session, the handler can encourage the dog to enthusiastically greet new visitors after which the handler would cue the dog to assume a more placid (i.e., calm) position for the remainder of the interaction.

The temperament and behavior of therapy dogs within individual sessions likely fosters or hinders the extent to which visitors to sessions perceive a connection between themselves and the therapy dog or a human–animal bond. As argued by Hill and colleagues (2020, p. 729), "The human-animal bond (HAB) has been found to contribute to positive characteristics offered in social support relationships, such as unconditional acceptance, love, stability, and a non-judgmental allegiance (Cobb, 1976; Collis & McNicholas, 1988; Hirschman, 1994; Levinson, 1969)." With regards to the findings of our study, the bond established between visitors to sessions and individual therapy dogs, especially for visitors who made frequent use of the within-detachment CAI, the human–animal bond can "provide a buffering effect to adversity" (Hill et al., 2020, p. 729). Repositioning our findings within the framework of the human–animal bond informs how programs and individual sessions ought to be structured – there must be a sufficiently low ratio of dog-to-visitors to allow interactions to cultivate such a bond. The strength of this bond, in turn, may facilitate well-being benefits for visitors such as the reduction of stress.

Finally, the present study sought to establish whether members perceived the CAI to have a place within the unique environment of a police detachment. Participants were overwhelmingly positive in their responses, both endorsing the program in general and stating that they would continue to attend in the future. Participants reported finding the program beneficial for stress reduction and improving their mood, amongst others. This aligns with the wealth of literature in the field that has established that CAIs can elicit well-being outcomes in visitors. In addition, the participants' testimonies demonstrate that there is an appetite for innovative, accessible, and enjoyable CAIs within the unique, high-stress context of a detachment. It is hoped that this will help to inspire other detachments to seek out CAIs to introduce as a well-being initiative within their workplace.

Limitations

Despite best intentions, this study is not without limitations. In this study, we captured the experiences of eight participants who participated in a CAI integrated into their workplace. It should also be noted that participants in this study were all obtained from a single, urban detachment in western Canada and self-selected for participation. The lived experiences of these RCMP members may not reflect the lived experiences of members from other detachments, such as those in rural areas or in other locations.

Data was also collected through interviews alone. It would have been beneficial to have used triangulation to gather more information. Triangulation can be achieved in a number of ways (Denzin, 2017). It may have been beneficial to have collected other information, such as feedback in individual sessions over time; measures of sleep quality, irritability, and other reported effects of stress; or reports from colleagues and/or family members.

Implications

There are several notable implications arising from the findings of this study. First, through this research we were able to gain insights into the views and experiences of female law-enforcement personnel. The literature in law enforcement is saturated with studies wherein participants were predominantly male, including many of the studies discussed in the literature review of this paper. Gershon et al. (2002) for example conducted a study wherein 98% of the participants were male and the findings incorporated the views of only two female participants. These studies, although informative, are dominated by the experiences of the male member. The sample from the current study was 75% female and 25% male. This allowed for an exploration into the experiences of female RCMP members. In addition, this study sample was largely representative of the population who make use of the B.A.R.K. program. The present study aimed to build upon the knowledge obtained in an earlier, quantitative study wherein a CAI was introduced within an urban RCMP detachment (Binfet et al., 2020).

This study also has high ecological validity, defined as "the extent to which the environment experienced by the subject in a scientific investigation has the properties it is supposed or assumed to have by the investigator" (Bronfenbrenner, 1977, p.516). The study sought to explore participants' experiences of an existing CAI within their detachment, a real-world, applied setting. The findings reflect strong ecological validity because the interviews were based on an existing CAI that occurs throughout the year and not artificially created for the purpose of the study. This program is also held within the RCMP detachment during a normal working day – it is integrated into the ebb and flow of this complex work environment.

The purpose of this study was to explore the lived experiences of a CAI within the context of law-enforcement which, despite the increasing popularity of CAIs, remains an under-utilized well-being resource. This, combined with the established need of law-enforcement personnel to reduce stress and the current concern over police stress and mental health demonstrates that this research is both worthy of exploration and timely. Furthermore, the researcher embedded quotations from the transcripts throughout the results section to allow for the participants' voice to be reflected and to substantiate findings. The present study also represents an important contribution to the literature as this study seeks to explore, for the first time, the lived experiences of law-enforcement personnel who participated in a CAI.

As the field of HAI advances, that task of researchers is not to simply find out if an intervention worked but to also uncover the circumstances within which interventions are situated and to explore the views of the participants asked to engage in interventions. As Fournier (2019, p. vii) posits, "There is very little study of just how humans and animals interact and which interactions with or features of the animal are therapeutic." As evidenced through the responses of participants in this study, therapy dogs played a key role in reducing barriers to accessing a well-being initiative introduced within the workplace and informed the broader research community's understanding of the role therapy dogs play in eliciting well-being outcomes in visitors to sessions. The responses of participants 4 and 6 summarize these sentiments in their descriptions:

> We've seen more people doing it and I've been surprised by some of the people who have attended the program – I think in some ways that's helped to draw others in as well, those that wouldn't normally [seek resources]. I think the ability to open people's minds to a new idea is a positive thing, and the program helps to do that (Participant 4).

> [The dogs] are a huge component to the program. It's their calm presence and that relaxed attitude that draws you in and it's a comforting thing. Just scratching a dog's ear or petting a dog's head gives them so much enjoyment that it comes right back to you (Participant 6).

Conclusion

The findings of the present study corroborate previous descriptions of law-enforcement as a profession in which organizational stress is a significant source of stress for members and serves to compromise employee well-being (Gershon et al., 2009; Terpstra & Schaap, 2013; White &

Robinson, 2014). When asked to describe the toll of this stress, consistent with prior research, participants described heightened irritability, disrupted sleep, and diminished mood. As such, compromised well-being positions employees poorly to perform their work responsibilities, certainly with regard to serving the public and interacting with members of the public who, are themselves, often stressed. Participants provided an insight into how they cope with workplace stress, including getting exercise or perspective, and taking breaks from work. Further, participants identified a variety of resources made available to them (including Psychologists and Medical services, exercise rooms, and peer-support programs) but also noted numerous barriers to making use of these (including stigma, trust, and accessibility) which are consistent with prior literature (Bryan & Morrow, 2011; Fox et al., 2012; Lauber & Rössler, 2007; Lucia and Halloran, 2019).

The present study demonstrated that RCMP members' perceptions of a CAI integrated within their workplace was an appealing and nonthreatening way to reduce their stress and enhance their well-being. In addition, members demonstrated overwhelming support for the program in general, appreciated management's efforts to integrate well-being within their routine workday experience, and felt strongly that CAIs have a place within the detachment setting. Participants also revealed that therapy dogs require nuanced skills to facilitate interactions and that the dogs played a key role within the CAI. It is hoped that the findings from the present study will encourage first-responder agencies and research organizations to explore the integration of CAIs more widely to foster well-being and reduce workplace stress.

References

Anshel, M. H. (2000). A conceptual model and implications for coping with stressful events in police work. *Criminal Justice and Behavior, 27*, 375-400. https:/doi.org//10.1177/0093854800027003006

Ayres, L., Kavanaugh, K., & Knafl, K. A. (2003). Within-case and across-case approaches to qualitative data analysis. *Qualitative Health Research, 13* (6), 871-883. https:/doi.org//10.1177/1049732303255359

Bano, B., & Talib, P. (2017). Understanding police stress towards a secure and sustainable society. *International Journal of Police Science & Management, 19*(3), 159-170. https:/doi.org//10.1177/1461355717713999

Beetz, A. M. (2017). Theories and possible processes of action in animal assisted interventions. *Applied Developmental Science, 21*(2), 139-149. https:/doi.org//10.1080/10888691.2016.1262263

Binfet, J. T. (2017). The effects of group-administered canine therapy on first-year university students' well-being: A randomized controlled trial. *Anthrozoös*, *30*, 397-414. https://doi.org/10.1080/08927936.2017.1335097

Binfet, J. T., Draper, Z. A., & Green, F. L. L. (2020). Stress reduction in law enforcement officers and staff through a canine-assisted intervention. *Human Animal Interaction Bulletin, 8*(2), 34-52.

Binfet, J. T., & Hartwig, E. K. (2019). *Canine-assisted Interventions: A Comprehensive Guide to Credentialing Therapy Dog Teams*. New York, NY: Routledge.

Binfet, J. T. & Passmore, H. A. (2016). Hounds and homesickness: The effects of an animal-assisted therapeutic intervention for first-year university students. *Anthrozoös*, *29*, 441-454. https://doi.org/10.1080/08927936.2016.1181364

Binfet, J. T., Passmore, H. A., Cebry, A., Struik, K., & McKay, C. (2018). Reducing university students' stress through a drop-in canine-therapy program. *Journal of Mental Health, 27*(3), 197-204. https://doi.org/10.1080/09638237.2017.1417551

Blum, L. N. (2000). *Force Under Pressure: How Cops Live and Why They Die*. New York, NY: Lantern Books.

Bronfenbrenner, U. (1977). Toward an experimental ecology of human development. *American Psychologist, 32*(7), 513. Retrieved from https://s3.amazonaws.com/

Braun, C., Stangler, T., Narveson, J., & Pettingell, S. (2009). Animal-assisted therapy as a pain relief intervention for children. *Complementary Therapies in Clinical Practice*, *15*(2), 105-109. https:/doi.org//10.1016/j.ctcp.2009.02.008

Bryan, C. J., & Morrow, C. E. (2011). Circumventing mental health stigma by embracing the warrior culture: Lessons learned from the defender's edge program. *Professional Psychology: Research and Practice, 42*, 16-23. https:/doi.org//10.1037/a0022290

Cairney, J., Kwan, M. Y., Veldhuizen, S., & Faulkner, G. E. (2014). Who uses exercise as a coping strategy for stress? Results from a national survey of Canadians. *Journal of Physical Activity and Health, 11*(5), 908-916. https://doi.org/10.1123/jpah.2012-0107

Carleton, N. R., Afifi, T. O., Turner, S., Taillieu, T., Duranceau, S., LeBouthillier, D.M, Sareen, J., Ricciardelli, R., MacPhee, R. S., Groll, D., Hozempa, K., Brunet, A., Weekes, J. R., Griffiths, C. T., Abrams, K. J., Jones, N. A., Beshai, S., Cramm, H. A., Dobson, K., Asmundson, G. J. G. (2018). Mental disorder symptoms among public safety personnel in Canada. *The Canadian Journal of Psychiatry, 63*, 54-64. https:/doi.org//10.1177/0706743717723825

Cobb, S. (1976). Social support as a moderator of life stress. *Psychomatic Medicine, 38*(5), 300-314. https:/doi.org//10.2307/2136404

Cohen, S., Kamarck, T., & Mermelstein, R. (1983). A global measure of perceived stress. *Journal of Health and Social Behaviour, 24*(4), 385-396. https:/doi.org//10.2307/2136404

Collis, G. M., & McNicholas, J. (1998). *A theoretical basis for health benefits of pet ownership: Attachment versus psychological support.* In C. C. Wilson & D. C. Turner (Eds.), *Companion Animals in Human Health* (p. 105–122). Sage Publications, Inc. https://doi.org/10.4135/9781452232959.n6

Creswell, J.W. (2007). *Qualitative Inquiry and Research Design: Choosing Among Five Approaches.* Thousand Oaks, CA; London: SAGE Publications, Inc.

Crossman, M. K., & Kazdin, A. E. (2015). Animal visitation programs in colleges and universities: An efficient model for reducing student stress. In A. Fine (Ed.), *Handbook on Animal-Assisted Therapy: Theoretical Foundations and Guidelines for Practice* (4th ed., pp. 333–337). Burlington, MA: Academic.

Crouch, R. S. (2014). Wellness and fitness in law-enforcement: We need to do better. *Available from ProQuest Dissertations & Theses Global.* Retrieved from http://ezproxy.library.ubc.ca/login?url=https://search-proquest- com.ezproxy.library.ubc.ca/docview/1651234266?accountid=14656

Deb, S., Chakraborty, T., Chatterjee, P., & Srivastava, N. (2008). Job-related stress, causal factors and coping strategies of traffic constables. *Journal of the Indian Academy of Applied Psychology, 34*(1), 19-28.

Dell, C. A., Chalmers, D., Gillett, J., Rohr, B., Nickel, C., Campbell, L., Hanoski, R., Haugerud, J., Husband, A., Stephenson, C., & Brydges, M. (2015). PAWSing Student Stress: A pilot evaluation study of the St. John ambulance therapy dog program on three university campuses in Canada. *Canadian Journal of Counselling and Psychology, 49*(4), 332-359. Retrieved from https://dev.journalhosting.ucalgary.ca/index.php/rcc/article/download/61079/2821

Dell, C. A., Stempien, J., Broberg, L., Husband, A., Jurke, L., Rohr, B.,; Smith, J., Rubin, J., Tupper, S., Goodridge, D., Fornssler, C., & Fele-Slaferek, L. (2019). A case study of the patient wait experience in an emergency department with therapy dogs. *Patient Experience Journal, 6*(1). https:/doi.org//10.35680/2372-0247.1306

Denzin, N. K. (2017). *The Research Act: A Theoretical Introduction to Sociological Methods*. New Brunswick, US; London, UK: Transaction Publishers

Downs, M., & Eisenberg, D. (2012). Help seeking and treatment use among suicidal college students. *Journal of American College Health, 60*, 104-114. https:/doi.org//10.1080/07448481.2011.619611.

Fournier, A. K. (2019). *Animal-Assisted Intervention: Thinking Empirically*. Cham, Switzerland: Palgrave MacMillan.

Fox, J., Desai, M. M., Britten, K., Lucas, G., Luneau, R., & Rosenthal, M. S. (2012). Mental health conditions, barriers to care, and productivity loss among officers an in urban police department. *Connecticut Medicine, 76*(9), 525-531. Retrieved from https://www.ncbi.nlm.nih.gov/

Gershon, R. R. M., Barocas, B., Canton, A. N., Li, X., & Vlahov, D. (2009). Mental, physical and behavioural outcomes associated with perceived work stress in police officers. *International Association for Correctional and Forensic Psychology, 36*(3). https:/doi.org//10.1177/0093854808330015

Gershon, R. R. M., Lin, S., & Li, X. (2002). Work stress in aging police officers. *Journal of Occupational and Environmental Medicine, 44*(2), 160-167. Retrieved from https://journals.lww.com/joem/

González-Ramírez, M. T., Ortiz-Jiménez, X. A., & Landero-Hernández, R. (2013). Cognitive-behavioral therapy and animal-assisted therapy: Stress management for adults. *Alternative & Complementary Therapies, 19*(5), 270-275. https:/doi.org//10.1089/act.2013.19505

Guest, G., Bunce, A., & Johnson, L. (2006). How many interviews are enough? An experiment with data saturation and variability. *Field Methods, 18*(1), 59-82. https:/doi.org//10.1177/1525822X05279903.

Hamilton, L., & Corbett-Whittier, C. (2013). *Using Case Study in Education Research.* Retrieved from http://methods.sagepub.com.ezproxy.library.ubc.ca/book/using-case-study-in-education-research

Hill, L., Winefield, H., & Bennett, P. (2020). Are stronger bonds better? Examining the relationship between the human–animal bond and human social support, and its impact on resilience. *Australian Psychologist, 55*, 729-738. https:/doi.org//10.1111/ap.12466

Hirschman, E. C. (1994). Consumers and their animal companions. *Journal of Consumer Research, 20*(4), 616-632. https://www.jstor.org/stable/2489763

Hoffmann, A. O. M., Lee, A. H., Wertenauer, F., Ricken, R., Jansen, J. J., Gallinat, J., & Lang, U. E. (2009). Dog-assisted intervention significantly reduces anxiety in hospitalized patients with major depression. *European Journal of Integrative Medicine*, *1*, 145–148. https:/doi.org//10.1016/j.eujim.2009.08.002

Hsieh, H.G., & Shannon, S.E. (2005). Three approaches to qualitative content analysis. *Qualitative Health Research, 15*(9), 1277-1288. https:/doi.org//10.1177/1049732305276687

Joseph, S., Williams, R., & Yule, W. (1995). Psychosocial perspectives on post-traumatic stress. *Clinical Psychology Review, 15*(6), 515-544. https:/doi.org//10.1016/0272-7358(95)00029-O

Karaffa, K. M., & Koch, J. M. (2016). Stigma, pluralistic ignorance, and attitudes toward seeking mental health services among police officers. *Criminal Justice and Behavior*, *43*(6), 759-777. https:/doi.org//10.1177/0093854815613103

Kazdin, A. E. (2017). Strategies to improve the evidence base of animal-assisted interventions. *Applied Developmental Science, 21*(2), 150-164. https:/doi.org//10.1080/10888691.2016.1191952

Kjellstrand Hartwig, E. (2017) Building solutions in youth: evaluation of the human–animal resilience therapy intervention. *Journal of Creativity in Mental Health, 12*(4), 468-481, https://doi.org/10.1080/15401383.2017.1283281

Kline, J. A., VanRyzin, K., Davis, J. C., Parra, J. A., Todd, M. L., Shaw, L. L., Haggard, B. R., Fisher, M. A., Pettit, K. L., & Beck, A. M. (2020). Randomized trial of therapy dogs versus deliberative coloring (art therapy) to reduce stress in emergency medicine providers. *Academic Emergency Medicine*, *27*(4), 266-275. https:/doi.org//10.1111/acem.13939

Kloep, M. L., Hunter, R. H., & Kertz, S. J. (2017). Examining the effects of a novel training program and use of psychiatric service dogs for military-related PTSD and associated symptoms. *American Journal of Orthopsychiatry*, *87*(4), 425-433. https:/doi.org//10.1037/ort0000254

Krause-Parello, C. A., & Friedmann, E. (2014). The effects of an animal-assisted intervention on salivary alpha-amylase, salivary immunoglobulin a, and heart rate during forensic interviews in child sexual abuse cases. *Anthrozoös*, *27*(4), 581-590. https:/doi.org// 10.2752/089279314X14072268688005

Kuehl, K. S., Elliot, D. L., Goldberg, L., MacKinnon, D. P., Vila, B. J., Smith, J., … McGinnis, W. (2014). The safety and health improvement: Enhancing law- enforcement departments study: Feasibility and findings. *Frontiers in Public Health*, *2*(38), 1-7. https:/doi.org//10.3389/fpubh.2014.00038

Kuehl, K. S., Elliot, D. L., MacKinnon, D. P., O'Rourke, H. P., DeFrancesco, C., Miočević, M., Valente, M., Sleigh, A., Garg, B., McGinnis, W., & Kuehl, H. (2016). The SHIELD (safety & health improvement: Enhancing law-enforcement departments) study: Mixed methods longitudinal findings. *Journal of Occupational and Environmental Medicine, 58*(5), 492-498. https:/doi.org//10.1097/JOM.0000000000000716

Liakopoulou, D., Tigani, X., Varvogli, L., Chrousos, G. P., & Darviri, C. (2020). Stress management and health promotion intervention program for police forces. *International Journal of Police Science & Management*, *22*(2), 148-158. https:/doi.org//10.1177/1461355719898202

Lang, U. E., Jansen, J. B., Wertenauer, F., Gallinat, J., & Rapp, M. A. (2010). Reduced anxiety during dog assisted interviews in acute schizophrenic patients. *European Journal of Integrative Medicine*, *2*, 123–127. https:/doi.org//10.1016/j.eujim.2010.07.002

Lauber, C., & Rössler, W. (2007). Stigma towards people with mental illness in developing countries in Asia. *International Review of Psychiatry*, *19*(2), 157-178. https:/doi.org//10.1080/09540260701278903

Levinson, B. (1969). *Pet-oriented Child Psychotherapy*. Springfield, Illinois: Charles C Thomas, Bannerstone House.

Lucia, D. G., & Halloran, M. J. (2019). An investigation of the efficacy of programs to prevent stress in law-enforcement officers: a program manager's perspective. *Journal of Police and Criminal Psychology*, 1-13. https:/doi.org//10.1007/s11896-019-09341-6

Macauley, B. L. (2006). Animal-assisted therapy for persons with aphasia: A pilot study. *Journal of Rehabilitation Research & Development, 43*(3), 357-366. https://doi.org/10.1682/JRRD.2005.01.0027

Marmar, C. R., McCaslin, S. E., Metzler, T. J., Best, S., Weiss, D. S., Fagan, J., Liberman, A., Pole, N., Otte, C., Yehuda, R., Mohr, D., & Neylan, T. (2006). Predictors of posttraumatic stress in police and other first responders. *Annals New York Academy of Sciences, 1071*, 1-18. https:/doi.org//10.1196/annals.1364.001

Mazzola, J. J., Schonfeld, I. S., & Spector, P. E. (2011). What qualitative research has taught us about occupational stress. *Stress and Health, 27*, 93-110. https:/doi.org//10.1002/smi.1386.

McCraty, R., & Atkinson, M. (2012). Resilience training program reduces physiological and psychological stress in police officers. *Global Advances in Health and Medicine, 1*(5), 42-64. https:/doi.org//10.7453/gahmj.2012.1.5.013

McCullough, A., Ruehrdanz, A., & Jenkins, M. (2016). The use of dogs in hospital settings. *HABRI Central Briefs*, 1-9. www.habricentral.org

McIntosh, M. J., & Morse, J. M. (2015). Situating and constructing diversity in semi- structured interviews. *Global Qualitative Nursing Research*, 1-12. https:/doi.org//10.1177/2333393615597674

Menard, K. S., & Arter, M. L. (2013). Police officer alcohol use and trauma symptoms: Associations with critical incidents, coping, and social stressors. *International Journal of Stress Management, 20*, 37-56. https:/doi.org//10.1037/a0031434

Moreto, W. D. (2015). Introducing intelligence-led conservation: Bridging crime and conservation science. *Crime Science, 4*(15), 1-11. https:/doi.org//10.1186/s40163-015-0030-9

Mornement, K. (2018). Animals as companions. In: *Animals and Human Society* (pp. 281-304). Academic Press.

Morse, J. M. (1994). *Designing qualitative research.* In Y. Lincoln & N. Denzin (Eds.), *Handbook of Qualitative Inquiry* (pp. 220-235). Menlo Park, CA: SAGE publications, inc.

Mumford, E. A., Taylor, B. G., & Kubu, B. (2015). Law-enforcement officer safety and wellness. *Police Quarterly, 18*(2), 111-133. https:/doi.org//10.1177/1098611114559037

Nagengast, S. L., Baun, M. M., Megel, M., & Leibowitz, J. M. (1997). The effects of the presence of a companion animal on physiological arousal and behavioral distress in children during a physical examination. *Journal of Pediatric Nursing*, *12*(6), 323-330. https:/doi.org//10.1016/S0882-5963(97)80058-9

Naz, S., Gavin, H., Khan, B., & Raza, M. S. (2014). Cross cultural variations in attitude towards use of psychological support among police officers. *Pakistan Journal of Criminology, 6*(1), 31. https://s3.amazonaws.com/

Patterson, G. T., Chung, I. W., & Swan, P. W. (2014). Stress management interventions for police officers and recruits: a meta-analysis. *Journal of Experimental Criminology, 10*(4), 487-513. https:/doi.org//10.1007/s11292-014-9214-7

Pendry, P., Carr, A. M., Roeter, S. M., & Vandagriff, J. L. (2018). Experimental trial demonstrates effects of animal-assisted stress prevention program on college students' positive and negative emotion. *Human-Animal Interaction Bulletin, 6*(1), 81-97. Retrieved from https://www.apa-hai.org/human-animal-interaction/haib

Prati, G., & Pietrantoni, L. (2010). The relation of perceived and received social support to mental health among first responders: A meta-analytic review. *Journal of Community Psychology, 38*(3), 403-417. https:/doi.org//10.1002/jcop.20371

Queirós, C., Passos, F., Bártolo, A., Marques, A. J., da Silva, C. F., & Pereira, A. (2020). Burnout and stress measurement in police officers: Literature review and a study with the operational police stress questionnaire. *Frontiers in Psychology, 11.* https:/doi.org//10.3389/fpsyg.2020.00587

Ranta, R. S., & Sud, A. (2008). Management of stress and burnout of police personnel. *Journal of the Indian Academy of Applied Psychology, 34*(1), 29-39. Retrieved from http://medind.nic.in/jak/t08/i1/jakt08i1p29.pdf.

Robinson, O. C. (2014). Sampling in interview-based qualitative research: A theoretical and practical guide. *Qualitative Research in Psychology, 11*(1), 25-41. https:/doi.org// 10.1080/14780887.2013.801543

Serpell, J. (1996). *In the Company of Animals: a Study of Human-Animal Relationships* (2nd ed.). Cambridge; New York, NY: Cambridge University Press.

Serpell, J., McCune, S., Gee, N. & Griffin, J. A. (2017). Current challenges to research on animal-assisted interventions. *Applied Developmental Science, 21*(3), 223-233. https://doi.org/10.1080/10888691.2016.1262775

Spruin, E., Mozova, K., Franz. A., Mitchell, S., Fernandez, A., Dempster, T., & Holt, N. (2019). The use of therapy dogs to support court users in the waiting room. *International Criminal Justice Review*, *29*(3), 284-303. https:/doi.org//10.1177/1057567719827063.

Statistics Canada (2017) *Kelowna [Population centre], British Columbia and Alberta [Province]* (table). *Census Profile*. 2016 Census. Statistics Canada Catalogue no. 98-316-X2016001. Ottawa. Retrieved from https://www12.statcan.gc.ca/census-recensement/2016/dp- pd/prof/index.cfm?Lang=E (accessed April 30, 2021).

Stevens, P., Kepros, J. P., & Mosher, B. D. (2017). Use of a dog visitation program to improve patient satisfaction in trauma patients. *Journal of Trauma Nursing, 24*(2), 97-101. https:/doi.org//10.1097/JTN.0000000000000272

Schwarzer, R., Bowler, R. M., & Cone, J. E. (2014). Social integration buffers stress in New York police after the 9/11 terrorist attack. *Anxiety, Stress & Coping, 27*(1), 18-26, https:/doi.org//10.1080/10615806.2013.806652

Syed, M., & Nelson, S.C. (2015). Guidelines for establishing reliability when coding narrative data. *Emerging Adulthood*, *3*(6), 375–387. https:/doi.org//10.1177/2167696815587648

Tanielian, T., & Jaycox, L. H. (2008). *Invisible Wounds of War: Psychological and Cognitive Injuries, Their Consequences, and Services to Assist Recovery*. Santa Monica, CA: RAND.

Tellis, W. M. (1997). Application of a case study methodology. *The Qualitative Report, 3*(3), 1-19. Retrieved from https://nsuworks.nova.edu/tqr/vol3/iss3/1

Terpstra, J., & Schaap, D. (2013). Police culture, stress conditions and working styles. *European Journal of Criminology, 10*(1), 59-73. https:/doi.org//10.1177/1477370812456343

Tracy, S. J. (2010). Qualitative quality: Eight "big-tent" criteria for excellent qualitative research. *Qualitative Inquiry, 16*, 837–851. https:/doi.org//10.1177/1077800410383121

Tracy, S. J., & Hinrichs, M. M. (2017). Big tent criteria for qualitative quality. *The International Encyclopedia of Communication Research Methods,* 1-10. https:/doi.org//10.1002/9781118901731.iecrm0016

Trammell, J. P. (2017). The effect of therapy dogs on exam stress and memory. *Anthrozoös, 30*(4), 607-621. https:/doi.org//10.1080/08927936.2017.1370244

Tsai, C. C., Friedmann, E., & Thomas, S. A. (2010). The effect of animal-assisted therapy on stress responses in hospitalized children. *Anthrozoös*, *23*(3), 245-258. https:/doi.org//10.2752/175303710X12750451258977

Tucker, J. M. (2015). Police officer willingness to use stress intervention services: The role of perceived organizational support (POS), confidentiality and stigma. *International Journal of Emergency Mental Health and Human Resilience, 17*(1), 304-314. http://digitalcommons.wcupa.edu/crimjust_facpub/4.

Waite, T. C., Hamilton, L., & O'Brien, W. (2018). A meta-analysis of animal assisted interventions targeting pain, anxiety, and distress in medical settings. *Complementary Therapies in Clinical Practice, 33*, 49-55. https:/doi.org//10.1016/j.ctcp.2018.07.006

Ward-Griffin, E., Klaiber, P., Collins, H. K., Owens, R. L., Coren, S., & Chen, F. S. (2018). Petting away pre-exam stress: The effect of therapy dog sessions on student well-being. *Stress and Health*, *34*(3), 468-473. https:/doi.org//10.1002/smi.2804

Westmarland, L. (2017). Putting their bodies on the line: police culture and gendered physicality. *Policing: A Journal of Policy and Practice*, *11*(3), 301–317. Retrieved from https://doi-org.ezproxy.library.ubc.ca/10.1093/police/pax019

White, V., & Robinson, S. (2014). Leading change in policing: Police culture and the psychological contract. *Police Journal: Theory, Practice and Principle, 87*, 258–269. https:/doi.org//10.1350/pojo.2014.87.4.675

White, A. K., Shrader, G., & Chamberlain, J. (2016). Perceptions of law enforcement officers in seeking mental health treatment in a right-to-work state. *Journal of Police and Criminal Psychology, 31,* 141-154. https:/doi.org//10.1007/s11896-015-9175-4.

Wilson, E. O. (1984) *Biophilia*. Cambridge, MA: Harvard University Press.

Wilson, E.O. (1992). *The Diversity of Life.* Massachusetts: Harvard University Press.

Wilson, E.O. (1993). Biophilia and the conservation ethic. In: S.R. Kellert & E.O. Wilson (Eds.), The *Biophilia Hypothesis* (pp. 31–41). Washington, DC: Island Press.

Wolcott, H.F. (2009). *Writing up Qualitative Research* (3rd ed.). Los Angeles, CA: SAGE publications.

Zimmerman, F. H. (2012). Cardiovascular disease and risk factors in law-enforcement personnel: A comprehensive review. *Cardiology Review, 20*, 159-166. https:/doi.org//10.1097/CRD.0b013e318248d631

Zimmerman, F. H. (2014). Cardiovascular risk in law-enforcement. In J. Violanti (Ed.), *Dying for the Job Police Exposure and Health* (pp. 41–56). Springfield: Charles C. Thomas Publisher.

Appendix

Semi-structured Interview Guide

The primary purpose of the individual interviews is to explore RCMP constables' perceptions of stress within the workplace. The interviews will be semi-structured. That is, the specific questions asked will depend upon the responses of each participant.
**Probes generated during the interview may be used to delve more deeply into the topic shared by participants.*

Category	Guiding Questions	Probes*	Justification
Levels of stress	As you are aware, this is a study about stress in RCMP members. Let me first begin by asking you to reflect over the past 30 days, and describe your stress level?	To clarify what you've said to me, could I describe you as low/ medium/ high stress?	• Evidence has suggested that police officers experience high-medium levels of stress (Bano & Talib, 2017). This question will seek to explore this from a qualitative perspective. • A 30-day period is used for the reflection on stress because this is deemed a sufficient length of time to take into account any events that are still influencing current stress (Cohen et al., 1983).
Perceptions of the effects of stress	Thank you for describing to me your stress level, I'm curious now to hear how you think stress affects you?	What else can you say about that? Tell me more.	• This question seeks to gather details as to the physiological and psychological effects of stress on RCMP. • This is asked because researchers have suggested that there are physiological and psychological effects to officers' well-being when they are stressed (Bano & Talib, 2017; Gershon et al., 2009; Terpstra & Schaap, 2013).
Coping mechanisms	In general, when you experience stress, do you do anything about it? When we're talking about workplace stress, whose responsibility is it to reduce stress? The precinct/organization, or the individual?	If so: Tell me about that? What makes you say that? Can you tell me more?	• These questions aim to establish what RCMP members are/are not doing to reduce their stress. • They also aim to explore whether officers take it upon themselves to reduce their stress, or if they are relying on organizational support.

Continued

Continued.

Category	Guiding Questions	Probes*	Justification
Sources of support	Many are concerned about member stress, describe for me what well-being resources are available to you? You have just described these opportunities; would you describe yourself as a low/med/high user of these opportunities? We've established that there are stress-reduction opportunities available to employees. What would you say are barriers that prevent you from making use of these?	If so: can you tell me about these? If they are using them: what is it about B.A.R.K. program that you find particularly valuable? Tell me more about your frequency of use?	• These questions aim to establish the barriers to seeking stress-reduction support. • This is asked because research has suggested that there are reasons why officers do not seek programs to reduce their stress (e.g. Karaffa & Koch, 2016).
Impact of the sessions	Participation in this study required you to have made use of a B.A.R.K. session here at the detachment. Would you describe yourself as a low/med/high user of the program? Why did you make use of the B.A.R.K. program? Did the B.A.R.K. sessions have any impact on you? You have described an impact of the B.A.R.K. session, how do you think this works? If you had to describe how this program works to someone else outside of the precinct, how would you describe the session?	Tell me more. What was it about this that made you feel that way? Why do you think the program impacted you in that way?	• These questions aim to explore the motivations for attending and what, if any, impact the CAI program had on members. • This is asked because research has established that this program was successful in reducing pre-to-post self-reports of stress (Binfet et al., 2020). Research has not explored whether there were any other perceived benefits to having attended.
Role of the dogs	How would you describe the role of the dogs in this program? What do they do exactly?	Tell me more. If so... How?	• Research has established the efficacy of CAIs within a variety of contexts (Binfet et al., 2018; Binfet & Passmore, 2016; Hoffman et al., 2009; Lang et al., 2010), however little is known about what aspect of the program fosters the beneficial effects.

Continued

Continued.

Category	Guiding Questions	Probes*	Justification
The potential of CAIs within law-enforcement	Do you think you will continue to attend B.A.R.K. sessions in the future? Do you think that canine-based interventions have a place in the detachment setting?	Why/Why not?	• This is asked because research has established that this program was successful in reducing pre-to-post self-reports of stress (Binfet et al., 2020). • As there is still very little research in this field, this question sought to establish whether participants would endorse the use of CAIs within their detachment.
Do you have any comments or anything else you would like to tell me?			

14 Therapeutic Horseback Riding as a Complementary Intervention for Military Service Members with PTSD

Beth A. Lanning[1]*, Amelia L. Wilson[2], Robert Woelk[3], and A. Alexander Beaujean[1]
[1]*Baylor University;* [2]*William Beaumont Army Medical Center;* [3]*Hope for Heroes Equine Therapy Consulting*

Abstract

The aim of this study was to examine the efficacy and potential effectiveness of an 8-week therapeutic horseback riding [THR] program for veterans with combat-related posttraumatic stress disorder [PTSD]. Eighty-nine military service members diagnosed with PTSD participated in either the THR group (n = 51) or the comparison group (n = 38). Group mean score differences in PTSD and depression symptoms, quality of life, functioning and disability scores were compared at baseline, 4 weeks, and post intervention. THR participants reported clinically meaningful improvement in PTSD (−13.02 points) and depression (−7.65 points) symptoms and mental health scores (+ 9.61 points) overtime. In comparison, change in comparison group mean scores indicated less improvement in the same variables. Group differences in PTSD and depression symptom scores and mental health scores increased pre to post intervention, resulting in a moderate to large effect size (g = −0.43 to 0.62). Two-month follow-up reflected sustained improvement in key variables. Outcomes of the study support the potential effectiveness of THR as complementary intervention for military service members with combat-related PTSD.

Keywords: combat, therapeutic horseback riding, depression, PTSD, quality of life

Author note

This project was made possible by funding from the Horses and Humans Research Foundation and from Baylor University. Additional in-kind support was provided by Ride On Center for Kids, Georgetown, Texas; Riding Equines to Achieve Confidence and Health, McGregor, Texas; Rainer Therapeutic Riding, Yelm, Washington; Triple H Equitherapy Center, Pipe Creek, Texas; and Texas A&M Systems Courtney Grimshaw Fowler Equine Therapeutic Riding Center (Courtney Cares), College Station, Texas. We especially want to thank all the staff and instructors at these facilities for their help and dedication to the project.

A very special thank you is extended to all the veterans who participated in the project for their service to our country and contributions to this project.

Nearly 17 years post 9/11 combat-related posttraumatic stress disorder (PTSD) and depression in our military service personnel remain a national concern. The exact point prevalence of combat-related PTSD is difficult to determine, but a recent review of PTSD studies reveals estimates of 2-17% in US military veterans (Richardson, Frueh, & Acierno, 2010). Further,

Corresponding author email: Beth_Lanning@baylor.edu.

mental health diagnoses among active duty military service personnel have increased by 65% during the past ten years with common diagnoses including adjustment disorders (26%), depression (17%), substance abuse/dependency (17%), anxiety (10%) and PTSD (6%) (Armed Forces Health Surveillance Center, 2012). These conditions often worsen in the months following deployment (Thomas et al., 2010) and diagnoses may actually increase during this time.

PTSD is classified as a trauma and stress-or-related disorder that occurs when one is exposed to a traumatic or stressful event. Individuals suffering from PTSD tend to avoid places and people that remind them of the traumatic experience, are overly sensitive to normal life experience (hyperarousal), relive the experience, and have feelings of self-blame and estrangement (American Psychiatric Association, 2013). To be diagnosed with PTSD, a person must have been exposed to a traumatic or stress event and have one the following for at least one month: 1) one re-experiencing symptom (flashbacks, bad dreams, frightening thoughts) 2) one avoidance symptom (staying away from people and places, avoiding feelings), 3) two arousal and reactivity symptoms (on edge, difficulty sleeping, angry outbursts), and 4) two cognitive and mood symptoms (negative thoughts, loss of interest in life activities, blame, guilt) (American Psychiatric Association, 2013).

While intervention and treatment options for PTSD, both within and outside of the Veterans Affairs (VA) healthcare system exist, many veterans do not access help or do not complete the course of treatment for a variety of reasons (Elbogen et al., 2013). Cornish, Thys, Vogel, and Wade (2014) conducted focus groups to determine help seeking barriers among military veterans. Emerging themes were difficulty relating to others, anxiety, depression, irritation and anger. Anxiety was most often cited and may be attributed to the fear of talking about traumatizing events and/or opening up to unfamiliar people. Many soldiers find themselves accustomed to non-stop, high-stress operational tempos and living in daily danger while deployed. This often leaves them feeling wired and at a loss for purpose once they return to a non-combat environment. They are concerned that they will not fit in with civilians and others whose lives continued as usual while they were deployed. These findings were similar to those reported by Kessler (2000) in an earlier study. Kessler (2000) reported that veterans expressed internal and external stigmatization related to mental health treatment, a concern that therapy would not be helpful, not being ready to engage in therapy when it is offered, and concern that therapists will not understand their emotions and experiences. Kessler (2000) suggested including more information about available treatment options and normalizing the process of seeking help as possible methods to reduce barriers to access. Additionally, having a wide variety of services available was perceived as helpful.

Although several therapies appear to be efficacious, PTSD remains a difficult mental health issue to treat (Cukor, Spitalnick, Difede, Rizzo, & Rothbaum, 2009). Bradely, Greene, Russ, Dutra, and Western (2005) conducted a meta-analysis of 26 PTSD studies including 44 treatment conditions. The researchers reported that overall 56% of individuals enrolled in treatment no longer met the criteria of PTSD after treatment. They noted that while this rate was encouraging, the failure rate of PTSD treatment programs is still high and encouraged inclusion of alternative and complementary treatment options.

Complementary and alternative medicine (CAM) or treatments are interventions that either augment tradition therapies or replace some or all parts of traditional therapies. CAMs span a variety of methodologies and can include virtual reality to yoga to acupuncture to animal assisted activities and therapies. The majority of CAMs have been used clinically to treat various forms of mental health disorders, including PTSD (Wynn, 2015). While these treatments provide additional options for clinicians, many lack research as to their efficacy and effectiveness.

Animal assisted activities and therapies, specifically equine assisted activities and therapies (EAAT) are emerging as efficacious interventions for mental and physical health issues in various populations (Griffin, McCune, Maholmes, & Hurley, 2011; McCune, Kruger, Esposito, Freund, Hurley & Bures, 2014). EAAT is an umbrella term that includes both equine assisted activities (EAA) (e.g., therapeutic riding) and equine assisted therapies (EAT) (e.g., hippotherapy, equine facilitated psychotherapy) (Professional Association of Therapeutic Horsemanship,

International (PATH Intl.)). The two differ by intent. EATs require the presence of a licensed therapist and includes specific therapy goals, whereas EAAs, such as therapeutic horseback riding, are therapeutic but not classified as therapy and therefore, do not require the presence of licensed therapist. Riding goals replace specific therapy goals. Robust research on EAAT and veterans is sparse, but preliminary findings from several pilot studies point to possible therapeutic benefits of this type of intervention for veterans with physical and mental health issues (Ferruolo, 2016; Lanning & Krenek, 2013; Mattson, 2015; Monroe, Meyers & Sanchez, 2014).

In a recent systematic review of EAAT, Selby and Smith-Osborne (2013) acknowledged the existence of strong evidence for the use of hippotherapy to improve mobility in individuals with motor and neuromotor dysfunction, but noted a lack of methodologically sound EAAT studies examining the biopsychosocial effects of equine-centered interventions for individuals with mental health disorders. The researchers found only 14 out of 103 research articles that met their inclusion criteria of quantifying biopsychosocial benefits not related to hippotherapy. Further, most of the studies were designed to examine the intervention effects on adolescents and none included military service members.

Likewise, Anestis, Anestis, Zawilinski, Hopkins, and Lilienfeld (2014) conducted a systematic review of equine-related treatments for mental disorders. The researchers reported 14 studies meeting the inclusion criteria of equine-centered, treatment for mental illness, peer-reviewed, and including an experimental protocol (randomized control trial, quasi-experimental, single-case design). Only four studies included adults and none was specific for military service members.

While some equine-centered intervention studies were published in peer-reviewed journals and met inclusion criteria of the reviews, the authors of both reviews point to the need for more rigorous and methodologically sound studies. The authors suggest that future research include randomized control trials or the use of comparison groups receiving established interventions, independent objective measures, follow-up data, adequate sample size, and structured or standardized protocol (Anestis et al., 2014; Selby & Smith-Osborne, 2013). In addition, data from both reviews reveal the absence of peer-reviewed published EAAT studies that specifically examine the psychosocial effects of equine-related interventions for combat veterans and military service members; however, some studies can be found published outside of peer-review (e.g., Mattson, 2015; Krob, 2015: Gomez, 2016).

In this study, we aimed to assess the changes in PTSD and depression symptoms, quality of life, and function of combat veterans and service members who participate in therapeutic horseback riding. Further, we designed the study to address the following methodological concerns noted in previous reviews of EAAT studies: adequate sample size, comparison group receiving treatment as usual (TAU), structured protocol, follow-up data, and standardized self-assessments and proxy assessments. The following research questions were used to guide the study: 1) How does engaging in therapeutic horseback riding affect functional impairment, quality of life, depression and PTS symptoms in military service members with combat related PTSD? 2) Is there a difference in outcome variables among military service members diagnosed with PTSD who participate in therapeutic horseback riding and those who do not participate?

Method

Participants

The study was approved by the university Institutional Review Board and the Institutional Animal Care and Use Committee. One arm of the study was also approved by Brook Army Medical Center Institutional Review Board. Participants were recruited using flyers placed at therapeutic riding facilities, veteran centers, and veteran organizations. In addition, the study was advertised in local newspapers and during information sessions at veteran group meetings.

Participants were included if they met the following criteria: participated in any of three Iraq and Afghanistan war missions, had not participated in equine assisted activities or therapies in the past 6 months, and were diagnosed with PTSD. PTSD diagnosis was confirmed using the Posttraumatic Stress Disorder Checklist Military (PCL-M) or Diagnostic and Statistical Manual of

Mental Disorders, Fifth Edition (DSM-5) Posttraumatic Stress Disorder Checklist (PCL-5). Exclusion criteria included diagnosis of a bipolar disorder or schizophrenia, or having significant cognitive impairment to the extent they could not follow instructions. See Fig. 14.1 for the participant flowchart.

Study Design

We used a quasi-experimental design trial with repeated measures. Two groups formed for this study were a treatment group and a comparison group. The comparison group received or had received treatment-as-usual (TAU), which was defined as established therapy for PTSD (i.e., cognitive behavioral therapy, exposure therapy).

Originally, we planned to complete a randomized experimental design, but many participants indicated that they did not want to be part of a randomization process whereby they or their military comrades could potentially not receive the treatment. Researchers have found that veterans, in particular, are more likely to participate in clinical trials where everyone is able to receive the treatment (Campbell, Raisch, Sather, Warren & Segal, 2007). Consequently, there was some self-section involved in creating the groups, which can limit a study's internal validity (Shadish, Cook, & Campbell, 2002). We attempted to minimize internal validity threat by using the same inclusion criteria for both groups, recruiting from the same geographical locations, and preventing cross-contamination by minimizing opportunities for members in one group to interact with members or treatment protocol of the other group. We also examined the possible effects of self-selection bias in the data analysis by examining baseline group differences of key variables.

Sample Size. Sample size was determined using a Monte Carlo study (Beaujean, 2014; Muthen & Muthen, 2002). We used a model with four time points and 10% attrition (see Imel, Laska, Jakupcak & Simpson, 2013) by wave three (i.e., week 8), because that is when

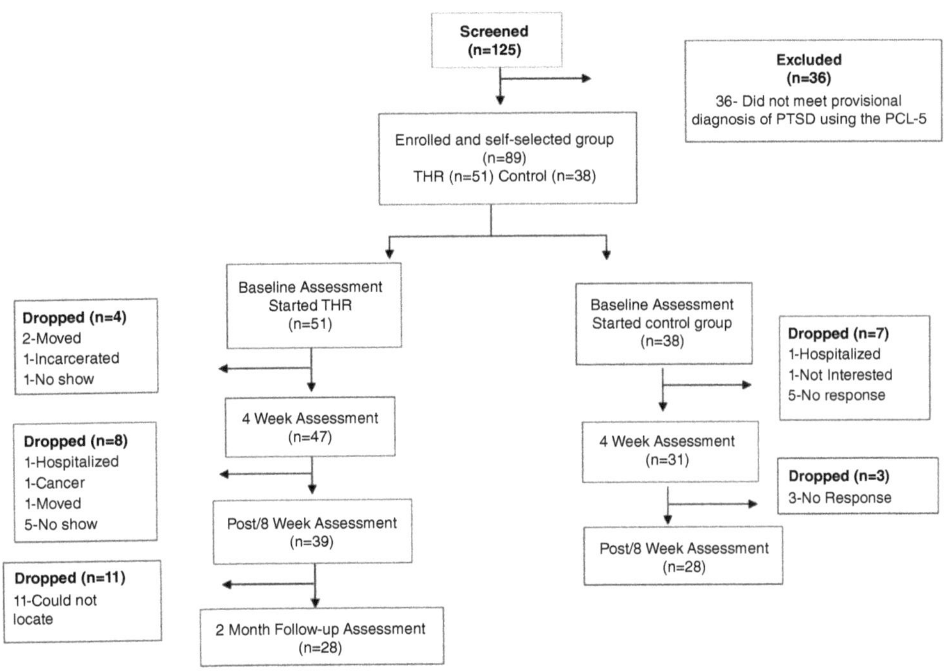

Fig. 14.1. Therapeutic horseback riding (THR) and veterans with combat PTSD: participant flowchart. Notes: PCL-5= Posttraumatic stress disorder checklist-5

the treatment ended. The main focus of this study was the difference in means between the first and third time point (i.e., week 8), which we specified to have an effect size (*d*) of 0.60 reflecting the effect size found in a recent study examining the effects of EAA with an at-risk population (Pendry & Roeter, 2013). Based on the results, we determined 75 participants was an adequate sample size for the study.

Group Assignment. Interested military service members meeting eligibility criteria were asked to sign an informed consent and self-selected either the treatment-as-usual (TAU) condition or therapeutic horseback riding (THR) treatment. The participants in the comparison group did not participate in any equine activities during the trial, but were given the opportunity to participate when the study was complete. All participants were asked to report if they were currently receiving or had received established treatment for PTSD (e.g., cognitive behavioral therapy, exposure therapy), but they were not asked to stop their current programs.

Fidelity. We used several procedures to ensure program fidelity across intervention sites. The same curriculum was used at all intervention sites, all instructors were PATH certified and were trained on how to implement the curriculum, and research team members completed field notes during site visits to monitor implementation.

Procedure and materials

Treatment was provided in one of five Professional Association Therapeutic Horsemanship (PATH) Premier Accredited therapeutic sites. Five sites were used in the study to ensure recruitment and treatment of an adequate number of participants. The comparison group continued treatment-as-usual outside of the therapeutic riding facilities. The participants were not asked to disclose the location of the treatment (e.g., private therapist, outpatient, Veterans Health Administration medical clinics).

Each participant completed a battery of self-assessments prior to the start of the study (baseline), after 4 weeks (mid-point), 8 weeks (end of the treatment). The participants in the treatment group also completed the assessments 2 months after the treatment ended. All participants were asked to identify a person who knew them well (e.g., significant other, close family member) and would be willing to complete an assessment of the participants' functioning and disability at the beginning and end of the treatment period.

The relationships between quality of life components, PTSD symptom clusters and functioning is complex and not clearly understood (Schnurr, Lunney, Bovin, & Marx, 2009); therefore, multiple assessments from various perspectives were used to understand the shared and unique features of each variable of interest. We chose the assessment instruments based on validity and reliability scores for measuring the behaviors outlined in this study, the linkage of constructs across instruments, and the ease of completing them by the participant, family member, or data collector.

Posttraumatic stress disorder symptoms. Posttraumatic Stress Disorder (PTSD) and PTS symptoms were assessed using the *PTSD Checklist Military* (PCL-Military) and *PTSD Checklist-5* (PCL-5) (Weathers et al., 2013). The PCL-Military assessment tool, reflecting DSM-IV symptoms of PTSD was used during the initial stage of the project because the PCL-5 was not available at the time. Provisional diagnosis of PTSD using the PCL-M and the PCL-5 served to confirm PTSD diagnosis for inclusion. A presumptive PTSD diagnosis can be made by treating each item rated as 2 = "Moderately" or higher as a symptom endorsed, then following the DSM-V diagnostic rule which requires at least: 1B item (question 1-5), 1 C item (question 6-7), 2 D items (question 8-14), 2 E items (questions 15-20). Total symptom severity scores range from 0-80. A 5-10 point change represents reliable change and a 10-20 point change represents clinically meaningful change (Monson et al., 2008).

Quality of life. Health related quality of life variables were assessed using the *Short Form-36 question version 2 Quality of Life Assessment* [SF36v2] (Ware, Kosinski, & Keller, 1994). This instrument provides an 8-scale profile of functional health and well-being. Raw scores are converted to norm-based scores, and a score of 50, with a standard deviation of 10 points is considered average for the U.S. population. At the group level, scores within 0.3 standard deviation, or 3 norm-based points, of the mean are considered within the normal range. Scores falling below 47 norm-based points indicate impaired functioning.

Functioning and disability. The *World Health Organization Disability Assessment Schedule 2.0* [WHODAS-2.0] was used to measure changes in functioning and disability (Ustun et al., 2010). Both the self-reported version and the proxy version were used in the study. The WHODAS-2.0 is a 36-item questionnaire that measures function and disability according to the International Classification of Functioning, Disability and Health [ICF]. Complex scoring (Item Response Theory –IRT) can be used for more in depth analysis. The summary score is converted into a metric ranging from 0 to 100, where 0 = no disability: and 100 = full disability. The WHODAS 2.0-Proxy 12-item form was used to measure change in functioning of the participant as observed by a person who knows the participant well. Each item was assessed using a 5-point Likert scale from 1 (none) to 5 (extreme or cannot do). Level of functioning summary scores, using simple scoring, range from 12-60.

Depression Symptoms. Depression symptoms were measured using the *Major Depression Inventory* [MDI] (Bech et al., 1997). The MDI includes 10 items with each item answered using a 6-point Likert scale. The scale range is 0 (the symptom has not been present) to 5 (the symptom has been present all the time). Total symptom severity scores range from 0-50. Compared to the Beck Depression Inventory, the MDI is unidimensional and can be used to distinguish changes in both typical and atypical depression (Bech, Christensen, Vinberg, Ostergaard, Martiny, & Kessing, 2013; Konstantinidis, Martiny, Bech & Kasper, 2011).

Therapeutic horseback riding intervention

The treatment condition consisted of an eight-week structured therapeutic riding curriculum, *Rainier Therapeutic Riding's Riding Through Recovery* (Rainier Therapeutic Riding, 2017). The curriculum consisted of eight 90-minute sessions that occurred once a week. Before the treatment, participants shared a meal together. The first four weeks included non-riding exercises (e.g., grooming, leading, working with the horse in a round pen, developing a relationship with the horse) and the last four weeks included riding and horsemanship exercises. Participants selected their own horse to work with throughout the program. The curriculum is based on a natural horsemanship philosophy of working with a horse's natural instincts and methods of communication. Emphasis is placed on developing a mutually respectful relationship with the horse both on the ground and while riding. The participants learned basic horse care and riding skills along with verbal and non-verbal communication skills needed to work with the horses.

To ensure safety, PATH International standards and guidelines (PATH Intl, 2017) were followed and each session was taught by PATH-certified riding instructors. Additionally, each horse–rider pair was accompanied by a trained volunteer who was a military service member not participating in the study.

Data analysis

For data analyses, we relied on effect sizes (ESs), their confidence intervals (CIs), and graphical displays of the variables of interest. This approach is consistent with modern data-analytic approaches (Cumming & Calin-Jageman, 2017) and preferred because there are many problems associated with the more traditional approach that relies solely on null hypotheses significant testing to determine if an effect exists or is meaningful (Wasserstein & Lazar, 2016).

To compare groups, we calculated the difference in means on the variables of interest. For all comparisons, we subtracted the comparison group mean from the treatment group mean; thus, positive values indicate the treatment group had higher scores, on average. We converted the raw mean differences into the g effect sizes (Borenstein, Hedges, Higgins, & Rothstein, 2009) and calculated its 95% confidence interval. g is a corrected version of the d effect size, so values are interpreted the same: mean differences in standard deviation units.

There was some attrition in both the treatment and comparison groups. Instead of removing observations with missing data, we used the total number of individuals available at a given time point for our comparisons. Because this might bias the results, we also conducted a sensitivity analysis to see if differences for the wave-complete data were similar to the differences for those who had completed information across all the waves.

Results

Sample

One hundred twenty-five veterans were recruited as possible participants. Of those, 89 met inclusion criteria and consented to participate. Fifty-one (57%) participated in the treatment and 38 (43%) were in the comparison group. Thirty-nine (77%) of the treatment group members completed all 8 weeks of the program and 28 (55%) also provided information two months post intervention. Twenty-nine (76%) of the comparison group members completed all 8-weeks.

Most of the participants had completed at least 2 tours of duty in at least one of the Operations Iraqi and Enduring Freedom (OIF/OEF) or Operation New Dawn (OND) conflicts. Seventy percent (n = 62) of the participants were male and 30% (n = 27) were female and ranged in age from 22 to 57 years (mean = 38.8 years; SD = 11.08). Overall, 69% (n = 61) of the participants indicated they completed and/or were currently in treatment for PTSD, and 17% (n = 15) did not answer questions related to therapy status. Seventy-five percent of the participants in the treatment group indicated that had completed and/or were currently receiving treatment, while 61% of the comparison group reported completing and/or currently receiving some type of established treatment for PTSD. See Table 14.1 for all descriptive data.

The number of participants at each of the five facilities was: Site A, 51; Site B, 13; Site C, 13; Site D, 11; and Site E, 1. There were minimal differences in outcome variables at baseline, so we do not consider facility further in our analyses.

Table 14.1. Descriptive data.

Variable	Number (Percentage)
Gender	
Male	62 (70%)
Female	27 (30%)
Age (years)	
Mean	38.8
Range	22-57
Rank	
Enlisted	46 (90%)
Officer	2 (4%)
Not stated	6 (6%)
Marital Status	
Married	47 (53%)
Divorced	21 (24%)
Not stated	5 (6%)
Treatment Status*	
Currently in therapy	50 (56%)
Completed therapy	29 (33%)
Both	17 (19%)
No therapy	8 (9%)
Did not answer	15 (17%)
Branch of Service	
Army	37 (73%)
Air Force	4 (8%)
Army National Guard	1 (2%)
Marine Corps	4 (8%)
Navy	1 (2%)
Not stated	4 (8%)
Current Status	
Active duty	21 (24%)
Retired or separated (veteran)	60 (67%)
Not stated	8 (9%)
Military Conflicts Served	
Operation Iraqi Freedom	46 (52%)
Operation Enduring Freedom	65 (73%)
Both	32 (36%)

*The percentages do not add to 100% because some participants did not answer all questions regarding current or past treatment.

Comparison of the Therapeutic Horseback Riding (THR) group and the comparison group data.

Baseline. Baseline results are displayed in Table 14.2. The ES CIs for all scores except SF36v2 Role-Emotion encompass zero, so it is likely that whatever differences that exist are due to error in sampling, measurement, or a combination of the two.

Between-group differences on the WHODAS 2.0 was minimal (ES between 0.02–0.04), likewise, for the MDI and PCl-5 (MDI ES = 0.04; PCL-5 ES: −0.04). Between-group difference on the WHODAS 2.0 proxy was greater than other measures (ES= 0.57), indicating family members perceived participants in the treatment group to have higher functional disability than participants in the comparison group. This difference should be interpreted with much caution, however, because not all participants had a family member who completed the forms.

Table 14.2. Baseline Results Mean, SD, effect size, and 95% confidence interval.

	Treatment			Control			Effect		
Variable	Mean	SD	n	Mean	SD	n	Raw dif	g	95% CI
WHODAS 2.0 Sum (32 items)*	50.28	17.69	50	49.50	17.70	38	0.78	0.04	[–0.37, 0.46]
WHODAS 2.0 Weighted (32 items)*	54.65	19.23	50	53.80	19.24	38	0.85	0.04	[–0.37, 0.46]
WHODAS 2.0 Sum (36 items)†	55.78	18.99	50	55.32	20.71	38	0.46	0.02	[–0.39, 0.44]
WHODAS 2.0 Weighted (36 items)†	52.62	17.92	50	52.18	19.53	38	0.44	0.02	[–0.39, 0.44]
WHODAS 2.0 (Proxy)	32.63	9.93	35	26.62	11.20	26	6.01	0.57	[0.06, 1.08]
SF36v2 (summary)	35.76	7.47	50	37.87	7.48	38	–2.11	–0.28	[–0.70, 0.14]
SF36v2.PF	43.58	10.36	51	43.17	10.29	38	0.42	0.04	[–0.38, 0.46]
SF36v2.RP	36.15	10.22	51	40.20	9.68	38	–4.04	–0.40	[–0.82, 0.02]
SF36v2.BP	39.62	10.30	50	37.85	7.90	38	1.77	0.19	[–0.23, 0.61]
SF36v2.GH	41.73	9.92	51	43.70	9.66	38	–1.97	–0.20	[–0.62, 0.22]
SF36v2.VT	35.94	8.82	51	36.73	9.12	38	–0.79	–0.09	[–0.50, 0.33]
SF36v2.SF	31.78	9.47	51	32.67	8.44	38	–0.89	–0.10	[–0.51, 0.32]
SF36v2.RE	28.79	11.38	51	34.54	11.54	38	–5.75	–0.50	[–0.92, –0.08]
SF36v2.MH	31.07	10.20	51	31.87	11.23	38	–0.80	–0.07	[–0.49, 0.34]
SF36v2.PCS	44.99	9.87	51	44.95	8.87	38	0.04	0.00	[–0.41, 0.42]
SF36v2.MCS	27.74	10.95	51	30.76	10.62	38	–3.02	–0.28	[–0.70. 0.14]
PCL-5	56.07	14.09	43	56.62	12.28	37	–0.55	–0.04	[–0.48, 0.39]
MDI	36.02	12.02	51	35.55	12.57	38	0.47	0.04	[–0.38, 0.45]

Note. Effects are calculated as Treatment group – Control group.
*Indicates scores from individuals not in school or working.
†Indicates scores from individuals attending school or working.
SF36v2.PF= Physical Functioning; SF36v2.RP= Role-Physical; SF36v2.BP= Bodily Pain; SF36v2.GH= General Health; SF36v2.VT= Vitality; SF36v2.SF= Social Functioning; SF36v2.RE= Role-Emotion; SF36v2.MH= Mental Health; SF36v2.PCS= Physical Component Summary; SF36v2.MCS= Mental Component Summary.

The group differences in SF36v2 composite scores varied. Between-group differences for the physical and mental health composite scores (SF36v2 PCS, SFv236 MCS) were relatively small (ESs of 0.04 and –0.28, respectively). ESs for group difference on the subscales ranged in size from –0.50 to 0.19.

Midpoint. Midpoint results are displayed in Table 14.3. While the between-group differences increased for many of the measures, the ES CIs all contain 0 so the differences are likely due, at least in part, to error. Nonetheless, the patterns in the ESs are generally consistent with the treatment working. The between-group differences on the WHODAS 2.0, MDI, and PCL-5 were larger than at baseline, with the comparison group having higher means (i.e., reporting more impairment). Group differences on the SF36v2 composite and subscales scores changed relative to baseline as well, with the treatment group showing higher means (i.e., reporting better quality of life).

End of intervention. Results from the end of intervention period are displayed in Table 14.4. As with the mid-point results, the ES CIs contain 0 for many between-group comparisons, but the magnitude of the ES tended to increase and the patterns in the ESs are generally consistent with the treatment working. See Figs. 14.2 and 14.3 for a graphic display of between-group changes in scores and ES over time.

For the WHODAS, PCL-5, and MDI, group differences were negative and larger than at baseline and midpoint, indicating that the treatment group participants reported less functional disability, fewer PTSD symptoms, and fewer depression symptoms than the comparison group. The ES for the WHODAS 2.0 proxy was positive, indicating family members still perceived participants in the treatment group to have higher functional disability than participants in the comparison group. Nonetheless, the magnitude of the group difference was smaller than at baseline. Again, these differences should be interpreted with much caution because not all family members completed this form.

On the SF36v2, treatment group participants' summary scores continued to be higher

Table 14.3. Midpoint Results Mean, SD, effect size, and 95% confidence interval.

	Treatment			Control			Effect		
Variable	Mean	SD	n	Mean	SD	n	Raw dif	g	95% CI
WHODAS 2.0 Sum (32 items)*	49.00	17.90	45	52.63	16.82	30	−3.63	−0.21	[−0.66, 0.25]
WHODAS 2.0 Weighted (32 items)*	53.26	19.46	45	57.21	18.29	30	−3.95	−0.21	[−0.66, 0.25]
WHODAS 2.0 Sum (36 items)†	54.71	20.47	45	58.40	19.05	30	−3.69	−0.18	[−0.64, 0.27]
WHODAS 2.0 Weighted (36 items)†	51.61	19.31	45	55.09	17.98	30	−3.48	−0.18	[−0.64, 0.27]
WHODAS 2.0 (Proxy)	—	—	—	—	—	—	—	—	—
SF36v2 Summary	38.89	8.05	46	36.82	7.23	31	2.07	0.27	[−0.19, 0.72]
SF36v2.PF	45.00	8.80	47	41.86	9.05	30	3.14	0.35	[−0.11, 0.81]
SF36v2.RP	41.01	10.65	47	36.27	9.62	30	4.73	0.46	[0.00, 0.92]
SF36v2.BP	40.17	10.15	45	37.10	8.39	30	3.08	0.32	[−0.14, 0.78]
SF36v2.GH	43.29	9.55	47	41.38	10.51	30	1.91	0.19	[−0.26, 0.65]
SF36v2.VT	38.78	9.61	46	37.25	8.37	30	1.53	0.17	[−0.29, 0.62]
SF36v2.SF	34.78	10.77	46	32.27	9.22	30	2.51	0.24	[−0.21, 0.70]
SF36v2.RE	33.35	11.61	47	32.84	10.55	30	0.51	0.05	[−0.41, 0.50]
SF36v2.MH	36.08	11.27	46	32.30	10.10	30	3.79	0.35	[−0.11, 0.80]
SF36v2.PCS	46.06	9.44	46	42.45	8.88	30	3.61	0.39	[−0.07, 0.85]
SF36v2.MCS	32.68	12.12	46	31.14	9.86	30	3.14	0.35	[−0.11, 0.81]
PCL-5	48.72	17.89	39	50.27	14.08	30	−1.55	−0.09	[−0.56, 0.38]
MDI	29.91	13.12	45	34.35	11.08	31	−4.44	−0.36	[−0.81, 0.10]

Note. Effects are calculated as Treatment group – Control group. —: Data not collected.
*Indicates scores from individuals not in school or working.
†Indicates scores from individuals attending school or working.
SF36v2.PF= Physical Functioning; SF36v2.RP= Role-Physical; SF36v2.BP= Bodily Pain; SF36v2.GH= General Health; SF36v2.VT= Vitality; SF36v2.SF= Social Functioning; SF36v2.RE= Role-Emotion; SF36v2.MH= Mental Health; SF36v2.PCS= Physical Component Summary; SF36v2.MCS= Mental Component Summary.

than those from the comparison group participants, indicating those in the treatment group continued to perceive they had a higher level of quality of life. This pattern applied to all subscale scores as well, except for the effect of physical limitation on quality of life (PF) and the physical health composite score (PCS).

Two-month follow-up. Two month follow-up assessments were administered to the treatment group only to determine if change in scores were sustained over time. For treatment group participants who provided information two months after the intervention, there was some within-group change from the end of the intervention although the ES CIs all contained 0 (see Table 14.5). Scores on the PCL-5, MDI, and WHODAS 2.0 increased, while scores on the SF36v2 decreased. This reflects a small increase in perceived functional disability, PTSD, and depression symptoms, and a small decrease in perceived quality of life in treatment participants two months after the intervention ended. The comparison group did not completed the 2 month post intervention assessments.

Sensitivity Analysis

Table 14.6 contains the baseline values for those who completed and did not complete the entire 8-week treatment protocol. On the WHODAS 2.0, PCL-5, and MDI the completers had higher scores indicating more PTSD symptoms, depression symptoms, and disability, while on the SF36v2 they had lower scores indicating worse overall health. Thus, completers appeared to have experienced more symptoms of poor health than the non-completers before the intervention started.

We attempted to contact everyone who did not complete the treatment protocol to see their reasons for not completing. We were able to contact 17 (52%). Interestingly, the reasons most of them provided for not completing the intervention had nothing to do with their mental or physical functioning. Instead, the most common reasons for withdrawing from the program included incarceration, not enough time, moving, change in work schedule, and change in job location.

Table 14.4. Post Results Mean, SD, effect size, and 95% confidence interval

	Treatment			Control			Effect		
Variable	Mean	SD	n	Mean	SD	n	Raw dif	g	95% CI
WHODAS 2.0 Sum (32 items)*	51.18	17.81	38	54.22	18.04	27	−3.04	−0.17	[−0.66, 0.32]
WHODAS 2.0 Weighted (32 items)*	55.64	19.36	38	58.94	19.61	27	−3.30	−0.17	[−0.66, 0.32]
WHODAS 2.0 Sum (36 items)†	56.21	19.17	38	61.59	20.93	27	−5.38	−0.27	[−0.76, 0.22]
WHODAS 2.0 Weighted (36 items)†	53.03	18.08	38	58.11	19.75	27	−5.08	−0.27	[−0.76, 0.22]
WHODAS 2.0 (Proxy)	32.36	8.70	28	29.47	12.23	19	2.88	0.28	[−0.30, 0.85]
SF36v2 Summary	39.13	8.66	38	36.21	7.26	27	3.10	0.38	[−0.11, 0.87]
SF36v2.PF	42.97	9.25	39	40.60	9.02	27	2.37	0.26	[−0.23, 0.74]
SF36v2.RP	37.36	10.23	38	37.94	9.53	27	−0.58	−0.06	[−0.55, 0.43]
SF36v2.BP	38.65	8.16	37	37.79	9.94	27	0.85	0.09	[−0.40, 0.58]
SF36v2.GH	42.36	10.71	39	39.75	9.21	27	2.61	0.25	[−0.23, 0.74]
SF36v2.VT	42.24	10.24	39	37.19	9.43	27	5.05	0.50	[0.01, 0.99]
SF36v2.SF	36.64	10.80	39	33.20	9.23	27	3.44	0.33	[−0.15, 0.82]
SF36v2.RE	34.64	12.48	38	30.77	10.35	27	3.87	0.33	[−0.16, 0.82]
SF36v2.MH	39.53	11.84	39	31.78	10.23	27	7.75	0.68	[0.18, 1.18]
SF36v2.PCS	42.40	8.33	38	42.82	8.56	27	−0.42	−0.05	[−0.54. 0.44]
SF36v2.MCS	37.35	12.58	38	30.27	9.18	27	7.08	0.62	[0.12, 1.12]
PCL-5	43.06	18.42	31	50.78	16.43	27	−7.71	−0.43	[−0.95, 0.08]
MDI	28.37	12.92	38	34.11	12.25	28	−5.74	−0.45	[−0.94, 0.04]

Note. Effects are calculated as Treatment group – Control group.
*Indicates scores from individuals not in school or working.
†Indicates scores from individuals attending school or working.
SF36v2.PF= Physical Functioning; SF36v2.RP= Role-Physical; SF36v2.BP= Bodily Pain; SF36v2.GH= General Health; SF36v2.VT= Vitality; SF36v2.SF= Social Functioning; SF36v2.RE= Role-Emotion; SF36v2.MH= Mental Health; SF36v2.PCS= Physical Component Summary; SF36v2.MCS= Mental Component Summary.

WHODAS 2.0 Informant Correlations

Correlation coefficients were computed between the WHODAS 2.0 self-administered summary scores and the WHODAS 2.0 proxy summary scores at baseline and post (8 weeks) to determine if the proxy assessment of functioning and disability was correlated with the self-assessment of functioning and disability. The summary scores were used because the proxy assessment was a shorter version of the self-administered assessment, which prevents the comparison of subscales. The baseline correlation coefficient was small-to-moderate ($r = 0.28$, 95% CI: 0.03–0.50). The post correlation coefficient was larger ($r = 0.47$, 95% CI: 0.21–0.67, but because the CIs overlap the difference is likely due to error. Thus, it appears that scores for self- and other-report forms for the WHODAS 2.0 are positively related, yet they each provide unique information about functional disability.

Discussion

Overall, the findings from this study point to the efficacy and potential effectiveness of therapeutic horseback riding as a complementary intervention for PTSD and depression in military service members. The magnitude of differences between group scores increased over time as well as the corresponding effect sizes, indicating a potential treatment effect. Further, the findings from this study provided the evidence needed to answer our research questions: 1) How does engaging in therapeutic horseback riding affect functional impairment, quality of life, depression and PTS symptoms in military service members with combat related PTSD? And, 2) Is there a difference in difference in outcome variables among military service members who participate in therapeutic horseback riding and those who do not participate?

Both of the research questions can be answered by examining the between and within

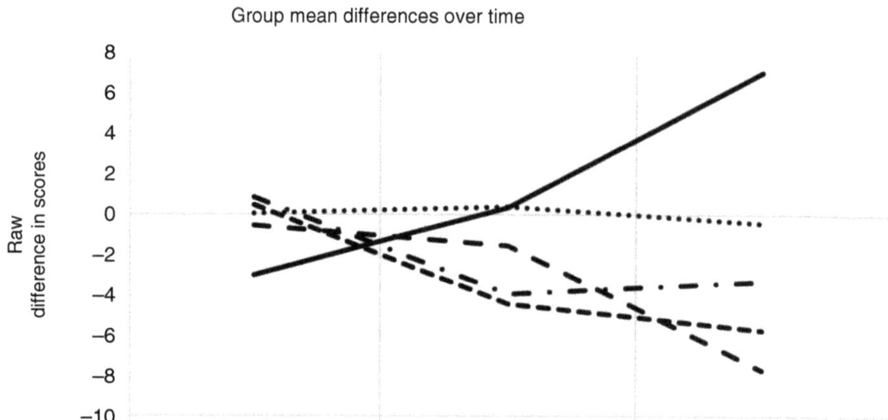

	Baseline	Mid	Post
PCL-5	−0.55	−1.55	−7.71
MDI	0.47	−4.44	−5.74
SF36v2 PCS	0.04	0.39	−0.42
SF36v2 MCS	−3.02	0.35	7.08
WHODAS2	0.85	−3.95	−3.3

Fig. 14.2. Group mean differences over time. Control group mean subtracted from therapeutic horseback riding [THR] group mean.
PCL-5: Posttraumatic Stress Disorder Checklist-5; MDI: Major Depression Inventory; SF36v2 PCS: Short Form 36 question 2nd edition health survey physical component summary score; SF36v2 MCS: Short Form 36 question 2nd edition health survey mental component summary score; WHODAS2: World Health Organization Disability Assessment Schedule 2.0 composite score.

group changes in PTS and depression symptoms, quality of life indicators, and functioning and disability scores over time. Participants in the treatment group (therapeutic horseback riding) demonstrated a 50% greater improvement in PTS symptoms than the participants who were in the comparison group. The participants in the treatment group demonstrated a clinically meaningful improvement in PTS symptoms (−13.02 points, 23% reduction) and depression (−7.65 points, 21% reduction) between pre and post assessment with the group differences between mean scores increasing over time resulting in a medium effect size. A 5-10 point change on the PCL-5 represents reliable change and a 10-20 point change represents clinically meaningful change (see Monson et al., 2008). These changes moderated two months post treatment, but were still clinically meaningful. In contrast, the comparison group participants experienced a 10% (−5.84 points) and 4% (−1.44 points) reduction in PTS and depression symptoms over the same time period. Likewise, the participants in the treatment group demonstrated marked improvement (+ 9.61 points) in overall mental health as reflected in the mental composite summary score of the SF36v2 resulting in a moderate to large ES (g = 0.62). A change of 3-normed based points on the mental health composite score is considered a minimally important difference (MID) (Ware et al., 2007). Thus, the over 9-point improvement (nearly one standard deviation, 10 points) in mental health of the treatment group is noteworthy. Two-month follow-up scores reflected that improvement was sustained after treatment.

Participants in both groups demonstrated little change in physical health (SF36v2 PCS) from baseline to post intervention and the difference between groups was minimal. Interestingly, the participants in the treatment group compared to participants in the comparison

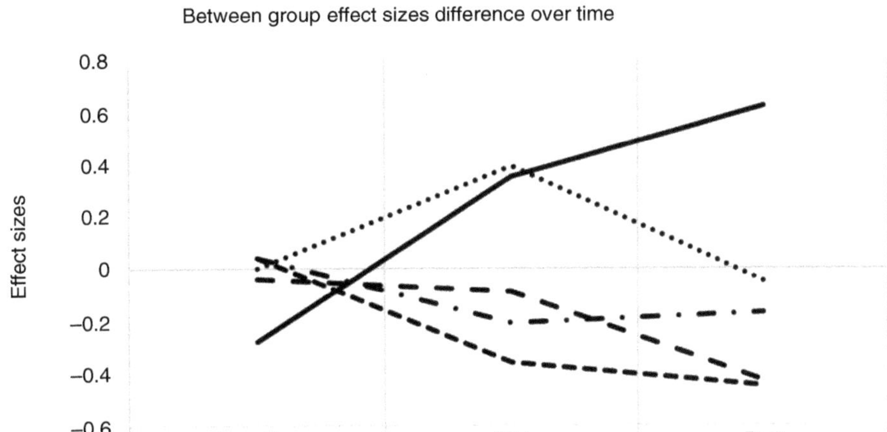

	Baseline	Mid	Post
PCL-5	−0.04	−0.09	−0.43
MDI	0.04	−0.36	−0.45
SF36v2 PCS	0	0.39	−0.05
SF36v2 MCS	−0.28	0.35	0.62
WHODAS2	0.04	−0.21	−0.17

Fig. 14.3. Between group effect size difference over time. Control group effect size subtracted from therapeutic horseback riding [THR] group effect size.
Effect size = Hedge g.
PCL-5: Posttraumatic Stress Disorder Checklist-5; MDI: Major Depression Inventory; SF36v2 PCS: Short Form 36 question 2nd edition health survey physical component summary score; SF36v2 MCS: Short Form 36 question 2nd edition health survey mental component summary score; WHODAS2: World Health Organization Disability Assessment Schedule 2.0 composite score.

Table 14.5. Two-month follow-up scores for therapeutic horseback riding group only.

	Post Scores		Two-month follow up			Effect
Key Variables	Mean (SD)	n	Mean (SD)	n	Raw diff	g [95% CI]
WHODAS 2.0 Sum (32 items)*	51.18 (17.81)	38	53.70 (16.30)	27	2.52	0.14 [−0.35, 0.64]
WHODAS 2.0 Weighted (32 items)*	55.64 (19.36)	38	58.37 (17.72)	27	2.73	0.14 [−0.35, 0.64]
WHODAS 2.0 Sum (36 items)†	56.21 (19.17)	38	58.70 (17.48)	27	2.49	0.13 [−0.36, 0.63]
WHODAS 2.0 Weighted (36 items)†	53.03 (18.08)	38	55.38 (16.49)	27	2.35	0.13 [−0.36, 0.63]
WHODAS 2.0 (Proxy)	32.36 (8.70)	28	___	3	___	___
SF36v2.PCS	42.40 (8.33)	38	41.00 (8.30)	28	−1.40	−0.17 [−0.66, 0.32]
SF36v2.MCS	37.35 (12.58)	38	33.67 (13.56)	28	−3.68	−0.28 [−0.77, 0.21]
PCL-5	43.06 (18.42)	31	47.90 (17.24)	20	4.84	0.19 [−0.44,0.83]
MDI	28.37 (12.92)	38	32.00 (16.50)	26	3.63	0.25 [−0.25, 0.75]

Raw difference and Hedges g calculated as Two-month scores – Post scores.
Two month scores for WHODAS 2.0 proxy were not calculated because only three participants returned the surveys.
*Indicates scores from individuals not in school or working.
†Indicates scores from individuals attending school or working.
SF36v2.PCS= Physical Component Summary; SF36v2.MCS= Mental Component Summary.

Table 14.6. Baseline Difference between completers and non-completers: Mean, SD, effect size, 95% confidence interval

	Completers			Non-Completers			Effect		
Variable	Mean	SD	n	Mean	SD	n	Raw dif	g	95% CI
WHODAS 2.0 Sum (32 items)*	53.23	17.95	39	39.82	12.46	11	13.41	0.78	[0.10, 1.45]
WHODAS 2.0 Weighted (32 items)*	57.86	19.51	39	43.28	13.54	11	14.58	0.78	[0.10, 1.45]
WHODAS 2.0 Sum (36 items)†	59.21	19.04	39	43.64	13.51	11	15.57	0.85	[0.17, 1.53]
WHODAS 2.0 Weighted (36 items)†	55.85	17.96	39	41.17	12.75	11	14.69	0.85	[0.17, 1.53]
WHODAS 2.0 (Proxy)	34.32	9.51	28	25.86	9.19	7	8.46	0.87	[0.04, 1.71]
SF36v2 Summary	41.59	10.33	39	50.05	7.76	12	−8.45	−0.85	[−1.51, −0.19]
SF36v2.PF	33.89	9.46	39	43.50	9.40	12	−9.60	−1.00	[−1.67, −0.33]
SF36v2.RP	36.50	8.43	38	49.50	9.68	12	−13.00	−1.46	[−2.17, −0.76]
SF36v2.BP	41.04	10.26	39	43.95	8.75	12	−2.91	−0.29	[−0.93, 0.35]
SF36v2.GH	34.54	8.55	39	40.47	8.45	12	−5.92	−0.68	[−1.33, −0.03]
SF36v2.VT	31.12	8.79	39	33.95	11.58	12	−2.83	−0.29	[−0.93, 0.35]
SF36v2.SF	27.15	11.64	39	34.12	8.95	12	−6.96	−0.62	[−1.27, 0.03]
SF36v2.RE	30.01	10.12	39	34.52	10.11	12	−4.51	−0.44	[−1.08, 0.20]
SF36v2.MH	42.71	8.91	39	52.38	9.48	12	−9.67	−1.05	[−1.72, −0.38]
SF36v2.PCS	27.06	10.88	39	29.96	11.37	12	−2.91	−0.26	[−0.90, 0.38]
SF36v2.MCS	34.55	7.63	39	41.24	6.35	12	−6.69	−0.90	[−1.56, −0.23]
PCL-5	58.65	14.58	31	49.42	10.54	12	9.23	0.67	[0.00, 1.33]
MDI	38.26	12.01	39	28.75	9.11	12	9.51	0.82	[0.16, 1.48]

Note. Effects are calculated as Completers – Non-Completers.
*Indicates scores from individuals not in school or working.
†Indicates scores from individuals attending school or working.
SF36v2.PF= Physical Functioning; SF36v2.RP= Role-Physical; SF36v2.BP= Bodily Pain; SF36v2.GH= General Health; SF36v2.VT= Vitality; SF36v2.SF= Social Functioning; SF36v2.RE= Role-Emotion; SF36v2.MH= Mental Health; SF36v2.PCS= Physical Component Summary; SF36v2.MCS= Mental Component Summary.

group reported little change in functioning and disability over time. Further, the two-month follow-up scores indicated a modest increase in functional disability. While worth noting, the findings are not surprising. The assessment for functioning and disability (WHODAS 2.0) includes measures of both mental and physical health, but is more weighted towards measuring physical aspects of health and disability. Further, physical health scores are related to the ability of the individual to complete everyday activities and the level of physical pain the person experiences. Many military service members experience combat related physical wounds. The participants in our study were ambulatory, but experienced bodily pain and physical limitation as evidenced in their baseline bodily pain scores (BP) and their scores related to the role of physical limitation in everyday activities (RP). These scores may actually underestimate the physical limitation of the participants because military members are trained to ignore pain and overcome physical limitation. Therapeutic horseback riding is a physical activity. While, participants reported they enjoyed working with a horse and riding the horse, the physical demands of the activity may have resulted in more physical discomfort. A longer intervention time (i.e. more weeks) may be needed to improve physical functioning of the participants. Research on hippotherapy (using the horse movements to provide motor and sensory input) supports the positive effects of equine interventions on balance, gait, and fatigue in participants with motor control deficits (Lee, Kim, Yong, 2015; Kwon et al., 2015).

The results from our study reflect meaningful change in several key variables and the between-group effect sizes were moderate indicating a potential treatment effect. Most of the participants (in both groups) had or were receiving established therapy for PTSD at the time of the study, yet participants in the treatment group experience additional therapeutic benefits not reported in the comparison group. As noted, the intervention effect sizes are modest, but they are similar to effect sizes reported for treatments for combat-related PTSD (Bradley et al., 2005). Moreover, we calculated the effect size using the Hedges g formula. Hedges g corrects for the bias found with effect size calculation for small sample sizes (Hedges, 1981). Most reported effect sizes in PTSD intervention studies were calculated using Cohen's d calculations, which may result in an overestimation of effect size, especially if the sample size is small (Grisson & Kim, 2005).

Limitation

The study is not without limitations. First, the participants were not randomized to the treatment group or comparison group. A randomized controlled trial (RCT) design is the 'gold standard' for determining effectiveness of a treatment or intervention, but a quasi-experimental design provides similar rigor when baseline difference between groups are considered. This type of design is frequently used when it is not logical or ethical to conduct a RCT. In the current study, many of the potential participants expressed concern about the randomization process and the potential that their comrades would be required to wait eight weeks to receive treatment. This concern may be reflective of PTS symptoms in general, but it may also be more common among veterans. Veterans and military service members tend to be altruistic wanting everyone to receive the same benefits (Campbell et al., 2007). The quasi-experimental design was the most logical and ethical design choice with this population. Moreover, the quasi-experimental design is appropriate for comparative effectiveness research especially in real-world settings (Abraham, Byrne, Young & Solomon, 2010).

We used several measures to address the threats to internal validity inherent with this type of design. First, we chose assessment instruments that had strong validity and reliability for detecting changes in the variables of interest. Second, we used specific inclusion/exclusion criteria to reduce selection bias. Third, we used the same assessment time intervals for both the comparison and intervention groups to reduce the effects of maturation and possible interactive effects between groups. Fourth, we monitored the fidelity of the intervention to ensure consistency across intervention sites. And fifth, we accounted for the effects of attrition by contacting and interviewing participants who dropped out of the study, however; we were unable to contact 17 participants. We also conducted a sensitivity analysis of difference between completers and non-completers. The completers reported more PTS and depression symptoms and lower mental health scores than the non-completers, yet the reasons for not completing the intervention appeared to be unrelated to the scores. We were unable to interview all non-completers so caution assessing the effects of attrition are still warranted.

Another limitation of the study is the use of self-administered assessments. While self-reports are commonly used in interventions studies, there is an inherent risk of over or under estimation on the part of the participant. In this study, participants were asked to complete several self-reports recalling the presence and severity of symptoms experienced in previous weeks. Social desirability is a potential bias. The participant might either over or under report symptoms depending on what he/she believes is socially acceptable (Plous, 1993). Military service members are acutely aware of the stigma associated with PTSD and depression and may underreport the severity for fear of professional repercussions. Other types of bias may include memory errors caused by either forgetting or telescoping, in which the participant remembers an event as occurring more recently than it did or with more severity (Bradburn, 1983). However, because participants in both the comparison and THR groups completed the same self-reports, it is possible to compare between group responses over time, with the assumption that the amount of bias in both groups is similar. In addition, a person who knew the participant well (e.g., spouse, parent, girlfriend, boyfriend) completed proxy surveys pre and post. These objective surveys were designed to assess the level of functioning and disability of the participant. We conducted a comparison of the self-report and proxy version to determine if the scores correlated. While only the post scores were significantly correlated, scores from the proxy forms indicated similar levels of disability as the scores from the self-report.

In the current study, we used an 8-week intervention protocol. PTSD is a complex mental health issue that is not typically alleviated with short duration interventions. While our findings indicated that military service members can experience less PTS and depression symptoms by participating in a short duration intervention program, participating in longer programs may provide additional or more substantial change. Future research should include programs of varying lengths to best determine optimal intervention dose. Research may also target the inclusion of family members in the intervention protocol. We included a proxy assessment, but the spouse and/or family member was not specifically involved in the THR intervention. Understanding the effects of combat-related PTSD on the family and including the family members in the treatment process may improve quality of life for all family members (Carlson & Ruzek, 2016).

Conclusion

Despite the limitations, the findings of this study provide evidence to support the efficacy and possible effectiveness of therapeutic horseback riding as therapeutic intervention for military service members. Further, this study adds rigor to the growing body of evidence supporting the use of complementary and experiential interventions for military service members diagnosed with PTSD and depression symptoms. Adding a comparison group enhances the ability to determine treatment effect and the quasi-experimental design provides a more realistic approach to inform future community based intervention programming.

References

Abraham, N. S., Byrne C. J., Young, J. M., & Solomon, M. J. (2010). Meta-analysis of well-designed nonrandomized comparative studies of surgical procedures is as good as randomized controlled trials. *Journal of Clinical Epidemiology, 63*(3), 238–245. doi: 10.1016/j.jclinepi.2009.04.005

American Psychiatric Association. (2013). *Diagnostic and Statistical Manual of Mental Disorders* (5th ed.). Washington, DC.

Anestis, M. D., Anestis, J. C., Zawilinski, L. L., Hopkins, T. A., & Lilienfeld, S. O. (2014). Equine-related treatments for mental disorders lack empirical support: A systematic review of empirical investigations. *Journal of Clinical Psychology, 70*(12), 1115–1132. Doi: 10.1002/jclp.22113

Armed Forces Health Surveillance Center. (2018). Mental disorders and mental health problems, active component, U.S. Armed Forces, 2001–2011. *Medical Surveillance Monthly Report, 19,* 11–17. Retrieved from http://www.dtic.mil/dtic/tr/fulltext/u2/a566014.pdf

Beaujean, A. A. (2014). Sample size determination for regression models using Monte Carlo methods in\ textbf{R}. *Practical Assessment, Research, and Evaluation, 19*(12), 1–16. Retrieved from http://pare-online.net/getvn.asp?v=19&n=12

Bradburn, N. M. (1983). Response effect. In Rossi, PH, Wright, JD, Anderson, AB, eds, *Handbook on Survey Research.* San Diego, CA: Academic Press, Inc., pp. 308–310.

Bradley, R., Greene, J., Russ, E., Dutra, L., & Westen, D. (2005). A multidimensional meta-analysis of psychotherapy for PTSD.[erratum appears in Am J Psychiatry. 2005 Apr; 162(4):832]. *American Journal of Psychiatry, 162*(2), 214–227. doi: 10.1176/appi.ajp.162.2.214

Bech, P., Christensen, M., Vinberg, M., Ostergaard, S. D., Martiny, K., & Kessing, L. V. (2013). The performance of the revised Major Depression Inventory for self-reported severity of depression—implications for the DSM-5 and ICD-11. *Psychotherapy and Psychosomatics, 82,* 187–188. Doi: 10.1159/000346456

Bech, P., Stage, K.B., Nair, N.P.V., Larsen, J.K., Kragh-Sørensen, P., Gjerris, A. (1997). The Major Depression Rating Scale (MDS). Inter-rater reliability and validity across different depression also fulfill the DSM-IV major depression settings in randomized moclobemide trials. *Journal of Affective Disorders, 42,* 39–48. doi: 10.1016/S0165-0327(96)00094-8

Borenstein, M., Hedges, L. V., Higgins, J. P. T., & Rothstein, H. R. (2009). *Introduction to Meta-analysis.* Hoboken, NJ: Wiley.

Campbell, H. M., Raisch, D. W., Sather, M. R., Warren, S. R., & Segal, A. R. (2007). A comparison of veteran and nonveteran motivations and reasons for participating in clinical trials. *Military Medicine, 172,* 1–27.

Carlson, E. B., & Ruzek, J. (2016). U.S. Department of Veterans Affairs; Professional Section PTSD and the Family. Retrieved from https://www.ptsd.va.gov/professional/treatment/family/ptsd-and-the-family.asp.

Cornish, M. A., Thys, A., Vogel, D. L., & Wade, N. G. (2014). Post-deployment difficulties and help seeking barriers among military veterans: Insights and intervention strategies. *Professional Psychology: Research and Practice, 45*(6), 405–409. doi: 10.1037/a0037986

Cukor, J., Spitalnick, J., Difede, J., Rizzo, A., & Rothbaum, B. O. (2009). Emerging treatments for PTSD. *Clinical Psychology Review, 29,* 715–726

Cumming, G. (2014). The new statistics: Why and how. *Psychological Science, 25,* 7–29.

Elbogen, E. B., Wagner, H. R., Johnson, S. C., Kinneer, P., Kang, H., Vasterling, J. J., & Beckham, J. C. (2013). Are Iraq and Afghanistan veterans using mental health services? New data from a national random-sample survey. *Psychiatric Services, 64,* 134–141. doi:10.1176/appi.ps.004792011

Ferruolo, D. M. (2016). Psychosocial equine program for veterans. *Social Work, 61*(1), 53–60. doi.org/10.1093/sw/swv054

Gerger, H., Munder, T., & Barth, J. (2014). Specific and nonspecific psychological interventions for PTSD symptoms: A meta-analysis with problem complexity as a moderator. *Journal of Clinical Psychology, 70*(7), 601–615. doi: 10.1002/jclp.22059

Gomez, I. B. (2016). *Evaluating a program of equine therapy for veterans with PTSD symptoms* (Order No. 10119467). Available from ProQuest Dissertations & Theses Global. (1805322272). Retrieved from http://ezproxy.baylor.edu/login?url=https://search.proquest.com/docview/1805322272?accountid=7014

Greger, H., Munder, T., Gemperli, A., Nuesch, E., Trelle, S., Juni, P., & Barth, J. (2014). Integrating fragmented evidence by network meta-analysis: Relative effectiveness of psychological interventions for adults with post-traumatic stress disorder. *Psychological Medicine, 44,* 3151–3164. doi: 10.1017/S003329174000853

Griffin, J., McCune, S., Maholmes, V., & Hurley, K. (2011). Scientific research on human-animal interaction. In: P. McCardle, S. McCune, J. A. Griffin, L. Esposito and L. Freund, editors, *Animals in our Lives: Human–Animal Interaction in Family, Community, and Therapeutic Settings*. Paul H. Brookes Publishing Company, Baltimore, MD. p. 227–236.

Grissom, R. J., & Kim, J, J. (2005). *Effect Sizes for Research: A Broad Practical Approach*. Mahwah, NJ: Erlbaum.

Hedges, L. V. (1981). Distribution theory for Glass's estimator of effect size and related estimators. *Journal of Educational Statistics, 6,* 107–128. doi:10.3102/10769986006002107

Imel, Z. E., Laska, K., Jakupcak, M., & Simpson, T. L. (2013). Meta-analysis of dropout in treatments for posttraumatic stress disorder. *Journal of Consulting and Clinical Psychology, 81*(3), 394–404. Doi: 10.1037/a0031474

Kessler, R. C. (2000). Posttraumatic stress disorder: The burden to the individual and to society. *Journal of Clinical Psychiatry, 61*(Suppl 5), 4–12 discussion 13-14.

Konstantinidis, A., Martiny, K., Bech, P., & Kasper, S. (2018). A comparison of the Major Depression Inventory (MDI) and the Beck Depression Inventory (BDI) in severely depressed patients. *International Journal of Psychiatry Clinical Practice, 15,* 56–61.

Krob, K. E. (2015). *Heroes and horses: Veteran and equine experiences with equine facilitated learning and therapy* (Order No. 3728954). Available from ProQuest Dissertations & Theses Global. (1734044791). Retrieved from http://ezproxy.baylor.edu/login?url=https://search.proquest.com/docview/1734044791?accountid=7014

Kwon, J. Y., Chang, H. J., Yi, S. H., Lee, J. Y., Shin, H. Y., & Kim, Y. H. (2015). Effect of hippotherapy on gross motor function in children with cerebral palsy: A randomized controlled trial. *Journal of Alternative and Complementary Medicine, 21,* 15–21.

Lanning, B. A., & Krenek, N. (2013). Examining effects of equine-assisted activities to help combat veterans improve quality of life. *Journal of Rehabilitation Research and Development. 50*(8): xv–xxii. http://dx.doi.org/10.1682/JRRD.2013.07.0159

Lee, C. W., Kim, S. G., & Yong, M. S. (2014). Effects of hippotherapy on recovery of gait and balance ability in patients with stroke. *Journal of Physical Therapy Science, 26*(2), 309–320, 11.

Maciejewski, M. L., Curtis, L. H., & Dowd, B. (2013). Study design elements for rigorous quasi-experimental comparative effectiveness research. *Journal of Comparative Effectiveness Research, 2*(2), p. 159. doi: http://dx.doi.org.ezproxy.baylor. edu/10.2217/cer.13.7

Mattson, L. (2015). The impact of equine assisted activities and therapies on trauma recovery: Stories of United States military veterans who have participated in equine assisted activities and therapies programs. Unpublished dissertation. Plymouth State University.

McCune, S., Kruger, K. A., Griffin, J. A., Esposito, L., Freund, L. S., Hurley, K. J., & Bures, R. (2014). Evolution of research into the mutual benefits of human-animal interaction. *Animal Frontiers, 4*(3), 49–57. Doi: 10.2527/af.2014-0022.

Monroe, M., Myers, C., & Sanchez, T. (2014). University of Central Florida study results: EAAT with veterans with PTSD. In Professional Association of Therapeutic Horsemanship Annual Conference 2014 (pp. 1–6). Orlando, FL: McCormick Research Institute.

Monson, C. M., Gradus, J. L., Young-Xu, Y., Schnurr, P. P., Price, J. L., & Schumm, J. A. (2008). Change in posttraumatic stress disorder symptoms: Do clinicians and patients agree? *Psychological Assessment, 20*(2), 131–138.

Muthen, L. K., & Muthen, B. O. (2002). How to use a Monte Carlo study to decide on sample size and determine power. *Structural Equation Modeling, 9*(4), 599–620. doi: 10.1207/S15328007SEM09048

Pendry, P. & Roeter, S. (2013). Experimental trial demonstrates positive effects of equine facilitated learning on child social competence. *Human-Animal Interaction Bulletin, 1,* 1–19.

Professional Association of Therapeutic Horsemanship International [PATH Intl.]. (2017). Retrieved from http://www.pathintl.org/

Plous, S. (1993). *The Psychology of Judgement and Decision Making*. New York: McGraw-Hill, Inc, pp. 191–204.

Rainier Therapeutic Riding. (2017). Rainier Therapeutic Riding's Riding Through Recovery. Retrieved from http://www.rtriding.org/horsemanship-programs.php

Richardson, L. K., Frueh, B. C., Acierno, R. (2010). Prevalence estimates of combat-related PTSD: A critical review. *Australian New Zealand Journal of Psychiatry, 44*(1), 4–19. doi: 10.3109/00048670903393597

Schnurr, P., Lunney, C.A., Bovin, M.J., & Marx, B.P. (2009). Posttraumatic stress disorder and quality of life: extension of findings to veterans of the wars in Iraq and Afghanistan. *Clinical Psychological Review, 29*(8), 727–735.

Selby, A. & Smith-Osborne, A. (2013). A systematic review of effectiveness of complementary and adjunct therapies and interventions involving equines. *Health Psychology, 32*(4), 418–432. Doi: 10.1037/a0029188

Shadish, W. R., Cook, T. D., & Campbell, D. T., (2002). *Experimental and Quasi-Experimental Designs for Generalized Causal Inference.* Boston, MA: Houghton Mifflin.

Thomas, J. L., Wilk, J. E., Riviere, L. A., McGurk, D., Castro, C. A., & Hoge, C. W. (2010). Prevalence of mental health problems and functional impairment among active component and National Guard soldiers 3 and 12 months following combat in Iraq. *Archives of General Psychiatry, 67,* 614–623. doi:10.1001/archgenpsychiatry.2010.54

Ustun, T. B., Chatterji, S., Kostanjsek, N., Rehm, J., Kennedy, C., Epping-Jordan, J., Saxena, S., von Korff, M., & Pull, C. (2010). Developing the World Health Organization Disability Assessment Schedule 2.0.

Ware, J. E., Kosinski, M., Bjorner, J. B., Turner-Bowker, D. M., Gandek, B., & Maruish, M. E. (2007). *User's Manual for the SF-36v2 Health Survey* (*2nd ed.*). Lincoln, RI: QualityMetric Incorporated.

Ware, J. E., Kosinski, M., & Keller, S. D. (1994). *SF-36 Physical and Mental Component Summary Measures: A User's Manual Boston*: The Health Institute.

Wasserstein, R. L., & Lazar, N. A. (2016). The ASA's statement on p-values: Context, process, and purpose. *The American Statistician, 70,* 129–133, doi:10.1080/00031305.2016.1154108

Weathers, F.W., Litz, B.T., Keane, T.M., Palmieri, P.A., Marx, B.P., & Schnurr, P.P. (2013). The PTSD Checklist for DSM-5 (PCL-5). Scale available from the National Center for PTSD at www.ptsd.va.gov.

Wynn, G. (2015). Complementary and alternative medicine approaches in the treatment of PTSD. *Current Psychiatry Reports, 17,* 62. doi: 10.1007/s11920-015-0600-2

15 Pets on Campus: Best Friend or Bad Decision?

Lauren Highfill* and Miranda Goodman-Wilson
Department of Psychology, Eckerd College

Abstract

This study explores the relationship between pet ownership and psychological benefits among college students. Sixty-six students either living with a pet on campus ($n = 32$; 16 dog owners, 16 cat owners) or not completed several assessments of stress and affective symptomatology during the first two weeks of an academic semester and again during the last two weeks. Overall there were no significant differences between students living with pets and students not living with pets on any of the measures. However, there was a significant interaction between pet ownership and stress in predicting students' somatic anxiety at Time 2. Although pet owning students reported similar levels of stress as their non-pet owning peers, this stress was not correlated with an increase to their bodily symptoms of anxiety. For the non-pet condition, however, stress and somatic anxiety were significantly, positively correlated. Overall, there was not strong quantitative support for pets reducing stress amongst college students. However, qualitative data from a pet owner questionnaire suggested that students greatly enjoy living with a pet on a college campus. Given the decidedly mixed findings, directions for future research more closely examining the impact of pet ownership on students are proposed.

Keywords: pet ownership, college students, stress, dogs, cats

Authors' note

This study would not have been possible without the invaluable assistance from Eckerd College Pet Life, especially Tonya Womack and William Clements. We would also like to thank research assistants, Amanda Balke and Carrie Shere for their help with data collection. We would also like to thank three anonymous reviewers for their helpful suggestions and edits to this manuscript.

Stress is a significant issue among college students (Towbes & Cohen, 1996). According to a recent survey of 70,000 students from 140 U.S. colleges and universities, the two most commonly acknowledged impairments to academic performance were stress (32.5%) and anxiety (23.4%) (American College Health Association, 2015). Furthermore, these same students were asked to rate the overall level of stress experienced and nearly 53% of students indicated "more than average" levels, whereas only 1.8% of students indicated "no stress" (American College Health Association, 2015). Also, 58% of students indicated that they "felt overwhelming anxiety" during the last 12 months. College students are also particularly vulnerable to psychiatric disorders. It is estimated that almost half

Corresponding author: email: highfile@eckerd.edu

of all college students experience a psychiatric disorder each year, with anxiety disorders and major depressive disorder being the most frequently diagnosed conditions (Blanco et al., 2008; Mistler, Reetz, Krylowicz, & Barr, 2012). In light of these data, effective methods for managing stress and affective symptomatology among college students are needed.

Colleges and universities are invested in creating stress-management interventions, and various programs have been implemented with moderate success (e.g., meditation: Oman, Shapiro, Thoresen, Plante, & Flinders, 2008; yoga: West, Otte, Geher, Johnson, & Mohr, 2004). It is also increasingly common for schools to bring therapy animals onto campus during stressful periods, such as finals week (Reynolds & Rabschutz, 2011). A recent exploratory study found that college students experienced a reduction in their perceived, but not physiological, stress after visiting with therapy dogs during final exam week (Barker, Barker, McCain, & Schubert, 2016).

A fairly novel approach for addressing stress and anxiety among college students is to allow students to bring their family pets to live on campus. To that end, a growing number of U.S. colleges have "pet-friendly" housing, which allow for companion animals such as dogs and cats to live with students in their dorm rooms (Huss, 2012). While anecdotal accounts of the benefits of having pets live on campus are often reported by students, no formal studies of the efficacy have been published. The current study is the first to explore whether living on campus with a pet is beneficial.

Studies on the impact of living with pets on human health and psychological well-being have produced mixed results (see Friedmann & Son, 2009 for review). There are a number of prior studies that support the benefits of living with a pet. Past research has suggested that pet owners have better cardiovascular health, make fewer doctor visits, and are less depressed than non-pet owners (e.g. Friedmann, Katcher, Lynch, Thomas, 1998; Headey & Grabka, 2007; Headey, Na, & Zheng, 2008; Siegel, Angulo, Detels, Wesch, & Mullen, 1999). One such study surveyed dog owners and non-dog owners residing in urban China where pets had been banned until 1992 (Headey et al., 2008). The data indicated that the dog owners exercised more, slept better, and made fewer visits to the doctor than the non-dog owners. Another study examined the effect of living with a pet during recovery from a heart attack (Friedmann et al., 1998). The data indicated that the mortality rate among non-pet owners was 28%, while only 6% for pet owners. The authors linked the positive effect to more physical activity (e.g., walking a dog) for the pet owners. A large-scale, longitudinal study examining over 10,000 Germans and Australians indicated that pet owners make roughly 15% fewer annual physician visits than non-pet owners (Headey & Grabka, 2007). Finally, a study of men with AIDS found that those who owned pets reported less depression than those who did not own a pet (Siegel et al., 1999).

While there are a number of studies which suggest that pet ownership has a direct influence on health outcomes, other research has revealed a more complex relationship. For example, a study of individuals suffering from hypertension randomly assigned patients to either take medication only or to take medication while also acquiring a pet dog or cat (Allen, Shykoff, & Izzo, 2001). While there were no significant differences in blood pressure between the two groups at rest, the pet owners had significantly lower physiological reactions to specific stressors (an arithmetic test and presenting a speech). Additionally, the pet owners increased their performance on the arithmetic task from 74% to 95% whereas the non-pet owners remained at 75% (Allen et al., 2001). The authors suggested that a possible explanation for their results was that pets were serving as a source of social support for participants, and that sense of support helped to buffer participants from the physiological stress of performing an evaluative task (Allen et al., 2001). It is, however, important to note that there have been several studies unable to find a beneficial relationship between human and pet (e.g. Grossberg, Alf, & Vormbrock, 1988; Straatman, Hanson, Endenburg, & Mol, 1997) and some even find a negative relationship (e.g. Parslow & Jorm 2003; Parslow, Jorm, Christensen, Rodgers, & Jacomb, 2005). For example, Straatman et al. (1997) examined the influence of an unfamiliar dog on anxiety before and after a speech task. While the speech task itself increased blood pressure, heart rate, and state-anxiety in all participants, the presence of a dog had no effect on any of these measures for the experimental group. The authors suggested that the speech task may have been too stressful of a measure to reveal any positive effects of the dog.

This indicates that there may be limits to the anxiety-reducing efficacy of animals. Revealing the possible downside of pet ownership, Parslow and Jorm (2003) found that pet owners had higher body mass indexes, had higher diastolic blood pressures, were more likely to smoke, and participated in less physical activity when compared to the non-owners, although the authors caution that the increased health risks may only be indirectly associated with owning a pet. Relatedly, another study of cardiovascular patients found that pet owners were significantly more likely than non-owners to be re-hospitalized or die due to a cardiac event in the year following their initial hospitalization. This was particularly true for cat but not dog owners (Parker et al., 2010). Given the inconsistency of the literature, it is critical to actually investigate the impact of allowing pets on a college campus, rather than assuming it will be positive.

Even when a beneficial relationship is found, it can be difficult to determine the causal direction. For example, it is possible that pet owners are already in better health than non-pet owners and thus have more energy to dedicate to the care of an animal, or that individuals with higher socioeconomic status are more likely to have the financial resources to support the care of both their own health and an animal. Studying animal ownership amongst college students may represent a promising strategy for addressing the above concerns, as college students are relatively homogenous in terms of age and current personal financial resources. Despite this fact, research investigating the potential positive impact of animal ownership has not yet been conducted with college students.

One explanation for the positive effects of living with a pet may be attributed to the increase in companionship (e.g., Allen et al., 2001; Headey et al., 2008; Siegel et al., 1999). Additional social support and companionship could be especially beneficial for college-aged students (Rayle & Chung, 2007). However, it is also possible that the unique challenges (financial, time management, etc.) of caring for a pet while in college could contribute to a more complex relationship than has been documented when pet ownership has been studied in older adults. For example, a previous study which examined the relationship between pet ownership and emotional distress among working women, found that there were no differences between pet owners and non-pet owners (Watson & Weinstein, 1993). The authors concluded that the typical therapeutic benefits of owning a pet may be lessened when the owner has insufficient time to spend with her pets. College students may be faced with a similar predicament due to attending classes, engaging in extracurricular activities, and participating in various social events. College is also a time of limited financial resources for students as recent data indicates that 85% of undergraduates in the United States are receiving some form of federal financial aid (U.S. Department of Education, 2014). The costs of animal ownership, some of which can be quite unpredictable in the case of illness or injury, may further contribute to the stress of animal ownership.

Eckerd College (St. Petersburg, FL) is a private, liberal arts institution which permits residential students to bring a family pet to live with them in designated pet-friendly dorms throughout the year (https://www.eckerd.edu/housing/pet-life/policy/). All pets must have previously resided in the family home for at least one year; thus students are prohibited from adopting new animals while living on campus. This means that students are living with animals with which they have an already established bond. In the current study we explored whether living with a family pet on a college campus affects student stress levels and overall psychological functioning. We compared the responses of pet owners and non-pet owners on several psychological scales, assessing perceived stress and affective symptomatology, which were administered at the beginning and end of an academic semester. Because of the conflicting findings from previous research, and the potentially unique challenges, but also benefits of a student bringing a pet to campus, no directional hypotheses were developed. Additionally, we had pet owners complete a questionnaire assessing their overall experience living with a pet as a college student.

Method

Participants

Seventy-five students (64 females; $M = 20$ years, $SD = \pm\ 0.94$) participated in the first wave of data collection. All students were residents of an Eckerd College dormitory. As freshmen were not typically allowed to bring their family pet to campus for their first semester, all participants were sophomores, juniors, or seniors. Sixty-six students completed both waves of data collection and, of them, 32 were registered owners of a cat (n = 16; 15 females) /dog (n = 16; 10 females) which resided with them on campus. This represented approximately 74% of the dog/cat owners living on campus. The remaining 34 students were living in traditional, non-pet dormitories. Owners of caged animals such as reptiles, rodents, and other non-cat/dog pets were not eligible for participation. Pet owners were significantly more likely to report being diagnosed with a pre-existing psychological disorder than non-pet owners (40% versus 17.5% respectively, $p < 0.05$, Fisher's exact test). All participants were awarded an Eckerd College Pet Life t-shirt and a five-dollar gift card to Dunkin Donuts for their participation.

Measures

Participants were asked to complete three questionnaires assessing their psychological well-being. The Center for Epidemiologic Studies Depression Scale (CES-D) (Radloff, 1971), asks participants to indicate the number of depressive symptoms they have experienced in the previous two weeks. It can be used to assess the risk of a participant receiving a clinical diagnosis of major depressive disorder. The CES-D has both excellent internal consistency (Cronbach's α = 0.88-0.91) and test-retest reliability (r = 0.87). The Perceived Stress Scale (PSS) (Cohen, Kamarck, & Mermelstein, 1983) captures participants' perceptions of stressors experienced in the previous month. The PSS has strong internal consistency (Cronbach's α = 0.74-0.91) and test-retest reliability (rs = 0.55-0.74 depending on time interval, which makes sense given the nature of the instrument). Finally, the trait measure from the State-Trait Inventory for Cognitive and Somatic Anxiety (STISCA) (Ree, MacLeod, French, & Locke, 2000) asks participants to rate how they generally feel with respect to common symptoms of somatic (bodily) and cognitive (mental) anxiety. Both the cognitive and somatic subscales of the trait inventory have strong internal consistency (Cronbach's α = 0.87). Additionally, students in the pet condition completed a questionnaire, developed for the purposes of this study, assessing their experiences living with a pet on campus during the second wave of data collection (Highfill & Goodman, unpublished). Sample questions included, "Has living with a pet on campus ever positively impacted your ability to fulfill your academic responsibilities?" and "Has living with a pet on campus ever negatively impacted your ability to attend social/extracurricular events on/off campus?" Questions also asked students how much time and money they spend caring for their pets and what impact overall living with a pet has on their stress level.

Procedure

All participants completed the questionnaires during the first two weeks and the last two weeks of the fall 2014 semester. Participants in the pet condition were recruited using a list of all 43 registered pet owners on campus. Quota sampling was used to select non-pet owners from a list of all dorm residents who fulfilled the other recruitment requirements (sophomore status or higher, not residing with any animal including non-dog/cat species). This was done to build a group that roughly reflected the same gender and class ranking ratios as the pet condition. Due to the fact questionnaires needed to be completed during a specific time during the semester, we were unable to match non-pet owners after the pet owners had completed their measures. Ultimately 66 students completed both waves of data collection and, of them, 32 were registered owners of a cat/dog and 34 were non owners.

Participation was solicited via email and questionnaires were completed online at the convenience of the participant. The CES-D, PSS, and TICSA assessments were completed by all participants during both waves of data collection. The pet owner questionnaire was completed by that group only, and was the final measure included in the second wave of data collection. The study protocol was approved by Eckerd College's Institutional Review Board and informed consent was obtained from all participants. Since no data was collected directly from the animals, approval from Eckerd College's Institutional Animal Care and Use Committee was not needed. The significance threshold for all statistical tests was set at $p = 0.05$.

Results

Psychological assessments

T-test analyses were run in order to compare the pet and non-pet groups in terms of academic standing (as measured by self-reported GPA at Time 1) and psychological functioning at both periods of data collection. Overall, there were no significant differences between students living with pets and students not living with pets on any of the measures administered. Students living with a pet and students not living with a pet did not significantly differ in terms of reported GPA. All students reported a marginal increase in stress ($t(65) = -1.89$, $p = 0.06$, $r^2 = 0.05$) and depressive symptomatology ($t(65) = -3.47$, $p = 0.001$, $r^2 = 0.16$) over the course of the semester; however, anxiety remained stable (see Table 15.1 for means). Stress and depressive/anxious overall symptomatology were positively correlated at both time points (see Table 15.2). However, regression analysis of the Time 2 data revealed there was a significant interaction between pet ownership and stress in predicting students' somatic anxiety at the end of the semester $R2 = 0.35$, $F(3, 62) = 11.16$, $p < 0.001$, $\beta = 1.08$, $p = 0.02$. For students in the non-pet condition, higher stress was associated with higher somatic anxiety ($r(32) = 0.69$, $p < 0.001$), but this relationship was not significant for students in the pet condition ($r(30) = 0.29$, $p = 0.103$).

Table 15.1. Means and Standard Deviations for Three Measurements of Psychological Well-being and GPA at Time 1 and Time 2.

Measure	*M*	*SD*
CES-D (Time 1)	28.86	9.77
Non-Pet	32.00	10.04
Pet	25.72	9.50
CES-D (Time 2)	32.74	11.28
Non-Pet	28.85	12.37
Pet	36.63	10.19
PSS (Time 1)	21.14	6.95
Non-Pet	24.28	7.65
Pet	18.00	6.25
PSS (Time 2)	22.62	8.01
Non-Pet	18.90	8.40
Pet	26.34	7.62
TICSA Total (Time 1)	36.77	10.54
Non-Pet	34.95	11.01
Pet	38.59	10.07
TICSA Total (Time 2)	36.68	11.02
Non-Pet	35.43	12.90
Pet	37.93	9.14
TICSA Cognitive (Time 1)	19.73	6.14
Non-Pet	18.55	6.15
Pet	20.91	6.12
TICSA Cognitive (Time 2)	19.65	6.78
Non-Pet	18.85	7.05
Pet	20.45	6.51
TICSA Somatic (Time 1)	17.46	5.85
Non-Pet	17.23	6.00
Pet	17.69	5.70
TICSA Somatic (Time 2)	16.95	5.48
Non-Pet	16.99	6.31
Pet	16.91	4.65
GPA (Time 1 only)	3.28	0.49
Non-Pet	3.20	0.52
Pet	3.38	0.45

Pet owner questionnaire data

The questionnaire given to pet owners revealed that students report great satisfaction with their decision to live with an animal on campus. A majority of respondents reported no daily stress associated with the routine care of their pet (71%) and little to no stress associated with the responsibility of paying for their pet (83.9%). Approximately 60% of the participants from the pet group reported that they spend an hour or less per day directly caring for their pet (e.g. grooming, walking, feeding, etc.), and 70% of students reported that they spent \$50 or less each month on the routine care for their pet (e.g., purchasing food, cat litter, grooming, etc.).

The majority of students (81%) cited companionship as the being the best part of having their pet on campus. A large number of students (77.4%) also reported that living with their pets positively impacted their ability to fulfill their academic responsibilities. Although pet owners did not differ significantly in their responses to the Perceived Stress Scale when compared to the non-pet condition, 67.7% of pet owners

Table 15.2. Bivariate Associations between Perceived Stress Scale and Psychological Symptomatology Measures, All Participants

	PSS Time 1	PSS Time 2
CES-D	0.79*	0.82*
TICSA: Overall	0.73*	0.73*

*p < 0.001

reported that on a daily basis living with a pet greatly decreased their stress. Finally, there were no questions in which a majority of students reported a negative impact of pet ownership.

Discussion

Results from this study suggest that the relationship between pet ownership and psychological well-being among college students is complex. Overall, there were no significant differences between the pet owners and students in the non-pet condition on the measures of affective symptomatology and stress. One interpretation of these findings is that the unique stresses of owning and caring for an animal while in college may detract from the benefits of living with a family pet. That interpretation does not, however, seem supported by our data. Student pet owners, on average, reported a low investment of both time and money in the care of their pet and little accompanying stress from the responsibility of ownership. Students reported spending only an average of four hours per day with their pets, and so, alternatively, it may be that they are not interacting with their animals enough to benefit from their presence (Watson & Weinstein, 1993). This is not necessarily inconsistent with previous research with adult populations, as not all studies have demonstrated a positive association between pet ownership and owner outcomes (Grossberg et al., 1988).

It is important to note that our data included an equal division of dogs and cats. Previous research has demonstrated a weaker positive effect of cat ownership on positive outcomes (Friedmann et al., 1998) and, in some cases, a higher likelihood of cats contributing to adverse outcomes (Parker et al., 2009). Although our dog and cat owners were not found to differ significantly in their responses to any of our psychological assessments, this may be due to low statistical power given the small size ($n = 16$) of each subgroup. It may be beneficial to focus exclusively on *dog* ownership amongst college students in future studies.

An alternative explanation, albeit one not testable with the current data, is that pet ownership may in fact be having a positive impact on students' psychological functioning but these findings are being obscured by a lack of baseline assessment. In order to qualify for participation in the pet condition students had to already be residing with an animal on campus, and thus we do not have measures of their psychological functioning prior to bringing their pet to school. We also do not have data on how many of the pet owners were residing with an Emotional Support Animal (ESA), although in the previous two years less than one-quarter of animals residing on campus were registered. However, it is potentially telling that in our sample, students in the pet condition were significantly more likely to have a pre-existing psychological disorder than those in the non-pet condition. We would thus anticipate the pet group to have elevated scores on the self-report assessments of depressive and anxious symptomatology. The fact that our pet and non-pet groups were equivalent on these measures may indicate that living with pets does in fact help students to lower their affective symptomatology to sub-clinical levels. This interpretation may also help to explain the fact that pet owners reported experiencing their pet as a daily source of stress relief, yet did not actually score lower on the Perceived Stress Scale than students in the non-pet condition. Assessing the psychological functioning of students both before and after they make the decision to live with a pet on campus represents a promising direction for future research.

Although pet ownership did not lead to any direct difference in depression or anxiety, it did serve to moderate the relationship between stress and anxiety. Even in the context of high stress, pet owners experienced fewer symptoms of somatic anxiety. This finding is consistent with previous research linking animal interaction to improved cardiovascular functioning, such as reduced blood pressure during stressful events (Allen, 2003; Allen et al., 2001; Friedmann, Thomas, & Eddy, 2000).

Qualitative results from the pet survey provide some insight into the students' experience of bringing a family pet to campus. While pet owners did not differ significantly in their responses to the Perceived Stress Scale when compared to the non-pet condition, a majority of pet owners indicated, via the pet owner questionnaire, that on a daily basis living with a pet greatly decreased their stress. This discrepancy between subjective and objective measures was previously reported in a study examining the benefits of pet ownership on a group of patients suffering from chronic fatigue syndrome (Wells, 2009). It raises the interesting question of what it actually means to benefit from living with an animal.

In terms of the positive effects of living with a pet, students were particularly likely to report their animals as being a meaningful source of companionship while at college. It was also common for students to report that their pets helped them to facilitate social ties with their peers. These comments, along with previous research indicating that dogs in particular act as a "social lubricant," helping to encourage interaction amongst strangers (Friedmann & Son, 2009, p. 294), suggest that allowing students to bring a pet to campus may serve as a valuable strategy for recruitment and retention for colleges and universities. Studies have demonstrated that social support is important for all students adjusting to college life (Rayle & Chung, 2007). For example, Dwyer and Cummings (2001) demonstrated that social support from family and friends allows college students to better handle their various academic stressors. It was also found that social support and less loneliness predicted more positive academic persistence decisions among college freshmen (Nicpon et al., 2006). While the current study did not include any freshmen due to Eckerd's policy, this rule has since changed, and students can now bring their animals to campus from their first day of enrollment. A follow-up study focusing on first year students who bring their pets to campus would be a promising next step.

Although there was no reported difference in GPA among the pet and non-pet owners in our sample, previous research suggests that the presence of animals may indeed enhance academic performance (Allen et al., 2001). Exams are a well-known stressor among college students, but our current findings indicate that pet ownership may help to reduce the association between stress and bodily manifestations of anxiety. Given the deleterious impact of anxiety on test performance (Seipp, 1991), it stands to reason that students may be able to use their animals as a direct source of academic, as well as emotional, support. Indeed, more than half of students from both our pet and non-pet groups indicated that they would like to have a dog/cat present while they take an exam. This would be another promising area for future investigation.

The college years represent a period of both significant transition and increased vulnerability. As colleges and universities seek new ways to best support their students, the results of this study suggest that allowing animals to live on campus has few drawbacks, but may also not have many quantifiable psychological benefits. However, given how positively students respond to the opportunity to bring their pets to school with them, it is worth future investigation of the potential physical, academic, or social benefits.

References

Allen, K. (2003). Are pets a healthy pleasure? The influence of pets on blood pressure. *Current Directions in Psychological Science*, *12,* 236-239.

Allen, K., Shykoff, B. E., & Izzo, J. L. (2001). Pet ownership, but not ACE inhibitor therapy, blunts home blood pressure responses to mental stress. *Hypertension*, *38,* 815-820.

American College Health Association. (2015). American College Health Association-National College. Health Assessment II: Reference Group Executive Summary Spring 2015. Hanover, MD: American College Health Association.

Barker, S. B., Barker, R. T., McCain, N. L, & Schubert, C. M. (2016). A randomized crossover exploratory study of the effect of visiting therapy dogs on college student stress before final exams. *Anthrozoös*, *29,* 35-46.

Blanco, C., Okuda, M., Wright, C., Hasin, D. S., Grant, B. F., Liu, S., & Olfson, M. (2008). Mental health of college students and their non-college-attending peers: Results from the National Epidemiologic Study on Alcohol and Related Conditions. *Archive of General Psychiatry*, *65,* 1429-1437.

Cohen, S., Kamarck, T., & Mermelstein, R. (1983). A global measure of perceived stress. *Journal of Health and Social Behavior*, *24,* 385-396.

Dwyer, A. L., & Cummings, A. L. (2001). Stress, self-efficacy, social support, and coping strategies in college students. *Canadian Journal of Counseling*, *35,* 208-220.

Friedmann, E., Katcher, A. H., Lynch, J. J., & Thomas, S. A. (1998). Animal companions and one-year survival of patients after discharge from a coronary unit. *Public Health Reports*, *95,* 307-312.

Friedmann, E., & Son, H. (2009). The human–companion animal bond: how humans benefit. *Veterinary Clinics of North America: Small Animal Practice*, *39,* 293-326.

Friedmann, E., Thomas, S., & Eddy, T. (2000). Companion animals and human health: Physical and cardiovascular influences. In A. L. Podberscek, E. S. Paul, J. A. Serpell (Eds.), *Companion Animals and Us: Exploring the Relationships between People and Pets* (pp. 125-142). Cambridge, UK: Cambridge University Press.

Grossberg, J. M., Alf, E. F., Jr., & Vormbrock, J. K. (1988). Does pet dog presence reduce human cardiovascular responses to stress? *Anthrozoös*, *2,* 38-44.

Headey, B., & Grabka, M. M. (2007). Pets and human health in Germany and Australia: National longitudinal results. *Social Indicators Research*, *80,* 297-311.

Headey, B., Na, F., & Zheng, R. (2008). Pet dogs benefit owners' health: A 'natural experiment' in China. *Social Indicators Research*, *87,* 481-493.

Huss, R. J. (2012). Canines on campus: Companion animals at postsecondary educational institutions. *Missouri Law Review*, *77*, 2, Article 5.

Mistler, B. J., Reetz, D. R., Krylowicz, B., & Barr, V. (2012). *The Association for University and College Counseling Center Directors annual survey*. Retrieved from http://files.cmcglobal.com/Monograph_2012_AUCCCD_Public.pdf

Nicpon, M. F., Huser, L., Blanks, E. H., Sollenberger, S., Befort, C., & Robinson Kurpius, S. E. (2006). The relationship of loneliness and social support with college freshmen's academic performance and persistence. *Journal of College Student Retention: Research, Theory & Practice*, *8,* 345-358.

Oman, D., Shapiro, S. L., Thoresen, C. E., Plante, T. G., & Flinders, T. (2008). Meditation lowers stress and supports forgiveness among college students: A randomized controlled trial. *Journal of American College Health*, *56,* 569-578.

Parker, G., Gayed, A., Owen, C., Hyett, M., Hilton, T., & Heruc, G. (2010). Survival following an acute coronary syndrome: A pet theory put to the test. *Acta Psychiatrica Scandinavica*, *121,* 65–70.

Parslow, R. A., & Jorm, A. F. (2003). Pet ownership and risk factors for cardiovascular disease: Another look. *Medical Journal Australia*, *179,* 466-468.

Parslow, R.A., Jorm, A.F., Christensen, H., Rodgers, B., & Jacomb, P. (2005). Pet ownership and health in older adults: Findings from a survey of 2,551 community-based Australians aged 60–64. *Gerontology*, *51,* 40-47.

Radloff, L. S. (1971). The CES-D scale: A self-report depression scale for research in the general population. *Applied Psychological Measurement*, *1,* 385-401.

Rayle, A. D., & Chung, K-Y. (2007). Revisiting first-year college students' mattering: Social support, academic stress, and the mattering experience. *Journal of College Student Retention: Research, Theory & Practice*, *9,* 21-37.

Ree, M. J., MacLeod, C., French, D., & Locke, V. (2000). The State-Trait Inventory for Cognitive and Somatic Anxiety: Development and validation. Poster session presented at the annual meeting of the Association for the Advancement of Behavior Therapy, New Orleans, LA.

Reynolds, J. A., & Rabschutz, L. (2011). Studying for exams just got more relaxing: Animal assisted activities at the University of Connecticut Library. *College and Undergraduate Libraries*, *18,* 359-367.

Seipp, B. (1991). Anxiety and academic performance: A meta-analysis of findings. *Anxiety Research*, *4,* 27-41.

Siegel, J. M., Angulo, F. J., Detels, R., Wesch, J., & Mullen, A. (1999). AIDS diagnosis and depression in the Multicenter AIDS Cohort Study: The ameliorating impact of pet ownership. *AIDS Care*, *11,* 157-170.

Straatman, I., Hanson, E. K., Endenburg, N., & Mol, J. A. (1997). The influence of a dog on male students during a stressor. *Anthrozoös*, *10,* 191-197.

Towbes, L. C., & Cohen, L. H. (1996). Chronic stress in the lives of college students: Scale development and prospective prediction of distress. *Journal of Youth and Adolescence*, *25,* 199-217.

U.S. Department of Education. (2014). *Financial aid*. Retrieved from https://nces.ed.gov/fastfacts/display.asp?id=31

Watson, N. L., & Weinstein, M. L. (1993). Pet ownership in relation to depression, anxiety, and anger in working women. *Anthrozoös*, *6,* 135-138.

Wells, D. L. (2009). Associations between pet ownership and self-reported health status in people suffering from chronic fatigue syndrome. *Journal of Alternative and Complementary Medicine*, *15,* 407-413.

West, J., Otte, C., Geher, K., Johnson, J., & Mohr, D. C. (2004). Effects of hatha yoga and African dance on perceived stress, affect, and salivary cortisol. *Annals of Behavioral Medicine*, *28,* 114-118.

16 The Effects of Dog–Owner Relationship on Perceived Stress and Happiness

Mónica Teresa González-Ramírez*, René Landero-Hernández and Minerva Vanegas-Farfano[2]

Universidad Autónoma de Nuevo León (UANL), Facultad de Psicología; Av. Universidad S/N Ciudad Universitaria San Nicolás de los Garza Nuevo León, C.P. 66451 México.

Abstract

The purpose of this study was to evaluate the role of the pet–owner relationship on the perceived stress and subjective happiness of the owner, using structural equation modeling. A sample of 483 residents of Mexico, men and women, owners of at least one dog participated in this study. Data collection included The Monash Dog Owner Relationship Scale, the Perceived Stress Scale, the Subjective Happiness Scale and some questions regarding the daily dog–owner interaction. Within its primary results, this study showed a higher level of interaction in dyads and adequate relationships according to owners' perception. The structural model revealed the owner–dog interaction as a predictor of the owner's perception of their relationship; stressors and the dog–owner relationship as predictors of the owner's perceived stress, and stress on subjective happiness. It is concluded that the benefits of the human–animal bond are mediated by the dog–owner relationships' quality and this relationship is determined by their shared activities.

Keywords: pet-effect, human–animal bond, dog-owners, stress, happiness.

Human–animal bond research includes the study of its social, psychological and physiological effects. These effects may come from the contact with different species of animals; or of the ownership and bonding with a pet (Meléndez, 2014).

Some research shows evidence about positive effects of pet's companionship to the human health (Gutiérrez, Granados & Piar, 2007). To a social and psychological level, it is also suggested the decline of depressive symptomatology and negative feelings; as well as the enhancement of self-esteem, physical workout, social interaction and the perception of its support (Meléndez, 2014).

Guastello, Guastello & Guastello (2017) indicates that, the benefits of human–animal bonding had also been compared between non-owners and pet owners. These authors found lesser levels of depression and loneliness in pet owners and higher levels of social interaction compared to non-owners. Other studies that also compared pet owners and non-owners have found differences in both positive and negative emotions; as well as with life's satisfaction; but not in happiness (Bao & Schreer, 2016). In Mexico, it was also found that dog owners perceived themselves as healthier and less stressed; but not happier that non-owners (González-Ramírez & Landero-Hernández, 2014).

The type of pet that a person owns also contributes to these results and, according to Bao &

Corresponding author: email:monygzz77@yahoo.com

Schreer (2016) having a dog is associated to a higher well-being compared to having a cat. Rehn (2013) in the other hand, concludes that, it is not the dog per se, but the type and quality of relationship with it. Thus, people that consider the dog as a family member, show better scores in their perceived health than those that consider them as guardians or pets (González-Ramírez & Landero-Hernández, 2011). In Mexico, the most common pet is the dog (84%) and nearly six out 10 households (58%) report having at least one pet (dog, cat, birds, fish, turtles or rodents) (Campos & Hernández, 2011), consequently it would come from the contact with different species of animals; or of the ownership and bonding with a pet (Mélendez, 2014).

Explaining pet-effect has not been an easy research, different variables such as personality, emotional regulation styles and basic needs have been considered to understand the owner–dog relationship benefits (Bao & Schreer, 2016). Perceived needs support by a pet has been another variable considered to understand the pet-effect. Kanat-Maymon, Antebi & Zilcha-Mano (2016) found perceived needs support by a pet significantly predicted higher well-being but did not predict level of psychological distress.

Considering all these factors, the present research focused in some activities shared by humans and their dogs to evaluate its influence in the quality of their relationship. Perceived stress and happiness were measured, both variables are commonly included in the human–animal bond field and are related; also, avoidance of negative situations that produce stress is one of these mechanisms involved in happiness (Moyano-Díaz, Páez & Torres, 2016). Finally, this research's purpose is to evaluate the role of the dog–owner relationship on the perceived stress and subjective happiness of the owner; the main hypothesis was that dog–owner relationship has an effect over happiness and perceived stress, while perceived stress would be a mediator between the stressors' effect on subjective happiness.

Method

Participants

For this research, participants were recruited among dog owners with residency in Mexico, being this the sole criteria of inclusion. Surveys were distributed on line, via SurveyMonkey®; on social media and following a snow ball sampling method. Incomplete surveys were discarded. All surveys were voluntary and anonymous.

A total sample of 483 persons, with a mean age of 31.5 years (SD=8.8) participated in this research. The majority of them were women (82.2%, and 17.8% men). Slightly above the half of the sample identified themselves as single (51.6%), 33.3% as married, 11.8% in a relationship and the rest as separated or divorced. Of them, 47.2% reported to have only one dog, 26.9% two dogs, 14.3% three dogs and the rest between 4 and 9 dogs. For meeting this research purpose, people were asked to respond the questions thinking only about the dog with which they spend more time.

Regarding the dogs, 51.9% of them were females and 48.1% males; and presented a mean age of 4.1 years (SD=3.1). On average, the dogs had 3.7 years (SD=3.0) living with their owners. According to their owners, 17.6% of the dogs were mixed breed, the rest represent 63 different pure breeds. For a better description of this sample, people were asked to state the size that better represented their animal companion: 32.5% of them were reported as small dog (5 to 12 kilos); 25.3% as medium size (12 to 25 kilos); 17.0% as miniature size (3 to 5 kilos), 22.2% as large size (25 to 40 kilos) and 3.1% as giant size dogs (over 40 kilos).

Measures

In this research the **Monash dog owner relationship scale** (MDORS; Dwyer, Bennett, & Coleman, 2006) in its Mexican adaptation (MDORS-M; González-Ramírez, Vanegas-Farfano & Landero-Hernández, 2017) was used. This scale is based on the Social Interchange Theory, which explains that human relationships are only held when both costs and benefits seem balanced or when the perception of the benefits exceeds the costs; and it is considered as the more robust instrument for the evaluation of the human–dog relationship, from the perception of the human (Payne et al., 2015). This is a 28-item Likert scale, with options from 1 to 5. Arranged in three subscales: (1) dog–owner interaction; (2) perceived emotional closeness;

and (3) perceived costs. For scoring, the perceived costs scale items are reversed and summed to items of the other two subscales. The resultant score indicates the strength of the relationship according to the perception of the owner. In its Mexican adaptation, the MDORS-M scale presented a reliability of α=.082 in dog–owner interaction subscale; α=0.91 in the emotional closeness subscale and α=0.81 in the perceived costs subscale. This scale presents an adequate general reliability of α=0.88 (González-Ramírez et al., 2017).

To obtain information regarding the dogs' routine, participants were asked about the frequency in which play with their dogs, if the dogs could enter to the house and if owner take the dog with them whenever possible. Options to these questions range from 1=less frequently to 4=more frequently.

To measure happiness, we used the **Subjective Happiness Scale** (SHS; Lyubomirsky & Lepper, 1999) in its validated version for Mexican population (Quezada, Landero-Hernández & González-Ramírez, 2016). This is a 4-item Likert-type scale, which measures global subjective happiness by means of statements with which participants either self-rate themselves or compare themselves to others. Normative values of subjective happiness range from 4.55 to 6.65 in the group age of 25 to 34 years and 4.57 to 6.75 in the group age of 35 to 44 years old. The scale showed an adequate level of internal consistency by Cronbach's alpha coefficient=0.77 (Quezada et al., 2016). The Cronbach's alpha was 0.76 for the present study.

The **Perceived stress scale** (PSS; Cohen, Kamarak & Mermelstein, 1983) was used in its Mexican version (González-Ramírez & Landero-Hernández, 2007). The scale contains 14 Likert-type items with a score ranging from 0=never to 4=very often; there are 7 items that need to be reversed due to being in negative form (items 4, 5, 6, 7, 9, 10 and 13). The score ranges from 0 to 56 points, where a higher score corresponds to higher levels of stress. Reference values were proposed by González-Ramírez, Rodríguez-Ayán, & Landero-Hernández (2013) considering mean and standard deviation of their samples; thus, scores within one standard deviation of the mean for each group serve as reference values, describing average stress or expected values in general population. Expected values of perceived stress in this scale range from 12.16 to 29.70 for people with ages between 25 to 34 years and from 15.22 to 31.48 in people with ages ranging 35 to 44 years old (González-Ramírez et al., 2013). The scale exhibited a Cronbach's alpha of 0.83 (González-Ramírez & Landero-Hernández, 2007). The Cronbach's alpha of the present study was 0.86.

A question adapted from Sandin and Chorot's (1987) Life events questionnaire was also included. In its original form, the questionnaire includes 65 stressful situations; in this research only a question about its subescales: work (job), health, love, partner, family, children, social, legal, finance (economic), residence (for example, change of address or city), and academic. The following question was: In the last months, have you dealt with a difficult situation which you considered negative or that caused you stress, anxiety, or depression? In this research only those people that responded affirmatively to this question were included. It was also solicited to indicate to which of the areas correspond their answers and the number of stressful situations was the variable "number of stressors" included in the analysis.

Statistical analysis

Descriptive analysis of the variables was performed. The normal distribution was contrasted with the Kolmogorov-Smirnov test, indicating that scores of all variables were not normally distributed ($p<0.05$). Spearman correlational analysis evaluated associations between ordinal and interval variables. To identify group differences, Mann-Whitney U test was used. IBM®SPSS® Statistics 20 was used for the statistical analyses. Structural equation modeling was conducted in SPSS AMOS 18 (IBM Inc.). For the parameters in the model to be considered statistically significant, a *p* value of less than 0.05 was considered. To test the model fit, we followed the threshold levels recommended by Hooper, Coughlan, & Mullen (2008) with the following performance measures: for χ^2 divided by degrees of freedom [χ^2/df], values less than 3; for goodness of fit index, adjusted goodness of fit index, normed fit index, Tucker–Lewis index, and comparative fit index, values ≥ 0.95; and for root mean square error of approximation, values less than 0.07.

Results

Descriptive

Table 16.1 presents the means and standard deviations of each observed variable. As observed, the daily routine of the participants and their dogs showed a high level of interaction: the participants as a group play with their dogs frequently, let them stay in the house when the owner is in home and take them out whenever possible. No statistical differences were found between sexes. The MDORS-M score presented differences between men and women ($p<0.01$) the female subsample perceived a better relationship with their dogs. No differences were found in gender comparisons of number of stressors, stress or subjective happiness.

Correlations

Most of the evaluated variables presented significant correlation. The correlation between the *dog–owner relationship* with *play frequency* ($r_s=0.509$; $p=0.001$); with *allow the dog to be inside the house* ($r_s=0.481$; $p=0.001$); and with *take the dog with them whenever possible* ($r_s=0.542$; $p=0.001$) were among the strongest. Additionally, a negative and significant relationship was found between the perceived stress and the subjective happiness ($r_s=0.509$; $p=0.001$).

Structural equation model

Based on the theoretical model of González-Ramírez and Landero-Hernández (2006) to explain perceived stress and its consequences from transactional stress theory, and also taking into account the correlations presented in Table 16.2, a hypothetical model was evaluated presenting number of stressors as an exogenous and predictor variable of the perceived stress. In this model, we used the perceived stress as a mediator between the stressors' effect on subjective happiness. While this model also evaluated the dog–owner relationship over the stress; due to the weak correlations between the MDORS-M scale with the stressors and with subjective happiness, no other effects were tested. Thus, the present model includes the three questions concerning the dog–owner routine as predictor variables of the dog–owner relationship.

Standardized parameters (standardized regression weights and correlations) and its significance values are shown in Table 16.3. It is worth noticing that, by including the whole sample in this model, all regressions weights presented significant values; however, no significant correlations were found between the number of stressors and the play-time frequency.

The model showed that the routine questions explained 47% of the dog–owner variance, that is, their *play frequency*, to *allow the dog to be inside the house* and to *take the dog with them whenever possible* fully mediates the dog–owner relationship. Also, the direct effects of the dog–owner relationship and the number of stressors represented a 15% of the perceived stress' variance. The influence of number of stressors on perceived stress had a significant value on these participants: while incrementing this variable a standard deviation, the perceived stress variable incremented 0.384 standard deviations. The pet–owner relationship represented a negative effect over the perceived stress variable (an increment of one standard deviation of the dog–owner relationship represent a decrement of 0.184 standard deviations of perceived stress); which suggests that when the respondents experienced higher levels of dog–owner relationship, they experience much less perceived stress in their life. However, perceived stress represented a direct negative effect on happiness, which presented an explained variance of 29%; indirect effects over this last variable also margin from −0.186 to 0.098.

This study's aim was to evaluate the role of the dog–owner relationship on the perceived stress and subjective well-being of the owner. Considering the presence of statistically significance differences between men and women respondents (Table 16.3), two independent models were also tested. Table 16.4 presents selected goodness of fit indices of the whole sample, and men and women subsamples separately. As can be seen in this table, the three versions of this model present a reasonable fit to the data.

While the three versions of the model showed a good fit, only in the women's model the paths in the effect of the dog–owner relationship over the perceived stress was statistically significant (Table 16.3).

Table 16.1. Descriptive statistics and group differences according to the owner sex.

	Dog–owner daily shared activities			Dog–owner relationship		Stressors	Stress	Subjective happiness	
	Play with the dog	Allow the dog to stay in the house	Take the dog out as a companion when possible	MDORS-M total score	MDORS-M average scores	Number of stressors	Perceived stress scale (PSS) total score	SHS total score	SHS average scores
Total sample (n=483)									
Mean	2.84	3.49	2.60	110.01	3.93	1.72	19.97	21.31	5.33
Median	3.00	4.00	3.00	113.00	4.04	1.00	20.00	22.00	5.50
SD	0.87	0.84	1.01	14.58	0.52	1.19	7.67	3.86	0.97
Men (n=86)									
Mean	2.74	3.34	2.50	104.19	3.72	1.76	18.90	20.92	5.23
Median	3.00	4.00	2.50	107.00	3.82	1.00	18.00	22.00	5.50
SD	0.90	0.93	1.00	14.69	0.52	1.39	8.04	4.62	1.16
Women (n=397)									
Mean	2.86	3.53	2.62	111.27	3.97	1.71	20.20	21.40	5.35
Median	3.00	4.00	3.00	114.00	4.07	1.00	20.00	22.00	5.50
SD	0.86	0.82	1.01	14.27	0.51	1.40	7.58	3.68	0.92
Differences between men and women	Z=–1.151; p=0.250	Z=–1.980; p=0.048	Z=–1.019; p=0.308	Z=–4.278; p=0.001		Z = –0.596; p=0.551	Z=–1.698; p=0.090	Z=–0.626; p=0.531	

Table 16.2. Spearman correlations between the daily dog–owner routine and the scales.

	Play with the dog	Allow the dog to stay in the house	Take the dog out as a companion when possible	MDORS-M scale	Number of stressors	Perceived stress scale (PSS)
Allow the dog to stay in the house	0.351**					
Take the dog out as a companion when possible	0.371**	0.353**				
MDORS-M scale	0.509**	0.481**	0.542**			
Number of stressors	0.037	0.131**	–0.097*	–0.056		
PSS scale	–0.090*	0.013	–0.150**	–0.211**	0.372**	
SHS scale	0.117*	0.055	0.051	0.133**	–0.208**	–0.509**

**Correlation is significant at the 0.01 level (2-tailed).
*Correlation is significant at the 0.05 level.05 (2-tailed).

A new model was tested to understand if this difference in the effect of the dog–owner relationship over the perceived stress was explained by respondents' gender or by the quality of the dog–owner relationship. This fourth model included both respondents with the best and worst relationship (highest and lowest scores in the MDORS-M). Three groups were made considering, as cut-off points, means and standard deviations from study where Monash scale was translated and analyzed for Mexico (MDORS-M; González et al., 2017). Groups resulted are presented in Table 16.5. Thus, a hundred and thirty-two participants presenting the highest and lowest scores in the MDORS-M scale, those with score values falling over a standard deviation or above it (M=112, SD=14.1), were included in model 4.

As can be seen in Table 16.3, the explained variance of the dog–owner relationship and the perceived stress increased in model 4. Fig. 16.1 shows the model supported by the data of the participants with the highest and lowest scores on the MDORS-M scale showed an adequate goodness of fit (Table 16.4). Models 1 to 4 remain essentially unchanged. Routinely activities have a positive influence on the dog-relationship. Dog–owner relationship and the number of stressors have a direct and negative effect on the perceived stress. The more perceived stress experienced by participants, the less subjective happiness they reported.

Finally, differences of the perceived stress and subjective happiness values between men and women were evaluated on each MDORS-M subgroup. As seen in Table 16.5, the equivalency in most of their values supported that men and women were considered as a single group. Mann-Whitney U test was used to compare both, men and women; while Kruskal-Wallis test was used to compare the three MDORS-M dog-owners' quality of relationship, which confirms that both perceived stress and subjective happiness vary according to the dog–owner relationship.

Discussion

The main purpose of this research was to contribute to the explanation of the pet-effect, exploring its effect on the human happiness and stress; to achieve it, a model that included the variables of dog–owner relationship, stressors, perceived stress and happiness was performed. Testing this model is also a contribution in happiness study field, as Moyano-Diaz et al. (2016) indicates, is relevant to identify predictor variables of happiness that could be changed, in this study, perceived stress is an important predictor of happiness.

Participants were people who reported subjective happiness and perceived stress scores within the reference values for group aging suggested by Quezada et al. (2016) and González-Ramírez

Table 16.3. Parameter comparisons of the estimated models.

			Total sample (n=483)		Men (n=86)		Women (n=397)		Extreme values (n=132)	
			S	p	S	p	S	p	S	p
Dog–owner relationship	⇦	Take the dog out as a companion when possible	0.321	0.001	0.399	0.001	0.308	0.001	0.492	0.001
Dog–owner relationship	⇦	Allow the dog to stay in the house	0.307	0.001	0.212	0.020	0.323	0.001	0.197	0.002
Dog–owner relationship	⇦	Play with the dog	0.281	0.001	0.261	0.005	0.289	0.001	0.269	0.001
Perceived stress	⇦	Number of stressors	0.348	0.001	0.411	0.001	0.349	0.001	0.351	0.001
Perceived stress	⇦	Dog–owner relationship	–0.184	0.001	0.040	0.691	–0.256	0.001	–0.356	0.001
Subjective happiness (SHS average score)	⇦	Perceived stress	–0.534	0.001	–0.645	0.001	–0.511	0.001	–0.552	0.001
Take the dog out as a companion when possible	⇔	Allow the dog to stay in the house	0.371	0.001	0.398	0.001	0.362	0.001	0.554	0.001
Take the dog out as a companion when possible	⇔	Play with the dog	0.361	0.001	.432	0.001	0.343	0.001	0.570	0.001
Allow the dog to stay in the house	⇔	Play with the dog	0.345	0.001	0.472	0.001	0.310	0.001	0.495	0.001
Number of stressors	⇔	Take the dog out as a companion when possible	–0.097	0.035	–0.351	0.002	–0.030	0.547	–0.083	0.346
Number of stressors	⇔	Allow the dog to stay in the house	0.122	0.008	0.101	0.353	0.130	0.010	0.153	0.083
Number of stressors	⇔	Play with the dog	0.028	0.542	–0.041	0.704	0.048	0.343	–0.001	0.990
			Total Sample		Men		Women		Extreme scores	
Explained variance		Dog–owner relationship	47%		48%		47%		67%	
		Perceived stress	15%		17%		18%		25%	
		Subjective happiness	29%		42%		26%		27%	

S=Standardized estimates.
p=Statistical significance.

Table 16.4. Goodness-of-fit statistics of estimated models.

				Absolute Fit Index				Incremental Fit Index	
	X^2	Df	P	X^2/df	GFI	AGFI	RMSEA	NFI	CFI
Total sample	20.717	9	0.014	2.302	0.988	0.963	0.052	0.973	0.984
Men (n=86)	12.617	9	0.181	1.402	0.962	0.881	0.069	0.934	0.979
Women (n=397)	12.088	9	0.208	1.343	0.991	0.973	0.029	0.980	0.995
Extreme values (n = 132)	11.280	9	0.257	1.253	0.976	0.924	0.044	0.968	0.993

Table 16.5. Participant's distribution according to the dog–human relationship, and differences of perceived stress and subjective happiness.

			Subjective Happiness (SHS)				Perceived Stress (PSS)			
MDORS-M subgroups		n	Median	Mean	SD	Mann-Whitney U test	Median	Mean	SD	Mann-Whitney U test
Less than one SD	Men	27	22.00	20.96	4.34	Z=–0.526; p=0.599	18.00	19.30	7.78	Z=–2.691; p=.007
	Women	63	21.00	20.60	3.44		22.00	23.03	6.75	
	Total	90	21.50	20.71	3.71		21.00	21.91	7.23	
Within one SD	Men	58	22.00	21.02	4.73	Z=–0.264; p=0.792	18.00	18.55	8.19	Z=–1.606; p= 0.108
	Women	293	22.00	21.34	3.69		20.00	20.24	7.58	
	Total	351	22.00	21.28	3.88		20.00	19.96	7.7	
Over one SD	Men	1	14.00			Z=–1.711; p=0.087	28			Z=–1.614; p =0.106
	Women	41	22.00	23.07	3.51		14.00	15.59	6.62	
	Total	42	22.00	22.86	3.74		14.40	15.88	6.81	
Kruskal-Wallis test			H=9.058; p=0.011				H=16.456; p=0.001			

et al. (2013) respectively. Thus, findings could reflect what happens in people with average scores of these variables. Although, those who reported the highest levels of happiness and lowest levels of perceived stress, also presented the higher values in dog–owner relationship.

According to our research, men and women presented differences in their dog–owner relationship, as seen in the MDORS-M scale's values. In a previous research, Herzog (2007) found that responses between sexes are more similar than different; but also found that women, on average, show higher levels of positive behaviors and attitudes toward animals in many areas of human–animal interactions.

Based on theory and research, we did propose and test a mediation model of dog–owner relationship, perceived stress and subjective happiness to explain the human perception over the relationship with their own dogs. Three interaction activities were measured to meet this purpose: their play frequency, whether the dog can stay in the house if supervised and; if they take the dog with them whenever possible. These independent variables did not show significant differences between sexes, although showed significant correlation with dog–human relationship. This finding is not too surprising. In previous research, time spent as a dyad was related with emotional closeness or activities that require more owner engagement with the dog, like dog sports (Meyer & Forkman, 2014; Payne et al., 2015). Thus, routine interaction was likely to be perceived as a similarly positive experience that triggers emotional closeness responses.

The three independent variables used to measure the dog–owner quotidian interaction explained 47% of the total variance of MDORS, and reached 67% in the last model. In previous research where the variance in MDORS scores has been investigated, variables included in structural models have only predicted a small proportion of it. For example, in Meyer & Forkman (2014) research, where owner characteristics appeared to influence the dog–owner relationship more than the dog's personality traits, their

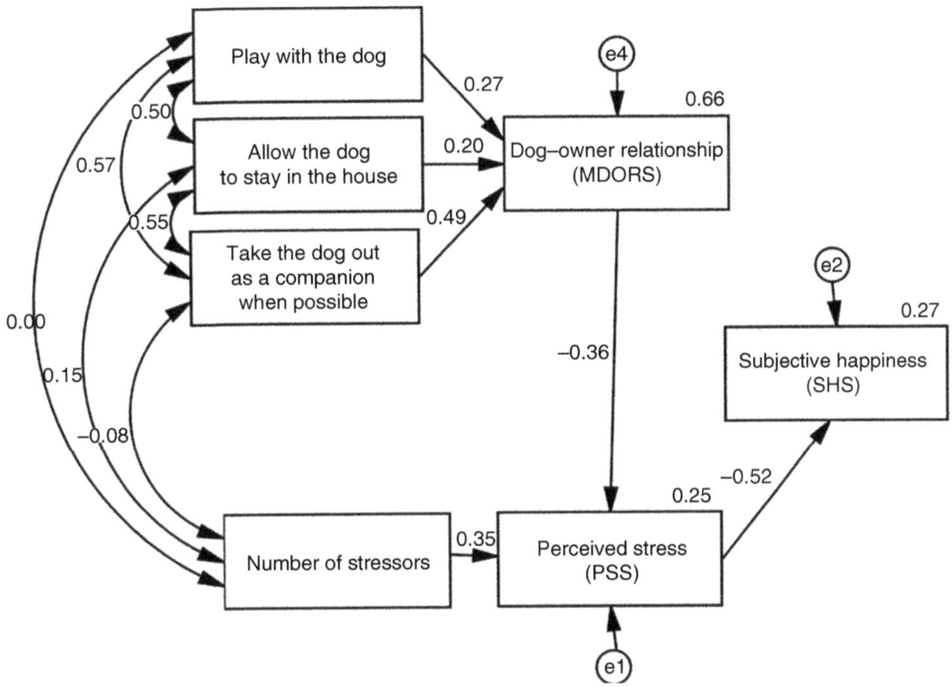

Fig. 16.1. Structural model of the dog–owner relationship effect on the owner's perceived stress and subjective happiness. Model includes participants with extreme values according to the MDORS–Mscores (± 1 SD).

estimated models could only explain 8% of the emotional closeness variance, and 6% of the total variance of the perceived cost using this same scale. Supported in this research and our data, it is possible to conclude that shared activities is the best predictor of the human perception of their pets' relationship. This idea has similarities to Dotson & Hyatt's (2008), who suggested that quantity and quality of time shared with the dog have a strong impact on the experience of the underlying dog-companionship dimensions.

A major contribution of our study is differences in explained variance of happiness between sexes. Men's subjective happiness reached a 42% of explained variance, while in women this value only represented 26%. This finding is relevant because it suggests the important role of the stress' perception as predictor of male subjective happiness; and that future research should add other variables to explain its difference to females.

This study found different effects of the human–dog relationship over the perceived stress, related to gender. While in the men's model this effect did not reach statistical significance, the women's one did. As mentioned early, in this research women had higher MDORS-M scores than men, which may possible relate to the quality of their relationship, and not to gender differences. Considering this possibility, a fourth model was tested including only those participants with extreme score values in their MDORS-M (± 1 SD). This model confirmed the observed effects of the previous three proposals and an increment in the explained variance of the perceived stress and dog–human relationship. It is necessary to notice that, in this model, the group that presented a better relationship with their dog only included one male respondent; a common occurrence in these kinds of studies where most of the participants are women (e.g., Bennett & Rohlf, 2007; González-Ramírez & Landero-Hernández, 2011).

According to the results, initial hypothesis was partially supported. Perceived stress is a mediator between the stressors' effect on subjective happiness. Dog–owner relationship has an effect over perceived stress, but not a direct effect on subjective happiness.

The resulting models and the differences shown in Table 16.5, suggest altogether that benefit of owning a dog, over perceived stress and subjective happiness, is determined by the quality of the dog–owner relationship. In other words, for achieving the pet-effect, having a pet is not enough; dog ownership must include quality and constancy in their interaction.

Conclusion

Dogs that spend more time with their owner in their house, as company in daily activities or playing, not only present a better relationship, they are also linked to a lesser perception of stress in the owners. According to social support theory, one of the theories commonly used to interpret the positive humans' health effects of pets, animals are considered a source of social support (Beck & Katcher, 2003). This perception of support provided by pets could explain that the dog–owner interaction helps human to relax, contributes to a lesser perception of stress, and the recognition of subjective happiness. This research results also support the notion that, what affects people are not the quantity of stressors they face, basic proposal of transactional stress theory (González-Ramírez & Landero-Hernández, 2006); but how they perceive those situations, and how this cognition influences subjective happiness.

As limitations of the study we have, most of the participants are women. Also, it should be considered that to perform this research, the main inclusion criteria was to be a dog–owner. Sampling method could influence that people participating were those who had best dog–owner relationship. A biasing effect of this restriction could make it unrepresentative of the population: the participants' desirability to report a high level of interaction with their dogs may threatened the generalizability of this data.

The present study concludes that the benefits of the human–animal bond are mediated by the quality of the relationship with the dog and, that this relationship is determined by the activities shared with the dog.

References

Bao, K. J. & Schreer, G. (2016). Pets and happiness: examining the association between pet ownership and wellbeing. *Anthrozoös, 29*(2), 283-296. doi: http://dx.doi.org/10.1080/08927936.2016.1152721

Beck, A. M., & Katcher, A. H. (2003). Future directions in human-animal bond research. *American Behavioral Scientist, 47*(1), 79-93. doi: http://dx.doi.org/10.1177/0002764203255214

Bennett, P.C., & Rohlf, V.I. (2007). Owner-companion dog interactions: relationships between demographic variables, potentially problematic behaviours, training engagement and shared activities. *Applied Animal Behaviour Science, 102*(1–2), 65e84. doi:https://doi.org/10.1016/j.applanim.2006.03.009

Campos, R. & Hernández, A.M. (2011). México: las mascotas en nuestros hogares. Encuesta nacional en viviendas. México, D.F.: Consulta Mitofsky.

Cohen, S., Kamarak, T., & Mermelstein, R. (1983). A global measure of perceived stress. *Journal of Health and Social Behavior, 24,* 385–396. doi: http://dx.doi.org/10.2307/2136404

Dotson, M. J., & Hyatt, E. M. (2008). Understanding dog–human companionship. *Journal of Business Research, 61*(5), 457–466. doi: http://dx.doi.org/10.1016/j.jbusres.2007.07.019

Dwyer, F., Bennett, P.C. & Coleman, G.J. (2006). Development of the Monash Dog Owner Relationship Scale (MDORS). *Anthrozoös 19,* 243–256. doi: http://dx.doi.org/10.2752/089279306785415592

González-Ramírez, M.T. & Landero-Hernández, R. (2006). Síntomas psicosomáticos y teoría transaccional del estrés. *Ansiedad y Estrés, 12*(1), 45–61.

González-Ramírez M. T., & Landero-Hernández, R. (2007). Factor structure of the Perceived Stress Scale (PSS) in a sample from Mexico. *The Spanish Journal of Psychology, 10,* 199–206.

González-Ramírez, M.T. & Landero-Hernández, R. (2011). Diferencias en estrés percibido, salud mental y física de acuerdo al tipo de relación humano-perro. *Revista Colombiana de Psicología, 20*(1), 75–86.

González-Ramírez, M.T., & Landero-Hernández, R. (2014). Benefits of dog ownership: comparative study of equivalent samples. *Journal of Veterinary Behavior: Clinical Applications and Research, 9*(6), 311–315. doi: http://dx.doi.org/10.1016/j.jveb.2014.08.002

González-Ramírez, M., Rodríguez-Ayán, M. & Landero-Hernández, R. (2013). The perceived stress scale (PSS): Normative data and factor structure for a large-sample in Mexico. *The Spanish Journal of Pyschology, 16*, E47, doi: http://dx.doi.org/10.1017/sjp.2013.35

Gonzalez-Ramirez, M.T., Vanegas-Farfano, M., Landero-Hernández, R. (2017). Versión mexicana de la escala Monash de relación del dueño con su perro (MDORS-M). *Alternativas en Psicología, 37*, 107–123.

Guastello, A.D., Guastello, D. D., & Guastello, S. J. (2017). Personality differences between dog people and cat people. *Human-Animal Interaction Bulletin, 5*(1), 41–57.

Gutiérrez, G., Granados, D. & Piar, N. (2007). Interacciones humano-animal: características e implicaciones para el bienestar de los humanos. *Revista Colombiana de Psicología, 16*, 163–184.

Herzog, H. (2018). The impact of pets on human health and psychological well-being fact, fiction, or hypothesis? *Current Directions in Psychological Science, 20*, 236–239.

Hooper, D., Coughlan, J., & Mullen, M. (2008). Structural equation modelling: Guidelines for determining model fit. *Electronic Journal of Business Research Methods, 6*(1), 53–60.

Kanat-Maymon, Y., Antebi, A., & Zilcha-Mano, S. (2016). Basic psychological need fulfillment in human–pet relationships and well-being. *Personality and Individual Differences, 92*, 69–73. doi: http://dx.doi.org/10.1016/j.paid.2015.12.025

Lyubomirsky, S., & Lepper, H. S. (1999). A measure of subjective happiness: Preliminary reliability and construct validation. *Social Indicators Research, 46*, 137–155. doi: http://dx.doi.org/10.1023/A:1006824100041

Meléndez, L. (2014). El vínculo humano-animal y sus implicaciones para la psicología en puerto rico. *Revista Puertorriqueña de Psicología, 25*(2), 160–182

Meyer, I., & Forkman, B. (2014). Dog and owner characteristics affecting the dog–owner relationship. *Journal of Veterinary Behavior: Clinical Applications and Research, 9*(4), 143–150. doi: http://dx.doi.org/10.1016/j.jveb.2014.03.002

Moyano-Díaz, E., Páez, D., & Torres, M. (2016). Propiedades psicométricas del cuestionario para medir estrategias de aumento de la felicidad (HIS) en versión castellana (CEA-EAP). *Terapia Psicológica, 34*(2), 143–154.

Payne, E., Bennett, P. C., & McGreevy, P. D. (2015). Current perspectives on attachment and bonding in the dog–human dyad. *Psychology Research and Behavior Management, 8*, 71–79 doi: http://dx.doi.org/10.2147/PRBM.S74972

Quezada, L., Landero-Hernández, R. & Gonzalez-Ramirez, M. T. (2016). A validity and reliability study of the Subjective Happiness Scale in Mexico. *The Journal of Happiness & Well-Being, 4*(1), 90–100.

Rehn, T. (2013) Best of Friends? Investigating the Dog-Human Relationship. Doctoral Thesis. Swedish University of Agricultural Sciences. Print: SLU Service/Repro, Uppsala.

Sandín, B. & Chorot, P. (1987). *Cuestionario de Sucesos Vitales (CSV)*. Madrid: Universidad Nacional de Educación a Distancia (UNED).

17 Conclusion

Lori Kogan
Colorado State University, USA

The chapters in this book reflect a rich, diverse sample of research that explores the impact of animals on human stress. Together, they provide a solid foundation suggesting that in a multitude of settings, with a variety of different populations, animal interaction offers a viable method for decreasing human stress and anxiety. However, these studies have only tapped the surface of what is possible. There are several important elements to highlight as we continue this line of research, including standardization of definitions, better-designed research studies that include a diversity of participants, and a clear commitment to the assessment and protection of animal welfare.

A recent article by Binder et al. (2024) highlighted the importance of consistent language to help both researchers and practitioners communicate effectively. Non-standardized terminology impedes the ability to compare studies and conduct meta-analyses. In Alfrey's chapter, which reviewed the literature to explore what effect dogs have on children's performance on cognitive tests, their search included "dog" OR "canine" OR "canine-assisted" OR "dog-assisted" OR "therapy dog" OR "assistance dog" OR "facility dog" OR "human–animal interaction" OR "animal-assisted". However, even with this extensive list of terms, they still felt the need to review the reference lists of relevant articles, and search digital research archives, the Human Animal Bond Research Institute (HABRI) research repository, and Google to ensure they did not miss any papers. The lack of consistent terminology can be witnessed even within this book's chapters, whereby a variety of terms are used for animal-assisted service, including human–animal interaction (HAI) (Thayer and Stevens), canine interaction (Banks et al.), and canine-assisted intervention (Manville et al. and Binfet et al.).

To address the issue of uniform terminology, two international organizations, Animal-Assisted Intervention International (AAII) and the International Association of Human–Animal Interaction Organizations (IAHAIO), formed an international task force, the International Consortium of Animal-assisted Interactions (IC-AAI). As a result of their extensive work, they proposed the use of the term animal-assisted service (AAS) to replace animal-assisted intervention (AAI) as the umbrella term for the full spectrum of practices in which animals are included in various roles for the benefit of humans (Binder et al., 2024). They defined AAS as "the mediated, guided or facilitator-led practices, programs and human services that incorporate specially qualified animals into therapeutic, educational, supportive and/or ameliorative processes aimed at enhancing the well-being of humans while ensuring the welfare of the animals involved in these practices." They categorize AAS as a component of HAIs, which are described as any relationship between people and animal(s). They went on to explain and define the three categories of AAS: animal-assisted treatment (AATx), animal-assisted education (AAE), and animal-assisted support programs (AASPs) (Binder et al., 2024).

Binder et al. defined AATx (and suggested that it replace animal-assisted therapy (AAT)) as "a class of mental or physical health professional treatment modalities for which the integration of animals, directly or indirectly, is a critical component of the treatment approach of the professional." They define AAE as "any educational program in which animals are integrated, directly or indirectly, as a critical component of an ongoing educational process" and AASPs (to replace animal-assisted activities) as "programs in which animals are engaged, directly or indirectly, in activities aimed at supporting and enhancing the well-being of humans" (Binder et al., 2024).

Another key element in helping advance the field involves assessing and minimizing biases. Although there is a commonly held belief that animals help improve people's physical and psychological health, numerous studies suggest that this impact is nuanced. The chapter by Martos-Montes et al., for example, found that a dog's presence significantly reduced students' anxiety and heart rate but not their blood pressure. Thayer and Stevens' chapter found that dog interaction had a positive effect on students' affect but no effect on executive functioning, and Banks et al. found that interacting with a dog was associated with lower levels of perceived stress and state anxiety but had no effect on sustained attention, mind wandering, or speed of processing. Several recent meta-analyses on AAS illustrate this point (Charry-Sánchez et al., 2018; Hu et al., 2018; Ribeiro et al., 2023; Zafra-Tanaka et al., 2019).

Inconsistent results seen within HAI studies are another issue that warrants attention. Certainly, variability in study results is seen in other fields (e.g., psychology, medicine) (Herrera-Perez et al., 2019; Open Science Collaboration, 2015), although attention to inconsistencies within research methods and design could help reduce this variability. While it is encouraging to see more randomized clinical trial (RCT) designs published in recent years, even RCTs can vary in terms of rigorousness. Many studies can inadvertently inject bias, may lack a control group, or may offer differing types of control groups (e.g., active control, no treatment, treatment as usual) that can influence results (Rodriguez et al., 2021).

Just as AAS studies illustrate the fact that animals do not help everyone uniformly, studies assessing the impact of pet ownership also suggest that the "pet effect" is not felt equally by all. While numerous studies suggest that pet ownership offers an array of benefits to humans (Hughes et al., 2020; Janssens et al., 2020), other studies have found that pets have no positive effect (or even a negative effect) on owners' mental and physical health (Gilbey & Tani, 2015; Herzog, 2011). For example, in this book, Highfill and Goodman-Wilson reported no significant differences between college student pet owners and non-pet owners when assessing depression or anxiety, and González-Ramírez et al. reported positive effects for female dog owners but not male owners. Regardless of whether one is studying AAS or pet ownership, clear operationalization of methods and standards and methodical evaluation are critical (Fine, 2019; Fine & Beck, 2015; Rodriguez et al., 2021).

Another challenge within HAI research is the lack of diversity among researchers, practitioners, and recipients (Jensen et al., 2023; Smith, 2019). One recent study involving HAI university-affiliated centers highlighted this fact. Jensen et al. (2023) found that the majority of these centers' faculty, staff, and students are white, non-Hispanic. In addition, all the center directors in the sample self-identified as white, predominantly non-Hispanic (89%) and female (72%). This need for increased diversity within HAI research has been highlighted in several recent studies (Applebaum et al., 2021, 2023; Hawes et al., 2023; Risley-Curtiss et al., 2006). This will likely involve concentrated efforts to reach a more diverse population. It is imperative to have knowledge pertaining to the targeted population to help ensure that recruitment strategies are culture sensitive (Liu et al., 2011). It is also worth noting that different ethnic groups may prefer different recruitment strategies, so a variety of recruitment methods, including both active and passive strategies, will need to be employed to help ensure a more representative sample in future studies (Ramirez et al., 2008).

The welfare of animals involved in AAS is another critical important topic. In the past,

AAS focused on the benefits for humans and paid little heed to the impact on the animals involved. As the field evolved, however, researchers and practitioners began to assess the stress levels of the animals involved to ensure they were not suffering negative effects. This early focus on animal welfare considered the animals' basic needs (freedom from hunger/thirst, discomfort, pain/injury/disease, fear, and distress, and the freedom to express normal behavior) (Webster, 2016). Advances in our understanding of animal cognition (Bekoff, 2007; Berns, 2020) and the fact that animals are sentient beings that experience an array of emotions, however, has led many to believe that a lack of suffering or stress is setting the bar too low. There is a growing sentiment that providers of AAS have a moral and ethical obligation to ensure that AAS is *mutually* beneficial and that the animals' needs are taken into account (Marinelli et al., 2009; Ng, 2021; Townsend & Gee, 2021; Winkle et al., 2020). It is increasingly understood that humans should benefit from HAIs only if the animals benefit as well (Enders-Slegers & Hediger, 2019; Fine et al., 2015; Glenk, 2017; Glenk et al., 2014; Hauben-hofer & Kirchengast, 2006; Ng, 2021; Wijnen & Martens, 2022; Winkle et al., 2020).

To this end, the One Health model has been proposed as a foundation for AAS research, providing a framework to help identify the benefits and risks for humans and animals (Animal-Assisted Intervention International, 2019; Fine & Griffin, 2022; Hediger et al., 2019; International Association of Human–Animal Interaction Organizations, 2018; Liguori et al., 2023; Menna et al., 2019; Pet Partners, 2018). The One Health concept recognizes that human health, animal health, and the environment are all interconnected. From a One Health perspective, AAS should benefit all participants, both humans and non-human animals (Glenk & Foltin, 2021), and it is not acceptable to obtain human benefits at the cost of animal health or well-being (Hediger et al., 2019; Menna et al., 2019). To help ensure the welfare of the animals involved in AAS studies, it is important to use established guidelines (e.g., American Veterinary Medical Association, n.d.; Fine, 2019; Lefebvre et al., 2008), including time limits, strictly reward-based, positive-reinforcement training and control methods, and regular evaluations for changes in behavior/temperament (Serpell et al., 2020).

Although there is growing consensus as to the importance of protecting animal welfare when conducting AAS, how best to assess animal welfare demands careful consideration. Animal welfare is the "state of an animal in its attempts to cope with changes in its environment" (Broom, 1991), a multidimensional construct comprised of good health, comfort, and expression of behavior (Botreau et al., 2007). Welfare assessment often involves an observer's subjective evaluation of an animal's response to change from the animal's perspective (Hiby et al., 2006). Because this can be challenging, multiple and varied objective assessments of welfare are suggested (Browning, 2022). This is typically accomplished with a combination of behavioral observation and noninvasive physiologic measurements. The most common physiologic parameter to assess stress and welfare is cortisol, often measured through the collection of saliva (Hennessy et al., 1998, 1998). Measuring cortisol levels requires attention to numerous factors in addition to stress including age, sex, breed, and disease state (Hennessy et al., 1998; Kirschbaum & Hellhammer, 2008). The timing of sampling is also an important factor, with researchers reporting a 15–20-minute delay in increased cortisol levels in the circulation after a stressful event (Handlin et al., 2012). Body temperature, heart rate, and respiratory rate are other indicators of stress that have been utilized in AAS research (Clark et al., 2020; Malinowski et al., 2018).

Behavioral observation is the easiest way to assess welfare, but it must be conducted in a structured and organized manner (Ng, 2021). An ethogram based on natural observation of the animal in the AAS session can be helpful (Winkle & Johnson, 2023). In addition, to help ensure animal welfare, it is important that handlers are knowledgeable about zoonotic diseases and infection-control practices (Howie, 2021). Handlers must also be able to accurately assess their animal's welfare, including the conditions that might place their animal at risk, and take action to either modify the intervention or remove the animal before welfare is compromised (Ng, 2021). This means that handlers must be willing to prioritize their animal's welfare, even if it means ending an AAS session prematurely (Howie, 2021). Handlers are their animal's protector; they must be able to monitor their animal's stress signals while maintaining awareness of the environment and interacting with those receiving AAS (Townsend & Gee, 2021).

In conclusion, the chapters in this book, together with a recent scoping review (Gandenberger et al., 2022), offer numerous examples of how animals can positively impact human stress. They provide a foundation from which to continue this important line of research. Future research in this area can benefit from the use of common terminology, clear descriptions of methodologies and operating protocols, the inclusion of ethnically and racially diverse participants, and a commitment to prioritize animal welfare. Attention to these factors can help the field move toward a more definitive answer as to how, and for whom, animals impact human stress.

References

Animal-Assisted Intervention International. (2019). *Animal-Assisted Intervention International Standards of Practice*. Animal-Assisted Intervention International. https://aai-int.org/wpcontent/uploads/2019/02/AAII-Standards-of-Practice.pdf

Applebaum, J. W., MacLean, E. L., & McDonald, S. E. (2021). Love, fear, and the human-animal bond: On adversity and multispecies relationships. *Comprehensive Psychoneuroendocrinology*, *7*, 100071. https://doi.org/10.1016/j.cpnec.2021.100071

Applebaum, J. W., Peek, C. W., & Zsembik, B. A. (2023). Examining U.S. pet ownership using the General Social Survey. *The Social Science Journal*, *60*(1), 110–119. https://doi.org/10.1080/03623319.2020.1728507

American Veterinary Medical Association. (n.d.). *Animal-assisted interventions: Guidelines*. American Veterinary Medical Association. https://www.avma.org/resources-tools/animal-health-and-welfare/service-emotional-support-and-therapy-animals/animal-assisted-interventions-guidelines

Bekoff, M. (2007). *The Emotional Lives of Animals: A Leading Scientist Explores Animal Joy, Sorrow and Empathy – and Why They Matter*. Dominican University of California. https://scholar.dominican.edu/cynthia-stokes-brown-books-big-history/96

Berns, G. (2020). Decoding the canine mind. *Cerebrum: The Dana Forum on Brain Science*, *2020*, cer-04-20.

Binder, A. J., Parish-Plass, N., Kirby, M., Winkle, M., Skwerer, D. P., Ackerman, L., Brosig, C., Coombe, W., Delisle, E., Enders-Slegers, M.-J., Fowler, J.-A., Hey, L., Howell, T., Kaufman, M., Kienast, M., Kinoshita, M., Ngai, D., & Wijnen, B. (2024). Recommendations for uniform terminology in animal-assisted services (AAS). *Human–Animal Interactions*, *12*(1). https://doi.org/10.1079/hai.2024.0003

Botreau, R., Veissier, I., Butterworth, A., Bracke, M. B. M., & Keeling, L. J. (2007). Definition of criteria for overall assessment of animal welfare. *Animal Welfare*, *16*(2), 225–228. https://doi.org/10.1017/S0962728600031390

Broom, D. M. (1991). Animal welfare: Concepts and measurement. *Journal of Animal Science*, *69*(10), 4167–4175. https://doi.org/10.2527/1991.69104167x

Browning, H. (2022). Assessing measures of animal welfare. *Biology & Philosophy*, *37*(4), 36. https://doi.org/10.1007/s10539-022-09862-1

Charry-Sánchez, J. D., Pradilla, I., & Talero-Gutiérrez, C. (2018). Effectiveness of animal-assisted therapy in the pediatric population: Systematic review and meta-analysis of controlled studies. *Journal of Developmental & Behavioral Pediatrics*, *39*(7), 580–590. https://doi.org/10.1097/DBP.0000000000000594

Clark, S. D., Martin, F., McGowan, R. T. S., Smidt, J. M., Anderson, R., Wang, L., Turpin, T., Langenfeld-McCoy, N., Bauer, B. A., & Mohabbat, A. B. (2020). Physiological state of therapy dogs during animal-assisted activities in an outpatient setting. *Animals*, *10*(5), Article 5. https://doi.org/10.3390/ani10050819

Enders-Slegers, M.-J., & Hediger, K. (2019). Pet ownership and human–animal interaction in an aging population: Rewards and challenges. *Anthrozoös*, *32*(2), 255–265. https://doi.org/10.1080/08927936.2019.1569907

Fine, A. H. (2019). *Handbook on Animal-Assisted Therapy: Foundations and Guidelines for Animal-Assisted Interventions*. Academic Press.

Fine, A. H., & Beck, A. M. (2015). Chapter 1 – Understanding our kinship with animals: Input for health care professionals interested in the human–animal bond. In A. H. Fine (Ed.), *Handbook on Animal-Assisted Therapy, 4th edition* (pp. 3–10). Academic Press. https://doi.org/10.1016/B978-0-12-801292-5.00001-8

Fine, A. H., & Griffin, T. C. (2022). Protecting animal welfare in animal-assisted intervention: Our ethical obligation. *Seminars in Speech and Language*, *43*(1), 8–23. https://doi.org/10.1055/s-0041-1742099

Fine, A. H., Tedeschi, P., & Elvove, E. (2015). Chapter 3 – Forward thinking: The evolving field of human–animal interactions. In A. H. Fine (Ed.), *Handbook on Animal-Assisted Therapy, 4th edition* (pp. 21–35). Academic Press. https://doi.org/10.1016/B978-0-12-801292-5.00003-1

Gandenberger, J., Flynn, E., Moratto, E., Wendt, A., & Morris, K. N. (2022). molecular biomarkers of adult human and dog stress during canine-assisted interventions: A systematic scoping review. *Animals*, *12*(5), Article 5. https://doi.org/10.3390/ani12050651

Gilbey, A., & Tani, K. (2015). Companion animals and loneliness: A systematic review of quantitative studies. *Anthrozoös*, *28*(2), 181–197. https://doi.org/10.1080/08927936.2015.11435396

Glenk, L. M. (2017). Current perspectives on therapy dog welfare in animal-assisted interventions. *Animals*, *7*(2). https://doi.org/10.3390/ani7020007

Glenk, L. M., & Foltin, S. (2021). Therapy dog welfare revisited: A review of the literature. *Veterinary Sciences*, *8*(10), Article 10. https://doi.org/10.3390/vetsci8100226

Glenk, L. M., Kothgassner, O. D., Stetina, B. U., Palme, R., Kepplinger, B., & Baran, H. (2014). Salivary cortisol and behavior in therapy dogs during animal-assisted interventions: A pilot study. *Journal of Veterinary Behavior*, *9*(3), 98–106. https://doi.org/10.1016/j.jveb.2014.02.005

Handlin, L., Nilsson, A., Ejdebäck, M., Hydbring-Sandberg, E., & Uvnäs-Moberg, K. (2012). Associations between the psychological characteristics of the human–dog relationship and oxytocin and cortisol levels. *Anthrozoös*, *25*(2), 215–228. https://doi.org/10.2752/175303712X13316289505468

Haubenhofer, D. K., & Kirchengast, S. (2006). Physiological arousal for companion dogs working with their owners in animal-assisted activities and animal-assisted therapy. *Journal of Applied Animal Welfare Science*, *9*(2), 165–172. https://doi.org/10.1207/s15327604jaws0902_5

Hawes, S., Gutierrez, L., Rojas, L., Cohen, R., Camacho, B., Taeckens, A., Hupe, T., & Ekholm Fry, N. (2023). Diversity, equity, inclusion, and belonging in human-animal interactions: Reflections on practice. In A. H. Fine, M. K. Mueller, Z. Y. Ng, A. M. Beck, & J. M. Peralta (Eds.), *The Routledge International Handbook of Human-Animal Interactions and Anthrozoology*. Routledge.

Hediger, K., Meisser, A., & Zinsstag, J. (2019). A One Health research framework for animal-assisted interventions. *International Journal of Environmental Research and Public Health*, *16*(4), Article 4. https://doi.org/10.3390/ijerph16040640

Hennessy, M. B., Williams, M. T., Miller, D. D., Douglas, C. W., & Voith, V. L. (1998). Influence of male and female petters on plasma cortisol and behaviour: Can human interaction reduce the stress of dogs in a public animal shelter? *Applied Animal Behaviour Science*, *61*(1), 63–77. https://doi.org/10.1016/S0168-1591(98)00179-8

Herrera-Perez, D., Haslam, A., Crain, T., Gill, J., Livingston, C., Kaestner, V., Hayes, M., Morgan, D., Cifu, A. S., & Prasad, V. (2019). A comprehensive review of randomized clinical trials in three medical journals reveals 396 medical reversals. *eLife*, *8*, e45183. https://doi.org/10.7554/eLife.45183

Herzog, H. (2011). The impact of pets on human health and psychological well-being: Fact, fiction, or hypothesis? *Current Directions in Psychological Science*, *20*(4), 236–239. https://doi.org/10.1177/0963721411415220

Hiby, E. F., Rooney, N. J., & Bradshaw, J. W. S. (2006). Behavioural and physiological responses of dogs entering re-homing kennels. *Physiology & Behavior*, *89*(3), 385–391. https://doi.org/10.1016/j.physbeh.2006.07.012

Howie, A. R. (2021). *Assessing Handlers for Competence in Animal-assisted Interventions*. Purdue University Press. https://muse.jhu.edu/pub/60/monograph/book/85602

Hu, M., Zhang, P., Leng, M., Li, C., & Chen, L. (2018). Animal-assisted intervention for individuals with cognitive impairment: A meta-analysis of randomized controlled trials and quasi-randomized controlled trials. *Psychiatry Research*, *260*, 418–427. https://doi.org/10.1016/j.psychres.2017.12.016

Hughes, M. J., Verreynne, M.-L., Harpur, P., & Pachana, N. A. (2020). Companion animals and health in older populations: A systematic review. *Clinical Gerontologist*, *43*(4), 365–377. https://doi.org/10.1080/07317115.2019.1650863

International Association of Human–Animal Interaction Organizations. (2018). *White Paper on Animal-Assisted Interventions*. International Association of Human–Animal Interaction Organizations. https://iahaio.org/best-practice/white-paper-on-animal-assisted-interventions/

Janssens, M., Eshuis, J., Peeters, S., Lataster, J., Reijnders, J., Enders-Slegers, M.-J., & Jacobs, N. (2020). The pet-effect in daily life: An experience sampling study on emotional wellbeing in pet owners. *Anthrozoös*, *33*(4), 579–588. https://doi.org/10.1080/08927936.2020.1771061

Jensen, C. L., Ogeer, J., Beck, A. M., & O'Haire, M. E. (2023). Exploring diversity, equity, and inclusion perceptions among leadership in the field of human–animal interaction. *Human–Animal Interactions*, *11*, 1. https://doi.org/10.1079/hai.2023.0012

Kirschbaum, C., & Hellhammer, D. H. (2008). Salivary cortisol in psychobiological research: An overview. *Neuropsychobiology*, *22*(3), 150–169. https://doi.org/10.1159/000118611

Lefebvre, S. L., Golab, G. C., Christensen, E., Castrodale, L., Aureden, K., Bialachowski, A., Gumley, N., Robinson, J., Peregrine, A., Benoit, M., Card, M. L., van Horne, L., & Weese, J. S. (2008). Guidelines for animal-assisted interventions in health care facilities. *American Journal of Infection Control*, *36*(2), 78–85. https://doi.org/10.1016/j.ajic.2007.09.005

Liguori, G., Costagliola, A., Lombardi, R., Paciello, O., & Giordano, A. (2023). Human-animal interaction in animal-assisted interventions (AAI)s: Zoonosis risks, benefits, and future directions – A One Health approach. *Animals*, *13*(10), Article 10. https://doi.org/10.3390/ani13101592

Liu, J. J., Davidson, E., & Sheikh, A. (2011). Achieving ethnic diversity in trial recruitment. *Pharmaceutical Medicine*, *25*(4), 215–222. https://doi.org/10.1007/BF03256863

Malinowski, K., Yee, C., Tevlin, J. M., Birks, E. K., Durando, M. M., Pournajafi-Nazarloo, H., Cavaiola, A. A., & McKeever, K. H. (2018). The effects of equine assisted therapy on plasma cortisol and oxytocin concentrations and heart rate variability in horses and measures of symptoms of post-traumatic stress disorder in veterans. *Journal of Equine Veterinary Science*, *64*, 17–26. https://doi.org/10.1016/j.jevs.2018.01.011

Marinelli, L., Normando, S., Siliprandi, C., Salvadoretti, M., & Mongillo, P. (2009). Dog assisted interventions in a specialized centre and potential concerns for animal welfare. *Veterinary Research Communications*, *33*(1), 93–95. https://doi.org/10.1007/s11259-009-9256-x

Menna, L. F., Santaniello, A., Todisco, M., Amato, A., Borrelli, L., Scandurra, C., & Fioretti, A. (2019). The human–animal relationship as the focus of animal-assisted interventions: A One Health approach. *International Journal of Environmental Research and Public Health*, *16*(19), Article 19. https://doi.org/10.3390/ijerph16193660

Ng, Z. (2021). Strategies to assessing and enhancing animal welfare in animal-assisted interventions. In J. M. Peralta & A. H. Fine (Eds.), *The Welfare of Animals in Animal-Assisted Interventions: Foundations and Best Practice Methods* (pp. 123–154). Springer International Publishing. https://doi.org/10.1007/978-3-030-69587-3_6

Open Science Collaboration. (2015). Estimating the reproducibility of psychological science. *Science*, *349*(6251), Article aac4716. https://doi.org/DOI: 10.1126/science.aac4716

Pet Partners. (2018). *Standards of Practice in Animal-Assisted Interventions*. Therapy Animal Standards Site. https://petpartners.org/standards/

Ramirez, A. G., Miller, A. R., Gallion, K., San Miguel de Majors, S., Chalela, P., & García Arámburo, S. (2008). Testing three different cancer genetics registry recruitment methods with Hispanic cancer patients and their family members previously registered in local cancer registries in Texas. *Community Genetics*, *11*(4), 215–223. https://doi.org/10.1159/000116882

Ribeiro, C. D. P. V., Alves, J. B., Kominami, P. A., Takeshita, E. M., Bezerra, A. C. B., & Massignan, C. (2023). Does use of animal therapy during dental care help to reduce anxiety in children and adolescents? A systematic review. *International Journal of Paediatric Dentistry*, *33*(2), 181–195. https://doi.org/10.1111/ipd.13033

Risley-Curtiss, C., Holley, L. C., & Wolf, S. (2006). The animal–human bond and ethnic diversity. *Social Work*, *51*(3), 257–268. https://doi.org/10.1093/sw/51.3.257

Rodriguez, K. E., Herzog, H., & Gee, N. R. (2021). Variability in human–animal interaction research. *Frontiers in Veterinary Science*, *7*. https://www.frontiersin.org/articles/10.3389/fvets.2020.619600

Serpell, J. A., Kruger, K. A., Freeman, L. M., Griffin, J. A., & Ng, Z. Y. (2020). Current standards and practices within the therapy dog industry: Results of a representative survey of United States therapy dog organizations. *Frontiers in Veterinary Science*, *7*. https://www.frontiersin.org/articles/10.3389/fvets.2020.00035

Smith, Y. (2019). Chapter 25 – Pets and human diversity: Toward culturally competent, culturally humble psychotherapy. In L. Kogan & C. Blazina (Eds.), *Clinician's Guide to Treating Companion Animal Issues* (pp. 477–496). Academic Press. https://doi.org/10.1016/B978-0-12-812962-3.00025-3

Townsend, L., & Gee, N. R. (2021). Recognizing and mitigating canine stress during animal assisted interventions. *Veterinary Sciences*, *8*(11), Article 11. https://doi.org/10.3390/vetsci8110254

Webster, J. (2016). Animal welfare: freedoms, dominions and "A life worth living." *Animals*, *6*(6), Article 6. https://doi.org/10.3390/ani6060035

Wijnen, B., & Martens, P. (2022). Animals in animal-assisted services: Are they volunteers or professionals? *Animals*, *12*(19), Article 19. https://doi.org/10.3390/ani12192564

Winkle, & Johnson, A. (2023). The importance of animal welfare in animal-assisted services. In L. R. Koga (Ed.), *Animal-assisted Interventions: Recognizing and Mitigating Potential Welfare Challenges*. https://doi.org/10.1079/9781800622616.0001

Winkle, M., Johnson, A., & Mills, D. (2020). Dog welfare, well-being and behavior: Considerations for selection, evaluation and suitability for animal-assisted therapy. *Animals*, *10*(11), Article 11. https://doi.org/10.3390/ani10112188

Zafra-Tanaka, J. H., Pacheco-Barrios, K., Tellez, W. A., & Taype-Rondan, A. (2019). Effects of dog-assisted therapy in adults with dementia: A systematic review and meta-analysis. *BMC Psychiatry*, *19*(1), 41. https://doi.org/10.1186/s12888-018-2009-z

Index

Note: The page numbers in *italics* and **bold** represents *figures* and **tables** respectively.

www.ingramcontent.com/pod-product-compliance
Lightning Source LLC
LaVergne TN
LVHW070829220926
848486LV00029B/164